bare reality:
100 women, their breasts, their stories

Acknowledgements and Thanks

Thank you to my family and friends for listening to me, encouraging me and advising me. I'm fortunate to have had the help, love and support of so many people. Special thanks and acknowledgements must go to John, Ethan and Cole for their patience and support. To my parents, for encouraging me to be a free thinker, and have confidence in myself.

I would like to thank the very generous Kickstarter supporters who made the original edition of this book happen. They pledged significant amounts of money to help conclude a two-year project fuelled on passion alone, into a beautiful, printed book. Not only did their financial pledges help make this book happen, their belief in the project honoured, humbled and motivated me.

I'm grateful that Breast Cancer UK gave me the opportunity to support such a worthwhile charity. And it was an honour to work with Stella McCartney to create the 'No Less a Woman' campaign to raise awareness of breast cancer.

An enormous and heartfelt thank you goes to the 100 women who took part in *Bare Reality*. You took a touching leap of faith when you let me photograph and interview you. That trust in me, and the stories you told, moved and inspired me. I hope that *Bare Reality* honours you and your courage in baring your bodies and hearts.

Editor's Note

Clothing and shoe sizes that appear in interviews refer to UK sizes. Please note all the stories in *Bare Reality* are personal opinion. No book can replace the diagnostic expertise and medical advice of a trusted physician. Please be certain to consult your doctor before making any decisions that affect your health, particularly if you suffer from any medical condition or have any symptom that may require treatment.

bare reality:
100 women, their breasts, their stories

Laura Dodsworth

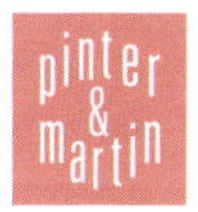

Bare Reality: 100 Women, Their Breasts, Their Stories

First published in 2015 by Pinter & Martin Ltd

This paperback edition featuring the 'No Less a Woman' campaign published 2019

Text and images copyright © Laura Dodsworth 2015, 2019

Laura Dodsworth has asserted her moral right to be identified as the author of this work in accordance with the copyright, designs and patents act of 1988.

All rights reserved.

ISBN 978-1-78066-319-7

Editor: Susan Last
Design: Blok Graphic, London

A catalogue record for this book is available from the British library.

Printed and bound in Poland by Hussar

Pinter & Martin Ltd
6 Effra Parade
London SW2 1PS

www.pinterandmartin.com
www.barereality.net

10p per book sold is paid to Breast Cancer UK,
a registered charity number 1138866
Registered Company Number 7348408

Contents

Foreword

There are few parts of human anatomy as provocative as a woman's breasts, which frequently exist, culturally, not as part of women's bodies, but as ideas defining an eternally shifting border between private and public.

The moment a girl's budding breasts make an appearance is the moment that her relationship to the world and the people in it begins to be redefined, even in her own imagination. As girls and women, we often learn to think about our changing breasts from the perspective of how they make other people feel – in particular, men and babies. In other words, beneath thoughts of bras and bathing suits, we think of ourselves in terms of sex or sacrifice, naked and exposed or comforting and nurturing. As the stories here attest, these lessons are filtered through class, race, sexuality, religion, illness, geography, politics and, too frequently, violence and war.

Images of bared female breasts have evolved as a primary symbol not just of what makes women valuable and important, but of what cultures think of themselves. In her book, *A History of the Breast*, Marilyn Yalom delightfully explores the manifold ways in which this part of our bodies has come to represent, visually, central ideas about women and what constitutes 'progress'. How the female breast is portrayed, and displayed, has illustrated gender relationships, changing political thought and dominant religious ideas. In addition, the regulation of these images, which varies tremendously across the globe, is related to the regulation of female freedom, sexuality and rights.

Breasts have been central to iconic depictions of women as sexually available fertility goddesses, as mothers who sacrifice their bodies for their children and as freedom-fighting avatars of national independence. If you are reading this, the chances are fairly high that you live in a place where naked breasts were, in the relatively recent historical past, associated with racialised and religiously-inspired ideas about the 'primitive' nature of women versus the 'superior' nature of others. Ideas about women's breasts were employed in colonialist mythologies about gender, sex and race. Among other things, 'good Christian women', light-skinned, had to be clothed – a signifier of a superior, 'civilised' culture. While we may not always be aware of these ideas, we live with their legacy nonetheless.

Rarely have women, like those in this volume, defined cultural ideas about our own bodies. It is an historical fact that, regardless of the particular symbolic meaning at any given time in history and art, images of and ideas about women's breasts have primarily been created by men. How women see themselves and public explorations of how we experience our female human bodies have been, until very recently, few and far between.

Idealised images of women's breasts have been, for the most part, created by men, from men's perspectives, for male purposes. To describe breasts, as writer Natalie Angier has, as 'modified sweat glands', is both an acknowledgement of some women's utterly unimpressed relationship with their breasts, and an almost hilarious affront to the Western male fixation on eroticising breasts to the point that the women they're part of can seem like nothing more than irritating appendages.

What a society chooses to allow of female toplessness, as with art, speaks volumes. It is entirely possible to see how a society's rules governing access to women's bodies continue, ultimately, to be rules governing what is considered a male property right. There are constant contestations over breastfeeding in public, toplessness on beaches, bare-breasted political protesting and what constitutes obscenity and pornography. In mainstream views and in social media, for example, female toplessness is largely prohibited, while barely camouflaged sexually objectifying pornography, that prioritises male sexual pleasure, is not.

This cultural norm goes a long way to explain why a common response to seeing 'real' women's breasts – messy, aged, damaged, asymmetrical, large, small, excised – is mystification. This mystification largely stems from two assumptions: one, that the male, breast-less body is the human standard and two, that breasts have to be 'doing something'. If women insist on being 'deviant', if their breasts must be exposed, they should, at the very least, serve a function: feeding, titillating, nurturing, providing solace. It's as though women's lives are mediated by our breasts' social value. What, after all, is the purpose of breasts if they are not idealised, perfect, feeding or entertaining someone? You might as well ask the same of women in general. It's an unsettling idea to fold into one's sense of self, the objectification of portions of your body. In point of fact, even though it's pervasive, it's absurd.

There are places in the world where the sight of the bare female chest is unfreighted by culture, where naked breasts evoke no sexual feelings in men, no neo-Victorian outrage in polite society, and no automatic, almost fetishistic, association with maternal sacrifice. As for restrictions on seeing women's naked breasts in public, which are rife, it's important to ask, what is it that is obscene in the end? Is it that female bodies are made visible, or, more fundamentally, that we dare to have them and insist they are not deviant, dangerous or subhuman? Why is it so threatening and taboo for us not only to have these bodies, but also to share them, publicly and with grace, as Laura Dodsworth has done here?

The stories collected here are both a striking counter-narrative to objectification and a loud renunciation of its effects. Each woman's story is its own quiet and brave rejection of the idea that her body is a public resource, a private tool, a thing divisible from her self. Each decided for herself, for her own reasons, to be here, to bare her self without shame, and share her story.

I, for one, am grateful to Laura for this refreshing, radical and revealing subjectification. Women who insist that we see their imperfect humanity and acknowledge their female human dignity, cause ripples in the universe.

Soraya Chemaly

Introduction

My breasts are simply part of my body, not the most important thing about me. Yet what they mean to me, and my experiences of them, provide insights into some of the most personal aspects of being a woman.

Women aged from 19 to 101 have taken part in *Bare Reality*, women with healthy breasts, cancer survivors, different ethnicities, women from all walks of life, all shapes and sizes, heterosexual, lesbian, bisexual, asexual and transwomen.

What will you gain from reading this book? If you are a man, you might not have seen as many 'real' breasts, or heard women be so frank. As a woman you might be interested in seeing what other women's breasts look like and take heart: no-one is perfectly symmetrical, many women perceive themselves to be too large, too small, too saggy. If you are younger and still developing, you might be curious to see 'real' breasts, learn about other women's experiences, and gain an insight into your own potential future.

The women in this book bare all. For the first time, 100 women share pictures of their breasts, along with their most personal, courageous and humorous stories about breasts, including growing up, sexual experience, breastfeeding, health problems, insecurities, surgery and ageing. Our breasts and our personal experiences of breasts can shape how we see the world. In turn, our breasts can shape how the world sees us.

I always knew that one aspect of creating *Bare Reality: 100 Women, Their Breasts, Their Stories* would be doing my part to provoke more awareness of breast cancer. But I couldn't have anticipated just how profoundly important it would be to me after meeting and interviewing the women who took part. Their stories were especially moving. Nothing puts your own problems, big or small, into perspective like someone else's life or death story.

The loss of a breast, or a scar, the diagnosis, treatment and recovery will mean different things to different women – we are individual, complex, nuanced. I wanted to tell these women's stories and share the brave, sad, painful, moving and sometimes even funny truth. This isn't about a pink-washed sugar coating, it's the truth.

I'm proud to include twelve additional stories and photos from a collaboration with Stella McCartney entitled 'No Less a Woman'

This is how we look. This is how we feel.

Laura Dodsworth

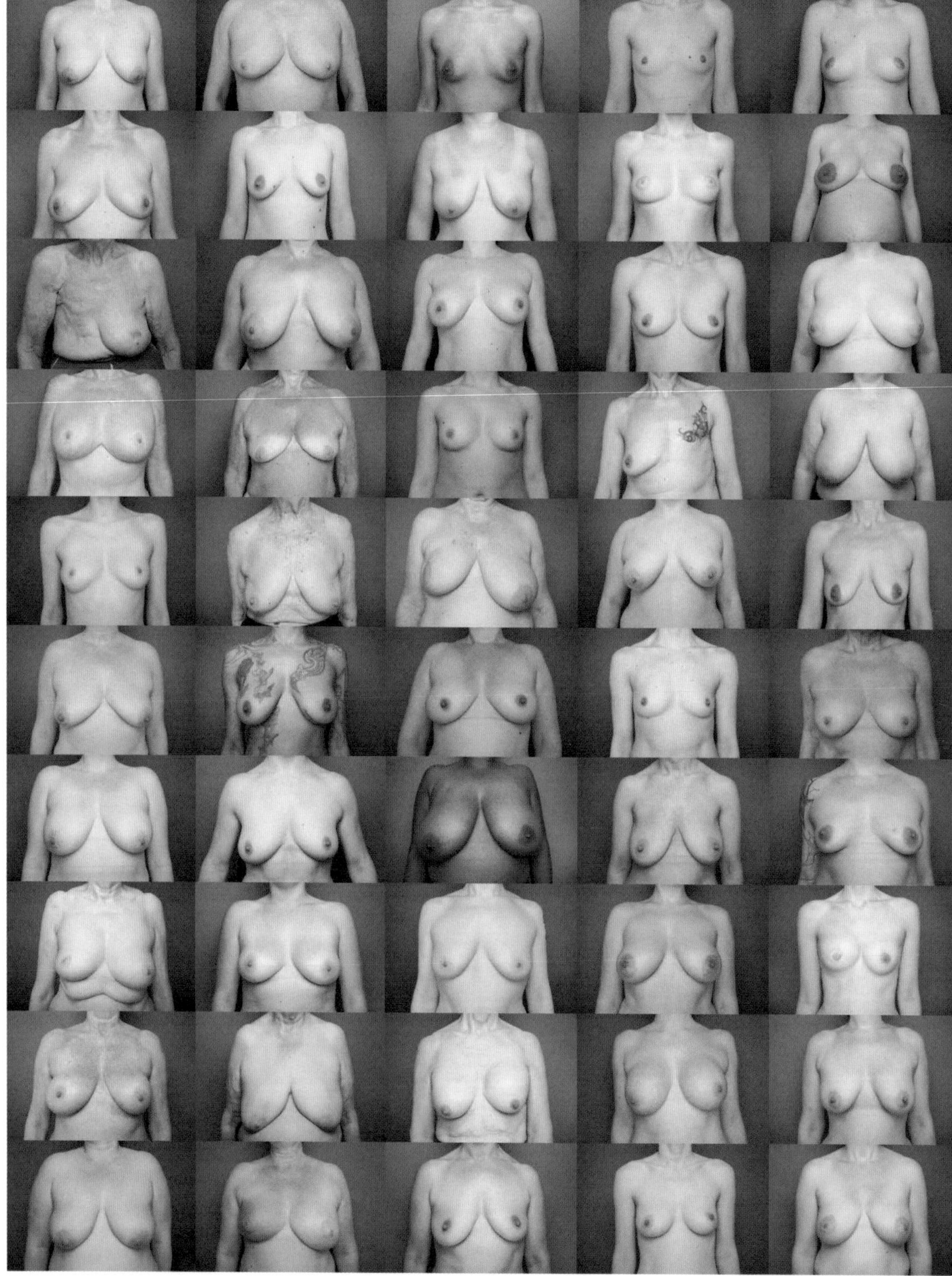

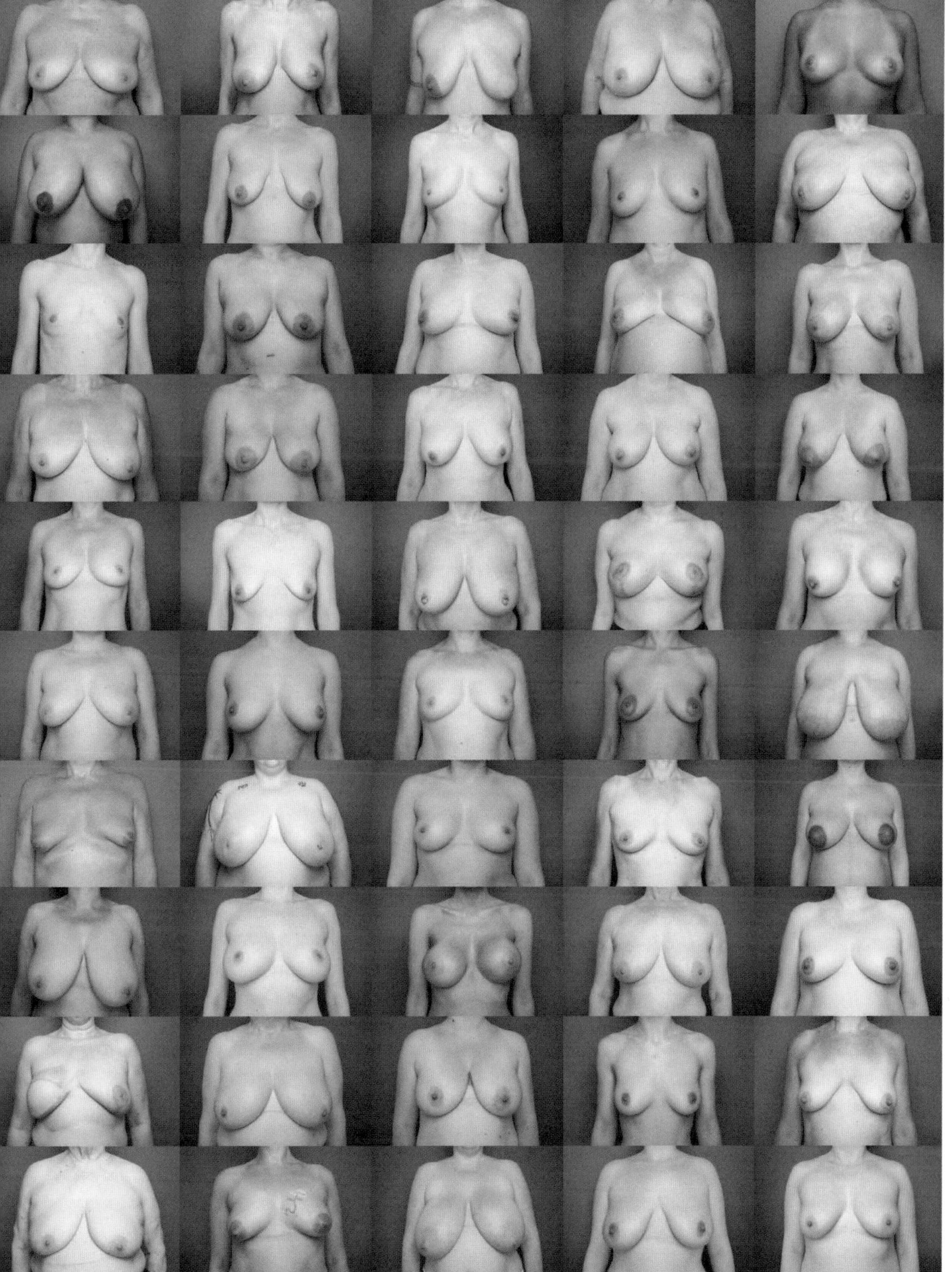

"I'm proud I decided to have a tattoo"

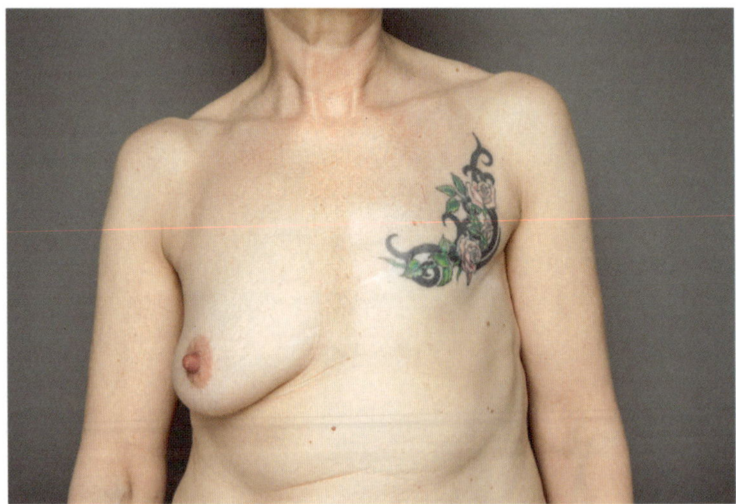

About 10 years ago I was diagnosed with breast cancer. First the lumps were taken out, but that didn't work, so I had a mastectomy. I came away with nothing but a horrible scar. It's bad enough having your breast off, but looking in the mirror and seeing the scar … I just thought, 'I have to make it look pretty!' I decided to have a tattoo with a little bit of colour. I liked the idea of flowers.

I had to wait about a year to heal, and there were a couple of bits of the scar which didn't heal as well and couldn't be tattooed. It took about four hours in two stages: first of all the outline, then the colouring. The tattoo artist made me feel comfortable, it wasn't embarrassing. For him it was just artwork. Funnily enough, because it was on the scarring it didn't hurt, it was numb.

I don't think I could have come to terms with my 'battle scar' as easily without the tattoo. It would have taken a lot longer to look in the mirror and feel okay about the scar where the boob was. It makes a statement and it's pretty to look at. I'm proud of it. I want people to realise you don't have to hide away just because you've had breast cancer.

I can't remember much about the operation. I remember dreading looking down. That frightened me, as it must for anyone who has had something removed, whether it's a breast or a leg. I cried. I remember seeing one boob but not the other, and it looked weird. The worst thing was having the drip out for removing the fluid. When that was pulled out it hurt all across my ribs.

At the time my partner had a brain tumour and was given two years to live. I had three children who were five, 12 and 14. I was offered a reconstruction but I didn't want my children to have to suffer any more, so I said no. I didn't have time to dwell on myself. After my partner died I went through a bad time. I had the children, and I had to keep it all together, but oh my God, I did go through a bad patch.

My partner was amazing, but the night before I went in for the mastectomy he went off and left me alone. I don't know if it was because of his brain tumour. I had the three children and had to come to terms with the fact I was going in the next day for the operation. He went out at lunchtime and came back about 10pm at night. Couldn't he cope? At the end of the day I needed someone. I was frightened, and my family don't live round here. He came into the hospital to see me. I showed him my chest when I got home, and I have to say he was good.

I do lack confidence since having the mastectomy, I don't feel a proper woman. Losing a breast is a massive thing because it's a big part of what makes you feel like a woman.

I have since wondered if I did the right thing about the reconstruction, especially now I am on my own. The only reason I would have a reconstruction would be for a potential partner. I was thinking about internet dating, but when do you tell someone you've had a mastectomy? Some men are boob men: the bigger the boobs, the better. If I met someone like that, they'd run. But then, would they be worth it? That's life, unfortunately. Some people can't handle a deformity. Someone is either going to accept me for who I am or they're not.

I was sexually involved with someone for a while and he wasn't bothered. When I told a male friend about my mastectomy he didn't run away either, but we aren't sexually involved. So, really, that should give me confidence. Everyone has accepted me for who I am, and it should be like that. If someone did run away I don't know how I would cope.

One day, a man I knew had a bit too much to drink and said, 'Phwoar, I've always thought you have a fantastic pair of boobs!' He's married so it really upset and annoyed me, and I thought, 'You slimy, dirty man'. I'd had my mastectomy, but he wouldn't have known that. I felt like getting the prosthesis out and plonking it down in front of him! If we hadn't been in a pub, maybe I would have. Some men look at women's boobs, and seem to think they are entitled to comment. It's totally out of order.

The prosthesis has got a nipple thing which is rather comforting, I have to say. I'll sit and touch it through my clothes. If I put my finger over it, it feels like a nipple. I find the prosthesis quite heavy, it's like a chicken fillet thing, so at night I take my bra off. I go braless most nights. On holiday recently, it was so hot I had to keep the prosthesis in the fridge. We'd go to the fridge for a drink and there was this boob sitting there! *(laughs)*

Unfortunately, a big thing is made of breasts in the media. Page 3 doesn't really bother me, but they're all 'perfect' breasts. I'd admire it if they put a mastectomy on Page 3, but they wouldn't, they'd worry people wouldn't buy it. But I think a lot of women would buy it, out of interest.

I do get a little bit upset when I see other women's breasts. I don't know if it is envy … A sense of loss. I do wish I had two.

It worries me when women have breast enlargements: how will they detect a lump? If they are huge and rock hard, how can you find a lump? Hopefully I am wrong.

My sister and nan had breast cancer. My daughter has to start mammograms once she reaches the age of 30. My other sister is higher risk too. I think my daughter is pleased she will be monitored. We don't really talk about it. I've never made a big deal of my breast cancer to my children, we all just forget I've had it.

My children all love my tattoo. I often wonder what my sons think about the mastectomy. My youngest one will only remember me with one breast. I wonder what they will think and feel about breasts as they grow older.

I feel lucky. I'm one of the lucky ones. (*cries*) There are people who don't get through it. I'm proud I decided to have a tattoo. The tattoo helped me get through it, and accept it.

———————————

Age 54 | Three children

"Breasts make you feel like a proper woman"

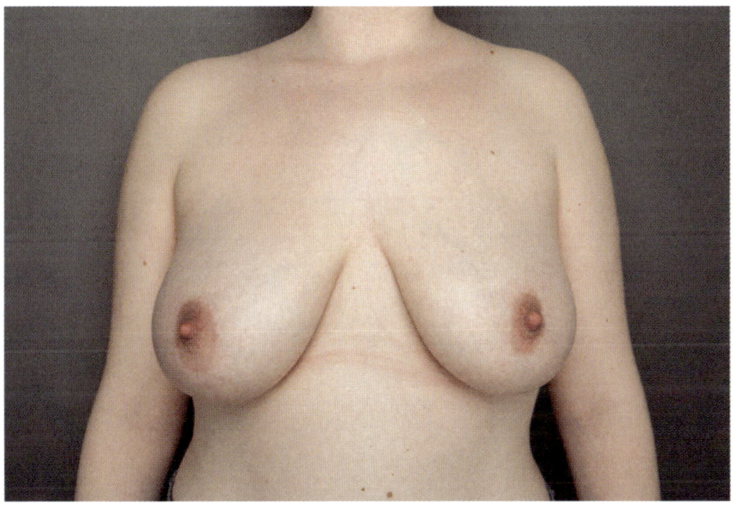

I think my breasts are alright looks-wise. They were a couple of corkers when I was a teenager, a nice pair. Then I had my first baby and fed her, then my next one, and they've gone a bit saggier and stretch-marked. But they're alright in a bra! *(laughs)* I'm very proud of them for being able to feed my children. I was very impressed with that.

I only go braless in the house. I would never go out without a bra on. They'd just look saggy, not attractive. And you know when you're cold and your nipples go hard and everyone looks?

I was pretty flat-chested till I was 15. All my friends had boobs. I was the last one. I was wearing a strappy top, and I put cotton wool bits in, and one day the cotton wool started protruding out of the bra, and all my friends were like, 'Oh, look at you with cotton wool in your bra!' It was so embarrassing.

I started my periods late as well. All my friends looked like women, and I looked like a little girl. I felt rubbish. When I grew, my friends didn't really say anything about it, but there was an impact on the boys, a little bit of attention: 'You've got big tits!' That kind of thing. It's pathetic really, but I was quite pleased everyone was noticing. *(laughs)* I've never been particularly shy, so I didn't mind that people were commenting on them.

I breastfed my first baby for six and a half months, and my second one for seven and a half months. It was easy and natural. I just whacked my boob out, on they went, and that was that. No problems at all. I was really lucky. 'Look at me, look at me feeding my child!'

I think breasts are amazing, they are so impressive. Magic. Yeah, my boobs are a bit saggier and stretch-marked now, but I don't care. I pretend I care. I'm like, 'Oh, my boobs, my boobs!' But I don't care, I'm proud of what they did. My kids survived off my breasts. They make me feel womanly and strong. Before I had kids, I just thought of them as boobs.

My partner absolutely loves them, just as much now as he did 10 years ago. On a date once, he made me get out of the car and he said, 'Can you do something to my car? Can you just bounce on the bonnet?' I later found out that bouncing was making my boobs go up and down, and that was why he was doing it. Pathetic. He'll kill me for saying that!

He still has a good old perv on them. He's happy with them, likes looking at them. They are a very big part of our sex life. He likes to spend a bit of time paying attention to them. I like attention in that area as well, it's important. I've got quite a lot of sensitivity in my nipples, so I do enjoy some fiddling. Breasts make you feel like a proper woman, and when you're having sex you want to feel like a proper woman. They are empowering.

I've noticed that a lot of my friends have been offended if they've had comments about their boobs or whatever. It never used to bother me. They are a symbol of being a woman. I've always been confident with my sexuality. This is me, I'm a woman, these are what I have.

When I was a barmaid, I had things like 'Get your tits out love!' or, 'Nice pair of melons!' You would think that would piss me off, but it didn't. I just used to laugh and make a joke of it. I'd say 'Don't be so rude!'

I think there's a time and a place for cosmetic surgery. Women have real insecurities about their breasts and if they want to do something about it for themselves, then there's nothing wrong with it. But I hate massive great big juggernauts on people's chests. They look horrible. They're grotesque, it's an awful fashion, 'Look at me being six stone with my enormous tits!' I think it comes from porn and glamour modelling. More and more girls aspire to it. When I was younger I remember thinking, 'Am I supposed to be that thin and tanned all the time with big boobs?' You do feel there is pressure to look like that. It's horrible, vile.

If I got to 40 or 50 and I wasn't happy with how they looked I might consider surgery. If I thought, 'These are crap, I could do with jazzing them up a bit!' For myself. For my partner as well, but for me really. I'd do other things as well. Would you like a list? *(laughs)* At the moment no, but I would certainly be open to stuff in the future, if the financial situation improves.

I work in a factory, I do the admin upstairs. Downstairs is chock-full of calendars of girls with their tits out. There was a time a few years ago when it used to really bother me and make me feel self-conscious. They're absolutely everywhere! It used to make me feel inadequate. Now I can be, like, 'There's your titty magazine', and it doesn't bother me.

When I started working there I was 21 and my youngest baby was still feeding. All my friends still had nice flat tummies, and I was going through a phase of thinking I had a wobbly tum and stretch marks. I'd see all these calendar girls with big boobs, and it made me feel a bit crap.

I don't have an awful lot of respect for these men. When I go down there, I'll be striding along because I need to talk to someone, and they'll be like, 'Phwoar, look at her boobs bouncing!' Honestly, genuinely! They're only mucking about. I'll just stick my finger up or whatever, 'Stop staring! Get on with your work!' It makes me feel like there's no respect, they're just pervy men.

Just after I'd had my first baby, there was a situation with my partner. Again, I was feeling low about my body, worried about stretch marks. I found some, shall we say, 'material' on the internet. I was absolutely disgusted, outraged. It got to the point where we nearly split up. I was so upset. And there were a few more situations over the next few years, and I would stress each time that I hated it, that it's degrading. Now I turn a bit of a blind eye. I haven't found any evidence of it, but I don't want to search for it. I don't want to know about it.

———

Age 26 | Two children

"There's a sense that breasts are for titillating men now"

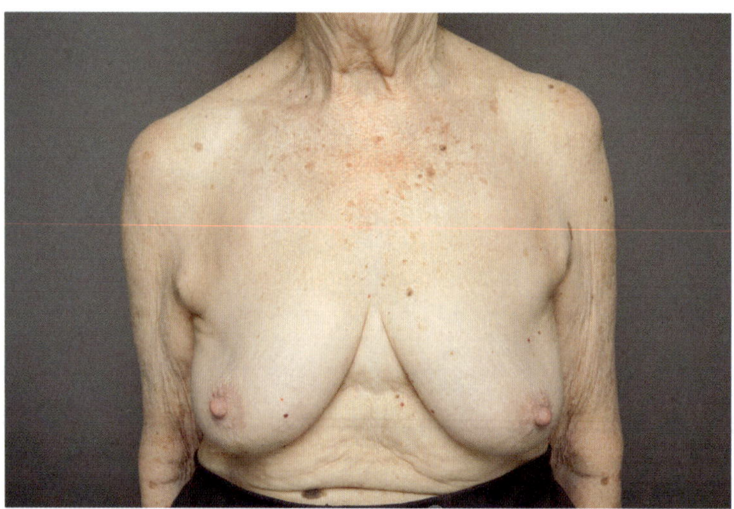

My breasts are my breasts. I don't think a lot about them. They are part of a female body. I've always thought that breasts were designed to feed the next generation.

I noticed my mother breastfeeding, because I had a sister four years my junior. Then the next time I took an interest in breasts, you might call it an interest, was when I had my 14th birthday in Paris. I can remember seeing all these ladies in restaurants breastfeeding their children, and I thought, 'Oh, how nice!' It was the first time I had ever seen that. They weren't exposing their breasts, they were very clever about using their jackets.

In England, you couldn't even take a child into a shop, you had to keep prams outside. And when you got inside, as I found out when I had children, there was nowhere to breastfeed or change a nappy. We were not a child-oriented society. In Britain people were, 'Eurgh, breastfeeding!' If you had breastfed in a cafe in Britain, you would have been told to go out. It was the 'yuck' policy.

I was disgusted when I learnt about history. I was aware of the feeling that breastfeeding is disgusting and unnatural. I learnt that in our blessed empire, the posh British were having their babies fed by wet nurses of the races they were living amongst, and yet they didn't rate these servants, they didn't deserve a vote, or equality, or anything. But the servants were feeding their baby, the most precious object they were ever going to have in their lives. I thought it was absolutely disgusting, very hypocritical. You have to be an 'animal' to do it, so the upper echelons of society employed someone else to do it.

At the hospital where I had my first baby they made you follow the rules. I went in because the pain was intense, but it was evening, the doctors weren't working in the evening, labour had to be suppressed in some way. They held it back and I had my baby in the morning. I delivered to coincide with the doctors' schedule. In this maternity ward, the men were kowtowed to by the nurses, particularly the sisters, they literally bent and bowed to them. They wanted to marry doctors.

You weren't allowed to get out of bed. They brought the baby to you for an hour, every four hours. If it didn't feed it was taken away from you, having not fed, and then they would take the milk from you for premature babies. The idea of having to get rid of my own milk, to be taken to someone else! He didn't want to breastfeed every time, he was always asleep. I have no idea if he was supplemented with formula. The book we were given in hospital was full of ads for formula milk. It was hard to establish breastfeeding like that. It was really wicked. I never saw my baby, except those hours, and neither did my husband. It still hurts me now, utterly.

I had my other two at home with a nurse and my husband. My husband told me, 'I'll be with you, I want to be a good father.' That was lovely, and they were much better experiences. I breastfed straight away. Because I was in my own house, I was sleeping cuddled by my husband that very night.

I breastfed all of my babies for nine months: six fully, and then you gradually move off for three months. I had been told to do that and it seemed to work.

We didn't have bras at school. I think my first one was when I was 16. Bras have changed. They've got built up ones now, there wasn't anything like that, they were merely to stop you wobbling about if you were very large. The cup sizes have changed. Shops hadn't organised the sizing regime then, the A, B, C bit came in quite late on.

There was a lot of talk about the difference between the women in the North and the women in the South, the ratio between their breasts, waists and hips. The women in the North had a greater percentage difference between the breasts and hips and the waist. We used to talk about an hourglass shape. I must say, I used to have a 22-inch waist.

We had a swimming pool, so sometimes I used to be topless, not sunbathing, but gardening, cutting grass and cleaning the pool. That's why my back is like a gravel patch now. My husband and I would swim naked when we fancied a swim on a hot summer's night, when it was dark.

I don't get magazines and newspapers anymore, I don't bother with them. It was lovely in the war when there were just two sheets, all about the war and important things. Now, newspapers are all about selling things, and are completely sexualised.

There's a sense that breasts are for titillating men now. I don't think it's a good idea at all. The sexualisation of the human body has gone too far. I think it's bad, wearing push up bras, deliberately showing the cleavage, the surgery that goes on, the money spent. It's sad. Why can't people accept what they are? It's a pathetic man if he needs all this to stimulate him. There's something wrong, it's a failure. I used to think men were making such a fuss because they weren't breastfed themselves. There's something in the brain that makes them want to suck, because their mothers denied them.

I think women are weakening themselves. It took years for women to get equality. There was no equality for females in my day. My mother didn't have a vote until she was 30. When I was at school, girls weren't taught to drive, only the sons, because women shouldn't have anything to do with engineering. Impressively, my father taught me to drive, showed me under the bonnet and I could take a wheel off. I also remember when I was at college my father had an argument with some men about sending me to university, they were saying, 'Why on earth are you sending a girl to university? What on earth for? How ridiculous!' He had five sisters and absolutely rated the female gender. One of the things he said was, 'The hand that rocks the cradle rules the world, don't you realise that?'

We were weak then, the rights weren't there. Now, women are

belittling themselves by turning themselves into sex objects. It's very dangerous. What's between the ears is more important. It's odd to have been part of the generation to observe a swing one way and then back again. If you're worrying about your appearance, your mind is distracted from important things.

———————————

Age 80 | Three children

"I tease my bra off"

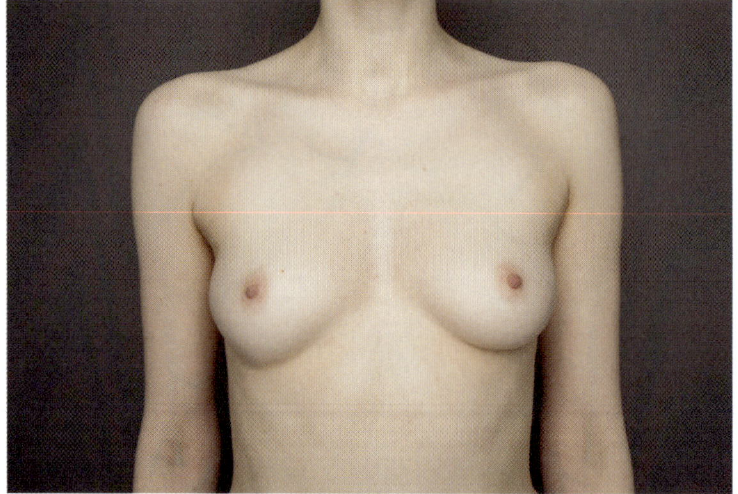

I love my breasts, I'm happy with them. Sometimes I look in the mirror, and think, 'I wish they were a little bit bigger' because of the whole stereotype of big boobs. But I like being a B. I love a little freckle on one boob by the nipple, it makes the boob mine. It's my freckle, on my breast.

I got teased for not having big breasts at school. I was called 'twig' and 'ugly'. I've kind of blocked it out. I hated high school, I got picked on so much. But then it all turned around. When I was 18 I started stripping. One night, some guys from school who used to pick on me came in. I was like, 'Hah! You're paying to see me naked! You called me all those names in high school, but look at me now!' They were quite surprised. Instead of calling me names, they were sleazeballs and called me sexual, dirty names. They treated me like an object. I wasn't going to do them any favours in the club, you know.

I started modelling to get attention, and going on the forum for *Nuts* magazine. I sent in pictures I took on a self-timer. I was 17. I got nice comments but I also got sleazy comments, talking about me like I was a piece of meat. But because I'd been bullied that was nice in a sense too.

I didn't start doing topless modelling straight away, but it wasn't long, about six months. I started with short skirts, then lingerie, then topless.

Guys seem to like me more when they fancy me. A friend told me the way I get people to like me is by being over-sexual.

I was doing childcare at the same time I was modelling and sending photos to *Nuts*. I got fired from the nursery for being in the magazine. I was young at the time, and I hated the job anyway. The funny thing was, they escorted me off the premises. What did they think I was going to do, run back in and flash my tits to all the kids? *(laughs)*

I was good at my job. I've never hurt a child in my life. Why does showing my breasts in a magazine make me not a good role model for children? They said if the children's parents saw, they wouldn't want me looking after their children. The manager's husband buys and reads *Nuts*, that's how he knew! He must have looked at it enough, to know it was me, but that was OK.

In the club, I don't get many comments about my breasts until I get them out. When I'm stood around in the main room I get more arse comments. A lot of the girls have a bust, and I don't, so the bosses let me wear see-through stuff. I struggle to wear a bra to push my boobs up because otherwise I get a line from the bra. I have to edge towards the guys and say things like, 'A handful is good enough' and talk about having tiny nipples. Words like 'tiny' sound nice and positive.

When I get into the room for a lap dance I get more comments. Some guys have said I have perfect breasts. A lot of guys don't realise what a good dance they are going to get. I tease my bra off. Eye contact is really important. Some guys stare into your eyes the entire dance. I've had that so many times. They love my eyes and it makes them think you're into it. Ah, they're so dim, aren't they!

Some people speak to you like you're a human being, and some speak to you like you're only boobs and bum. I can't stand it when guys talk really horrible to you. Some men like to feel superior, 'I've got all this money, and you've got to work for it!' I hate men like that.

Some guys try and lick my breasts when I'm dancing. I'm getting quite fast now! They're not supposed to touch you. You move towards them with your breast, you are this close to them (*indicates a couple of centimetres*) then I have this movement to get away! (*quick fluid backwards motion*)

It would be nice if they realised this girl comes with the body, but this is the job and it's going to happen. At the end of the night, sometimes we say, 'He was a dick!' We talk about the customers, what they're like. One guy might say to a girl, 'I love your big boobs'. then he might say to me, 'I love your small boobs'. Maybe they just love all boobs!

When the pub shuts guys come in just to carry on drinking, and to have a free look, they won't pay for it, it's so annoying. We don't get paid just for being there.

If I'm lying on my bed, and getting intimate with myself, I can get aroused touching my boobs. But while I'm dancing and touching my boobs and stuff like that, I never get aroused. It's so funny, I'm doing the exact same thing, and there's no sensation at all. I do touch my boobs when I'm masturbating, but not because I get pleasure from them, more because I like the way they feel. I like my nipples being touched, gently. As I'm sat here, I'm touching them! I do touch them quite a lot, I think it's a comfort thing. They don't give me much pleasure, it's in the head.

If a guy grabs them and starts squeezing them I don't get pleasure. I generally have quite tender breasts. Men can be quite heavy-handed, but you yourself know how much you like. My boyfriend knows I don't like it, so he doesn't do it. Men are obsessed with boobs, but when it comes down to sex, they're not bothered about them. They don't spend much time there at all.

I have a friend who is a very big boobs fan. Bless him, he's 40, and only slept with one girl. I met him when I was 18 on the *Nuts* forum. On his 35th birthday we went to Spearmint Rhino and at the end of the night I gave him a lap dance. I thought it would be a nice treat. His face! He loves boobs, and I think it's why he's single. He's got it set in his mind that he wants someone like a Page 3 girl. Bless him. He's like a big, clumsy, geeky giant. He likes the blonde, big-boobed girls. He likes his lap dances.

That's one of the problems with Page 3 and stuff like that. I'm not bothered about Page 3, I don't think it's a bad thing to make a woman a sexual object. Guys want to see it, so someone's got to do it. But it does make men live in a fantasy world, they think that's what a woman should look like and be like. There are lots of men like that. There are too many men waiting for the perfect girl, and I think it's all because of TV and magazines.

I definitely want to breastfeed one day, I don't even care if they don't look nice afterwards. I do believe that's what breasts are for, and it's healthier for the baby. It's one reason I wouldn't have pierced nipples or breast surgery. I love the fact that I'm natural.

I was at the Download festival eight years ago. There were maybe 10,000 people waiting at the big stage for a band to come on. Girls were literally getting on people's shoulders and pulling their tops off, and their boobs would be shown on the big screen. I thought, 'Right, I want to do this!' It's amazing, this huge group of people cheering for your boobs! It was funny seeing them on the big screen, because they were so small I thought, 'Can anyone tell?' But I did get a big cheer.

———————

Age 26 | No children

"This has been the year of the breast"

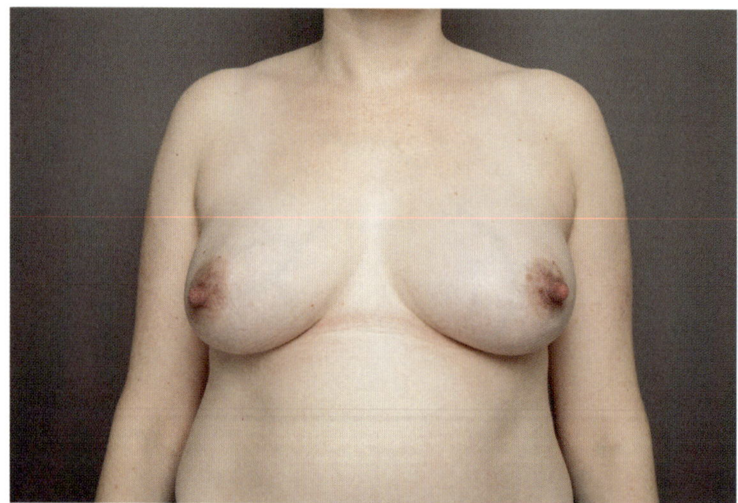

To tell you the truth, before my mum died of breast cancer, I hadn't thought of my breasts as anything more than inconveniences you had to put bras on. I hadn't even really thought of them in a sexual way. It's only since my mum died of and since having my baby, that my breasts have got a purpose. Your breasts can make you die, and they can give life. I think they are much more important now.

I found breastfeeding really natural. I think it's because I haven't stressed about it. Even if it had been painful I would have done it. For me, it's a pleasure to be able to give that to my daughter. I was adamant I wanted to breastfeed. After seeing what my mum went through, I wanted to do something good with my breasts.

The sexual side had gone, it wasn't what I was thinking about. That will come back. We have had sex since my mum died, before having the baby. My breasts were a no-go. I couldn't think of my breasts as sexual because of my mum, because of what her breasts had done to her.

My breasts grew when I was pregnant. Veins appeared and the nipples changed. I know some women say their breasts get saggier after breastfeeding, but I haven't really stood in front of the mirror and examined them. I'm not concerned if my breasts change permanently. My breasts are for feeding my daughter and giving her the best start in life.

Why do women have breasts? You should be proud if you are able to breastfeed, and I feel sorry for people who don't even try it, or put themselves and their breasts above the health of their children. I find that ludicrous.

I used to know someone who had a boob job. They didn't feel natural, they felt hard, almost like when your milk comes in. It was horrible! She had small breasts and she wanted bigger breasts. I find it strange because she can't breastfeed. She has put a boob job above feeding her kids in the future.

Mum didn't breastfeed. No one in our family really did, they all bottle-fed. My mum was always a very natural mum, but she never breastfed. I don't know why no one in my family did. I would love to be able to ask my mum, but because she died when I was still pregnant there are things I can never ask her.

My mum's tumour was big, half her breast. She was so calm, she wasn't bitter. She was really strong to protect my sister and me. If I have breast cancer in the future I will get strength from how she reacted.

She had a very rare, very aggressive form of cancer. I'm told I'm not at increased risk. I do feel to check the health of my breasts. But, it's interesting – they think earlier screenings can also increase the chance of getting breast cancer. So, do you start at an early age? The consultant recommended not to start until I am 40, so I'll wait till then.

Breastfeeding can reduce your risk of breast cancer. I now want as many people as possible to breastfeed, for their baby and also to reduce the amount of breast cancer. I would hate other people to go through what my mum went through.

Also, people don't check their breasts enough. I have to admit I had never properly checked my breasts. I work with people who have breast cancer and who die of it and even that was not enough to make me check my breasts. Maybe people won't listen to me, but I hope I can get through to a few people.

This has been the year of the breast. It's been hard. Breasts killed my mum, but my breasts give so much to my daughter. Just over a year ago I would never have known how important breasts would be to me. For me, the worst and the best things have happened.

———————

Age 35 | One child, breastfeeding 11-week-old

"My breasts are small and inconvenient for clothes"

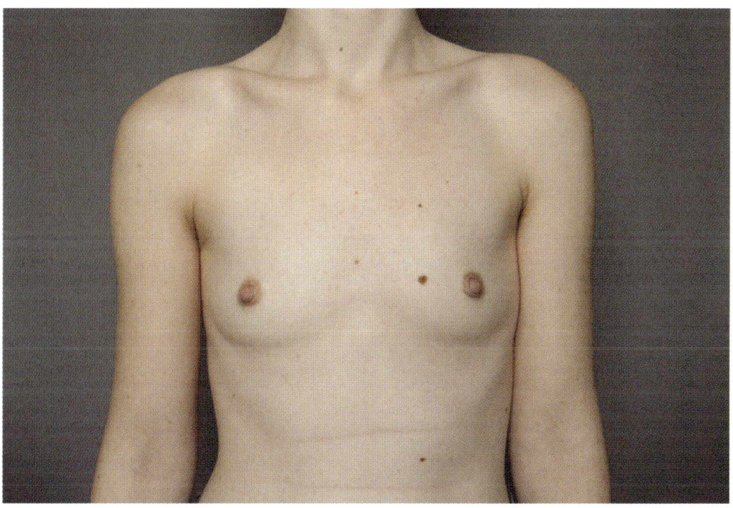

My breasts are small and inconvenient for clothes. I have to wear very high tops because otherwise there's a great gaping hole and people can see down my top. Even if I wear a bra people can see my nipples sometimes, because not only is the top so big it sits away from the bra, the bra is too big and will sit away from my boobs. So despite the top and the bra people can see my nipples!

I can live with my breasts happily, but I like other things better! Mine are an AAA or less. I wear a bra to bulk out the look of the boobs. The padding covers up the nipples. I would be uncomfortable if the nipples showed through, I wouldn't want people to see them, they're not theirs to see. It gives somebody something of yours to judge, they could laugh and it would draw attention.

They are so small and insignificant I barely noticed them developing. I definitely wanted bigger breasts when I was at school. Everything is so judged on looks at that age.

If I could pick the ideal pair of breasts for myself, I would have average-sized breasts that tops are made for. Clothes would look better because they would fit. The perfect breasts are out there, I've seen them! My friend at school had a lovely pair of boobs in comparison to mine, and I was always very jealous of them. Society's ideal breasts are B to C, perky, have cleavage, or possibility of cleavage, and no hair.

I loved my breasts when I was breastfeeding because they were bigger and I had cleavage. It was the only time I had the slightest hint of cleavage, which was just wonderful. Breastfeeding was a nice thing to do overall but it was painful at first. I would tap my foot with the pain, tap, tap, tap. There was a horrid sensation, a pulling, draining sensation through the boob.

I can tell you a story about when I was breastfeeding in front of two good friends of mine, a man and woman. When you're breastfeeding the nipple gets longer and the guy made a joke to say how my nipple looked like a slug. We laughed it off at the time, but I've never forgotten it. However, I do remember a very nice comment once when I was breastfeeding from a friend of a friend, 'What lovely neat little boobs you have'. That was nice.

I'm not sure what my partner thinks of my breasts. I don't think he has any problem with them being small. He's made reassuring comments, probably as a reaction to my lack of confidence. You know that they're small. I know that they're small. He knows that they're small. So, it doesn't even have to be acknowledged. They're not really important for me sexually.

I wouldn't seriously consider breast surgery. I think it would be nice, every now and then, but I would never have it done. You have to try and be happy with what you've got. If you start trying to change, it's a never-ending thing, you would never be happy.

I've got the chicken fillets, to fill the space in my clothes, but they're a pain. The big chicken fillets can make a difference to the look, but they are plastic so they don't feel nice to put in and they don't always sit quite right, or perhaps I just worry they don't look quite right.

I had an awful experience as a 16-year-old. I had some thin padded bits to put in bras. I was sitting around in a group and someone said 'What's that?' about this thing on the floor! And there it was, one of my padded bra things. Of course I had to pretend I had no idea what this thing was and left it there!

Recently my son asked me why men can take their tops off and women can't? And I really had no answer except, 'Isn't it ridiculous and unfair?' There's no reason why women should be prohibited from doing that.

I've been called flat-chested as an insult. I remember a couple of people saying that. Obviously I know I am, I don't need to be told. You know you are being told as an insult. There's no reason it should constitute an insult.

―――――――

Age 26 | One child

"I've got a great pair of melons!"

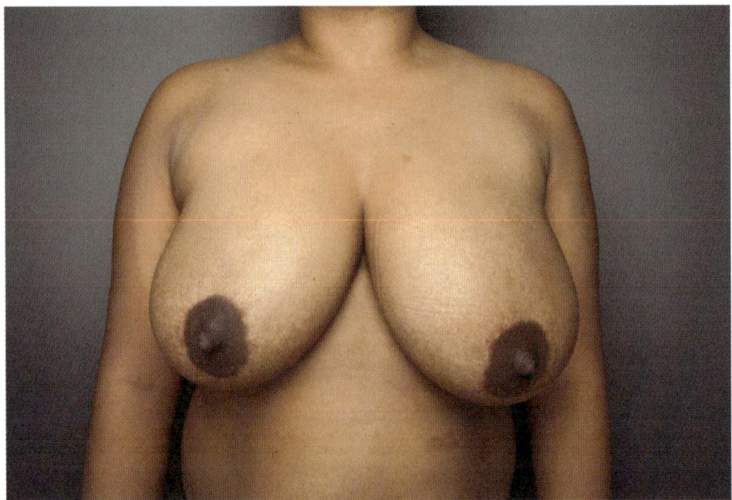

I absolutely adore my breasts. I think they're fantastic. I've always loved them and thought they are an amazing part of my body. They're big, so I've had to learn to be proud of them. I have a good relationship with my boobs. I've got a great pair of melons!

One of my breasts is bigger than the other, and I like that. I've always liked that they are perky and big and they look fantastic. The only thing about having big boobs on a small frame is it's all on your back and shoulders. I'm inclined to stoop my shoulders, not sit up straight.

Last weekend, I realised with horror that they are beginning to sag slightly. That was quite an interesting revelation. I wonder if it's because I've lost weight, or it could just be age-related? Now they're touching my stomach, and I don't like that feeling.

I always felt that because I love my boobs I would like to breastfeed. My boobs should be great for breastfeeding! I wanted to give them their natural job. When I had a child I was really excited about it, but unfortunately I could never fully breastfeed. I had to mix bottle and breast. Hospitals, midwives, breastfeeding experts ... no one ever identified the issue. There are just a small number of women who can't. There wasn't enough milk, and I'm not sure why.

Sadly, my daughter went into hospital and nearly died. Because she was born between Christmas and New Year at home, a lot of checks were lost. We asked if she was going to die, and no one would say yes or no. It was a horrific start. I became über-paranoid, so I would breastfeed for 45 minutes then give her a bottle. I did the best I could. But it took a long time to get over the guilt and grief of that scenario. I've always been a confident woman who is good with kids. I had an amazing pregnancy and an amazing home birth. I then failed at this, and it was really hard. I don't think I forgave myself until this Christmas.

Have you ever seen the electric milk extractors in hospital? They are literally like cow-milking machines. You attach one to each breast, it's a painful suck. One of my most poignant memories is doing that while fireworks went off on New Year's Eve, the machine taking the milk out of me. I remember being devastated that I didn't get enough milk in my bottle.

I have friends who are lesbian couples, heterosexual couples – not many gay couples – but all parenting different ways. One lesbian couple chose to bottle-feed from the beginning to equal up their relationship, which I thought was interesting. I don't advocate it, but it's interesting that when two women have the power to do that, they can go down that route. Normally female couples go the other way.

I'm single and I've had three years being single, and I think, 'Shit! What will a partner think of them? They didn't see them when they were perky and gorgeous'. That was the loss I was feeling when I noticed they were sagging.

I had a seven-year relationship with a man, then a seven-year relationship with a woman: they are my two long-standing relationships. I think a lesbian might apply the same judgements about breasts as a man, but it would depend on whether she's had children or not, and most lesbians don't have children. That's the reality. I share more commonality with single mothers first and foremost.

I remember a woman I dated had really saggy boobs. She hadn't had children, but she had been very big and lost weight so dramatically that her boobs sagged down to her belly button. I remember thinking, 'Wow, I've never seen that!' But it didn't matter, I fancied the pants off her. I'd like to think that someone could think of me like that, and understand. Sex is sex, and you can have great sex regardless of what they look like.

My boobs are important in a sexual relationship. I've got friends who can come if their breasts are touched!

I was the first in my school to develop. I didn't like developing when I was so young, it wasn't a proud celebration. They were very painful, even someone brushing past me, just like the pain when you are first pregnant. The boys teased me, they had a rhyme that had my name in and something about boobs – I think I've mentally erased it.

When I was about 16, I started to feel more confident about who I was. I started to understand the power of my body, and feminine wiles. Prior to that I was your average Asian girl in the 70s in a white area and I was in a minority. I had a strict upbringing and had no friends outside the family unit. My body and beauty were secondary. Then I got a 6ft 2in white boyfriend, and I started wearing jeans and showing my figure off. I look back at pictures now and think, 'Gordon Bennett!' I was stunning.

I've got brown skin and no wrinkles, I'm very lucky. Asian skin doesn't age as much. With my breasts, the elasticity's going, they're getting looser around the nipples, the skin is thinning. The rest of my body doesn't appear to have that.

I don't mind ageing, apart from not having a partner. What's it going to be like to go out there at 41? I've made a conscious decision not to have sex for the sake of it because I want to be mentally into somebody. And because of that, I feel I won't give a flying fuck about the physical variations. That's the theory.

I wouldn't, I couldn't, have any sort of breast enhancements. I'm too politically against changing yourself. No, no, God no. I do understand that people who've had horrific injuries might consider surgery, because society is cruel.

I'm 32H and my frustration with bras has been going on for nearly 33 years. I have finally found the right size, the right bra, and each one is a gobsmacking £35 to buy. That is the downside of getting special bras. Now it's almost like I am on a mission to find these bras everywhere I go!

I wore a nice dress to work, and everybody said, 'What are you doing hiding this beautiful body!' And I thought, 'Wow! That's powerful'. But I think my stomach sticks out. I will use my beauty, and a massive part of my beauty is my boobs. I wouldn't wear a low-cut dress to work because it wouldn't be appropriate, but I might wear a well-cut shirt. I don't want my boobs to be a dominating feature. I don't want people to stare at them.

Sometimes I change at the end of the evening, even for a short walk home. I don't flaunt it. I don't want men to look, and I don't want to feel unsafe. What I should be able to do is wear a beautiful dress with my boobs showing, but I won't. If I lived in a society of women I wouldn't feel that way. What that says about society is tragic.

———————

Age 40 | One child

"God gives life and creates, and as a woman you can connect with that"

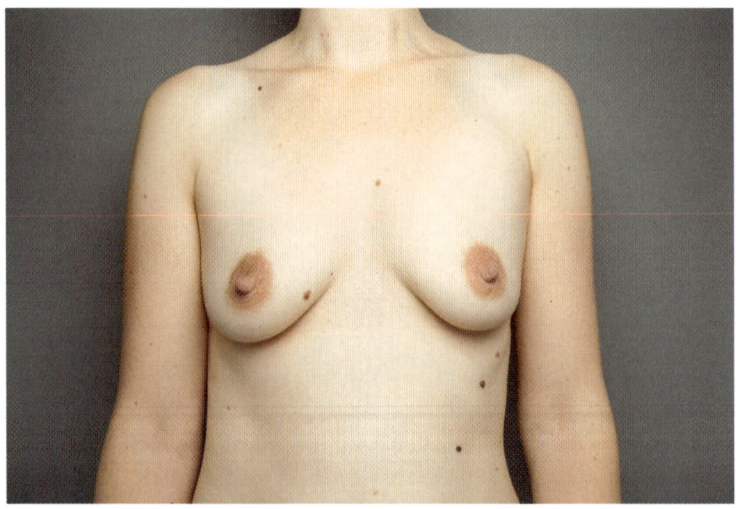

My breasts are smaller than they were a couple of months ago. I stopped breastfeeding my daughter when she turned one. They suddenly changed. I'm not sad about it, but it's been interesting.

The clothes I wear have changed, largely to do with my boobs. Things that looked nice before are baggy now because there is less filling them. In my role as a priest I have to wear clerical shirts which come right up to the neck, and there is no cleavage on show. On maternity leave I quite enjoyed wearing lower-cut tops in conjunction with bigger boobs. It was nice to get a suntan on my chest and feel a bit more feminine! *(laughs)*

The way the clergy dress is partly to diminish our individuality. The priest is vulnerable to quite a lot of projections and transference because we hold a particular, emotionally-loaded position; we deal with inner worlds and spirituality. I know women clergy who struggle with how to dress. Men's business dress has tended to be less exciting, but women are used to brighter colours, patterns and dressing to flatter their shape. Wearing a high-necked shirt is not flattering for me, yet that is what we are given in the tradition of denoting our role. I dress traditionally in black and I wear tailored trousers and skirts. I have a friend who wears her collar as a kind of choker above a lower-necked shirt. I think that was useful in the hot summer. That would be a step too far for me in terms of flamboyancy. It would stand out.

Because of this interview I've been thinking about my boobs. Mostly I think about breastfeeding when I think about my breasts because of having two small children who have breastfed for the best part of a year each.

I feel completely comfortable breastfeeding in church and I encourage other mothers to do so. I don't think people should feel embarrassed about it at all. In the Eucharist service there is a prayer at which the bread and the wine are offered to God and made holy. The words of Jesus are said during that prayer, about the bread, 'This is my body, broken for you, do this in remembrance of me'. And the wine, 'This is my blood, given for you'. As I was breastfeeding my baby with my body at that time, the image of Jesus feeding his friends at the last supper with his, and then the church for generations and generations, had a profound resonance for me.

I have found that quite sustaining when I have been trying to work out the spirituality of being a mum and being a priest, and how those significant things fit together in my life. It has been quite helpful in understanding how I can inhabit this world as a priest and how I can give those words meaning for the congregation.

Being a mother and being a priest are both roles which require you to be available to the people you care for. Because the two roles came quite close together in time for me, I've had to work out how to share myself between the two things. I can do both simultaneously, there is an overlap. When you are breastfeeding you are giving your body to sustain another person. That impacts on you because you have to think about what you are eating and drinking and physically where you are at any given time in case you are required. It's an interesting way of reflecting on how I am as a mother and how I give myself in the priesthood. Being there for someone can be physically limiting, or tiring, or enjoyable.

The Christian church has had a lot to do with women feeling negative about their bodies and ashamed of their sexuality. I think men are probably quite afraid of women's power to bring forth life and feed their babies. That's probably part of the reason women have been oppressed and made to feel ashamed.

We are told God gives life and creates. Jesus feeds us with his body. As a woman, if you have children, you can connect with that. There is not a lot in the Christian tradition that really picks up on that as a fruitful image. In the Old Testament there is imagery of God mothering, and in medieval times I think there was imagery of Jesus breastfeeding the church. There was a lot more freedom about using imagery like that in those times, life was more earthy.

There is an order of nuns I have been to on retreat. Their emblem is a breastfeeding Madonna and they have a statue of Mary breastfeeding Jesus. I find that image very powerful just before walking into a church.

A former bishop has used this image of Mary as an argument for having female bishops. His line is that a bishop's role is to feed and nurture the body of Christ, the church, and he says Mary was the first bishop because she nurtured and fed the body of Christ, in her son Jesus.

I try never to refer to God in the masculine if I can help it: I've always struggled with God being described as masculine, although I am given words to say in prayers which I cannot change. The experience of sustaining somebody has been helpful as an image of how God can sustain us. When I think of God as a parent, it's that kind of love and nurture, although I've never imagined being breastfed by God! *(laughs)* God isn't female or male.

There was a woman breastfeeding at the back of the church and I asked if she would like to receive communion there. She didn't want to come up with her baby latched on and she was missing out at the back. There was no reason for her to have to choose between breastfeeding her baby and receiving communion.

I encourage women to feel comfortable in church and I've led by example. Baring my breasts in my own church wasn't something I imagined I would be doing! *(laughs)* It doesn't sit uncomfortably with me though, it's natural and important, and not remotely embarrassing.

Age 33 | Two children

"Breasts are like psychic baubles"

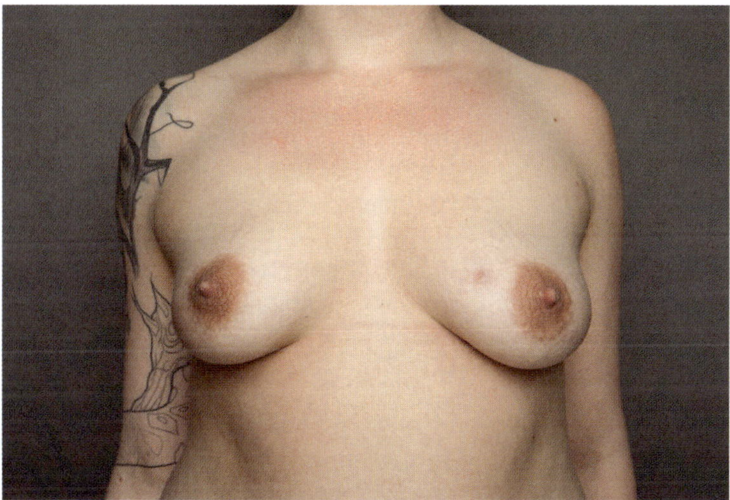

It's almost as though men are jealous of the capabilities of a woman's body. Girls and young women have absolutely no idea what their body is capable of until they become a mother. I went into motherhood wholeheartedly and breastfed my son.

I remember sometimes in the morning I'd get in the bath and, without me realising he was awake, the water would turn white. It was like my breasts knew he was awake, before he even whimpered. My milk would start and then he would whimper. Breasts are like psychic baubles.

Older people view women feeding their child with disgust. The looks of evil from older women! If my son is hungry, I am going to do what any other animal would do, because we are mammals. I'm not going to flaunt myself, but if my son is hungry I am going to feed him. I had comments like, 'How dare you do that in a public place', 'Disgusting', 'You slut', things like that, just for feeding my child.

I wasn't scared of having a baby. The way I saw it, it's the only time a woman can shit herself in public and get away with it. Three and a half hours of labour and then the best orgasm I've ever had. I loved it, absolutely loved it. You get a massive rush when the baby's shoulders go, and it's like, 'Woah!' The rush of endorphins, the orgasm, wow.

My son's first word was 'booby'. He still sees me topless but I wouldn't sit in a bath with him any more. He always used to poke my boobs, and say 'boobies!' I want him to just see my breasts as there, and not turn into one of those delightful cretins who buys the *Daily Star* going ape over women, 'Ooh ooh ooh!' (*monkey noise*) I want my son to be a decent human being.

Men are supposed to be hunter-gatherers, but I supported all of my exes while they sat scratching their arses. In my ideal world, as men don't really have any other purpose, they would be in a dairy farm, and you could choose which one you want to fertilise your egg without the trouble of court cases, or mind games, or the things they want to put you through. They would be serving their only function, to fertilise your egg.

I think it's awful how a woman getting out of a car makes the front page because you can see a flash of camel toe. It's demoralising for me as a woman. I want people to respect me for being a person, not for having body parts they want to do things to. It feels so hopeless sometimes. It's like men are being trained to be morons and treat women like pieces of shit.

It's hard, when you walk around the tube station, all you see is skinny girls in advertisements in their underwear with their breasts hanging out. The sexualisation and objectification of women ... Rather than celebrating what women are and can do ... I'm going to go feminist now: our bodies can do more than guys' bodies, they're merely there to fertilise eggs. But because of what we can do, they sexualise and objectify us. Maybe men never grow up and they desire to be breastfed by their mother.

Because of my dislike for the sexualisation of breasts I think I have a psychological block and I don't like them being played with, it does nothing for me. Some men grab breasts like they're trying to take money from a table, they don't have a clue about anything except how to play with their penis.

Women are better at knowing what to do with women. I'm 'hetero-flexible', I've played. I think it's very common for women to be bisexual because men aren't very good, to be fair. I remember when I had my first experience with a woman when I was 21, we didn't know what we were doing, but it was great and there was no pressure, no performance. I did to her what I would have wanted to be done to myself. You know how to take time with things, and there's a worship aspect to foreplay, that men tend to overlook massively. I masturbate myself better than a man can do.

I was a dominatrix for three years. I've always been fairly dominant. In so many respects women are more powerful than men. A very simple part of domination is don't give them what they want: 'Yeah, I know what you want, I have it right here, and you can't have it.' Men know we are more powerful and they hate that. I believe that a lot of how the media portrays women, not just breasts, but the overall vacancy of women's personalities, is because men are weak and they are afraid of us.

I was always fully clothed as a dominatrix, unless I really wanted to be nasty, and then I would tie them up and walk around in my lingerie. They weren't allowed to touch. But I would make good use of being feminine at that stage with under-bust corsets, classy clothes, a nicely-dressed, feminine woman. It's amazing seeing guys go from dominant man to weak. You can play with it: they can't touch and it frustrates the hell out of them, but they like that powerlessness.

I'm not vicious, I just make them do things that are going to humiliate them, and I sit there laughing at them. Occasionally I do something a bit more edgy, but nothing too harsh. You've got something they want, you use that energy, you don't have to be some scary thing. That's true domination.

Someone tried to grab my breasts once and he got the biggest backhand he's ever had in his life. And then he was sent out after paying. It's about worship of the female form, not grabbing. Occasionally you get men who try to overstep the line, but I've been incredibly lucky and had men who are very respectful.

I got out of it because I had my son. I would like to go back to it, because it rebalances my mind, the whole dom-sub thing. But it's very hard in this country for women to do anything that empowers them. It's not prostitution so it's not illegal, but if they don't like you they can try you for 'white feather laws'. If you leave a mark you can be done for assault, and if the mark lasts for more than an hour, they can be done for assisting assault. Of course, it doesn't happen the other way around. Men get away with hitting and raping women all the time. Women don't need to pay men to hurt them, they get it for free.

I prefer fighting men to fighting women. I know it sounds sexist, but women are more delicate. Men are thick and slow and I'd rather get the first punch in. Thankfully I haven't had to deal with it too many times. If men think you are more powerful than them, then wham, they're going to hit you to show you they are a man. Some girls will take it, they're brought up to believe they are supposed to take it. I've been hit, but I hit back. And I've been attacked by men I don't know. Once a man I didn't know tried to drag me to the toilets to rape me. I literally had his blood in my mouth and under my nails. I went mental, but I got away. The security guard threw me out, he said he didn't believe me. That's the protection we get as females.

———————

Age 30 | One child

"Naturism is a close and supportive community"

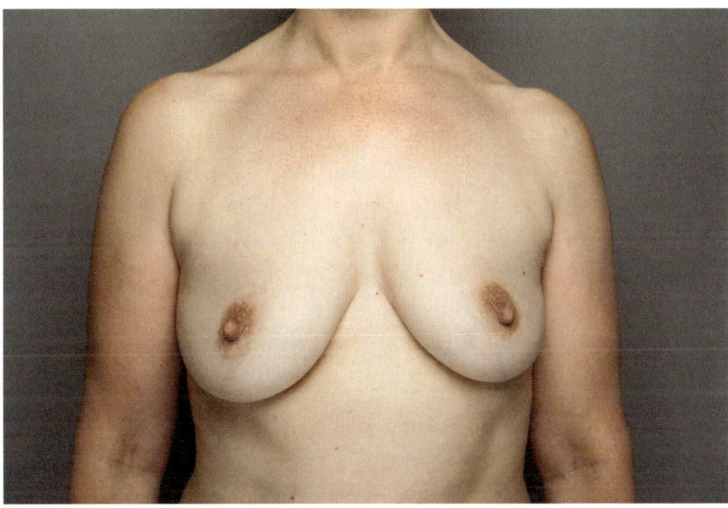

I know that one breast is larger than the other, but I'm quite happy with them. I would have liked larger breasts when I was younger, but I enjoy sport. When I'm at the upper end of my weight range they can be pendulous and then they're a hassle when I'm running. When I am not training I prefer not to wear a bra. As a naturist I prefer not to wear clothing wherever possible.

I have an issue with examining my breasts. I have a psychological hang-up because there's cancer in the family. I leave it to my doctor to do periodically. I had a mammogram, but I will pay for a private screening next time with a doctor who does early detection using thermal imaging, even though I am not on a high income. It's marvellous that the NHS screens breasts, but it was brutalising. They basically stick your boob between a couple of plates, compress it and take photographs. I'm not good with needles, speculums, blood, anything: I pass out. This nurse had obviously seen it all and was trained, but she didn't have a high degree of sensitivity. It was horrible. I was standing there, my breast was between these plates, and I passed out. I couldn't go through it again.

I had a vaginal exam once. There was a speculum and the nurse couldn't remove it. She told me to play with my nipples, and I thought, 'Are you joking?' She said, 'Yes, it will release the oxytocin'. Horrible. I was playing with my nipples on the examining couch to get the speculum out and I didn't even want it there in the first place. Women seem to have all the invasive procedures.

I've been a naturist for many years and am comfortable with the human body. My work is aligned to naturism as I deal with the human body doing massage therapy and Reiki.

When I was a child my mother was very comfortable with her body. She was my matriarchal role model and a naturist. My father was very coy. And ironically, in my marriage I was the one who was comfortable and my husband wasn't. I think that body acceptance and awareness has been passed to my children. Part of it is to do with being sporty; you change more regularly and you are more used to seeing the human body. The nice thing about naturism is the relaxation it confers, and it's a close and supportive community. You accept people for who they are without artifice and pretence, whatever size and shape they are. It doesn't matter if they've had a mastectomy, or have a disfiguring scar or an amputation. It's important to me as I work as a healer, and you are taught not to bring your judgements and assumptions into your work.

Women are wary of naturism because more men are involved with naturism. In fact, the men within the community are very protective and supportive of the women. The naturist community is ridiculed and pilloried; we're thought to be strange for wanting to live our lives clothes-free. Or we are lampooned, as the butt of seaside jokes, or we're bonkers, or whatever. In fact, we're normal grounded people from all walks of life who happen to like to be clothes-free. On a hot day like today it's nice not to wear clothes.

I'm a member of a club and we have good facilities. It's not illegal to be nude anywhere, but because of individual sensitivities you have to be discreet in some places, and you have to go where you know it will be OK. For me it's about relaxation, so I don't want to worry about it, unless I want to use it from an activist point of view. I have been to 'clothes optional' events where clothed members of the public are also present. I don't want to be clothes-free for the sake of it. I wouldn't want the media to use my comfort with nudity to take advantage, as 'sex sells'.

Breasts can have sensual and erogenous aspects. Then there's how breasts are portrayed in the media. For some people that's inappropriate, for some it's appropriate. Then there are the medical aspects of breasts. They are both private and public. Within a relationship they take on a different aspect because they are part of the lovemaking. As a naturist, that's just incidental, it's by the by, my body is in its entirety. But then I have to shroud my breasts to go into society. It's a hot day and outside there is a man walking down the street with no T-shirt on, but I can't take my T-shirt off because it's not acceptable in our society. In other cultures it's totally acceptable. There are so many taboos about breasts. They can give great pleasure and be the source of great torment, especially for those women and men who get breast cancer.

You know what's interesting, I didn't mention breastfeeding. I wanted to breastfeed my children as long as possible. I yearned for another child but sadly never had one. Now at the age of 51 and not in a relationship I don't think it will happen! *(laughs)* Breastfeeding was, and still is sadly, taboo in public. I used to feed my children with a shawl around myself, like they were encased within a little womb. It was a private moment between me and my child, and I shielded my breasts from prying eyes. Either I thought some men who can't disassociate the sexual aspects from breasts might see me and find it erotic, or someone might disapprove. I didn't want the stress hormones to flood my breastmilk so I kept it private. I would have liked to be able to breastfeed in public without recrimination, but you couldn't and you still can't. There should be signs everywhere reminding everyone that it's a breastfeeding friendly place: 'Public, like it or lump it, you will see a woman breastfeeding'.

This is what women do. We release and we share and we talk. It's cathartic. It's empowering.

Age 51 | Two children

"We are so fixated on them in our culture"

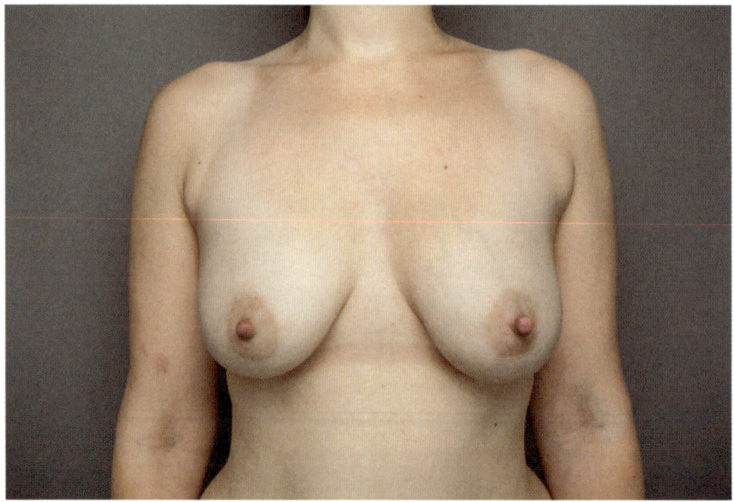

My breasts are mine now. I'm proud of them. They do a really important job, breastfeeding my baby. They are great. But they are mine, they are to do with me, not to do with other people, and that is a big shift.

When I was a teenager I would hoike them up in uplift bras. A friend said if you buy a bra that is a cup size too small and use a hair band to join the straps together at the top, you get an amazing cleavage. I'd pump them up as high as I could. We'd do everything we could to create gravity-defying breasts. Relatively recently at a modern jive event I was wearing a push-up bra that must have been an inch thick in places. I was dancing with one of my friends and he commented that my bra was like some sort of armour or weapon.

I think it's all about social programming and money. The reason a lot of women will spend money is to make themselves feel good. But the reason they feel good is the confidence they get through attention from men. And that's because their confidence is so undermined by companies trying to sell them stuff and make them feel bad about their body. I used to do all that, wear the make-up and the bras, for attention and sexual approval.

I have wonky boobs and different shaped nipples. I remember worrying about what men would think, but to be honest I don't think anyone ever noticed. I wasn't confident about my body with my first boyfriend when I was a teenager. I tried to hide under the covers and never really gave him an opportunity to actually see my body. He would see the boobs with a push-up bra, but not my body naked with none of that supporting stuff. I wanted to preserve the illusion. I wasn't happy about any of me.

My breasts didn't live up to the sexual images I saw and there was a certain amount of shame about that. My breasts weren't rock hard or symmetrical. They weren't sensitive in a good way. That all seemed to imply a lack of control. A lot of the beauty industry is about controlling your image. But in fact, good sex comes from a lack of control, from releasing your inhibitions.

Once I started to feel comfortable with myself I got more attention and respect. I feel like I have a duty to other women not to buy into all that image stuff. I wouldn't wear a bra now that makes me look not like myself.

I felt squeamish about my breasts for a long time. I think it came from the disparity between being bombarded by images of breasts as sexual things, but also knowing about breastfeeding and thinking they are for babies. Porn images of men playing with breasts aren't respectful, or sensual – it's to do with force a lot of the time, vulgarity. Therefore, gentle touch seemed like such an odd thing. The idea of touching my own breasts … I didn't want to do it. That lasted a long time. When I had my son I had breastfeeding problems, blockages in milk ducts, and you are supposed to massage them out. I found that really difficult because feeling my breasts and the lumps in them made my skin crawl.

I couldn't hand express till recently, but I finally feel 100 per cent comfortable with my breasts. Recently I had to hand express and I did it into a pint glass. It was pouring into the glass! I was proud and felt a sense of achievement. My husband was there and he was fascinated by the multiple jets. When I'd finished, I jokingly said, 'Right, who wants some milk now?'

He's tried my breastmilk. I do know women who are funny about trying it, although they drink cows' milk. He had a swig out of the glass and said it was really nice. We kept it in the fridge and he had some in his coffee the next morning. I'm really proud that we are like that as a family. He's totally into breastfeeding, it's what he sees my breasts as for, but he still finds them sexy. He's been more comfortable with the changes in my body than me.

I couldn't marry up the mum part of me with the sexual me from before, and I had to reinvent myself sexually after having a baby. My husband finds all of my body sexy, but breasts aren't really part of the sexual experience for him at the moment. He doesn't avoid them, but you can't risk going too near them or you have a let-down and milk goes all over the place. I don't want to include lactation in the sexual experience! He finds them sexy to look at but he doesn't quite know what to do with them.

I've wondered what it would be like if he tried milk from my breast, but I'm a bit scared after nipple damage and feeding problems to start with. A good latch makes all the difference and it's been a long time since he breastfed! *(laughs)* I think it's the only thing that puts me off actually.

I have a breastmilk keepsake necklace. Some people think it's weird, but a pearl necklace is made by an oyster. I felt that I wanted something to commemorate getting through the difficult breastfeeding times.

I've been thinking about breasts a lot lately. I find it odd that we are so fixated on them in our culture. Women have always been sexual. We've been celebrated for our fertility. But as a culture we've moved away from breasts being about babies and sexualised them in an exaggerated money-driven way. It's really sad and I worry about the way my child will view women's bodies. It's partly why I won't go back to wearing make up and push-up bras. I want him to know what women actually look like. We should be proud of how we look.

If I look rubbish it's because I'm feeling rubbish. If I've had three hours sleep, why should I have to cover it up with make up? I'm tired because I'm a mum. I think we should be nicer to each other about our bodies.

I'm pretty OK with toplessness now, due to breastfeeding. I don't mind lifting my whole top up to breastfeed, but it's cold in this country. I don't have a problem with being naked but I do have a problem with other people viewing my nudity in a certain way.

I originally thought I would breastfeed till my son is one, and that breastfeeding babies till they were two was all about the women not the babies. Then I did some reading and I realised it wasn't weird and they still get a lot out of it. (*son is currently breastfeeding and making 'mmm-yum' noises*) I'm now hoping to get to at least two years old. If I tell people I see a look in their eyes. They say it seems weird, but they can't say why. The only thing they ever come up with is, 'Isn't it confusing for them?' But children don't hit one year old and suddenly become open to sexual stimulus and subject to all of these influences that we've had about breasts being sexual. Babies see breasts as comfort and food.

More and more women are extending breastfeeding. I met a woman who still feeds her seven-year-old at bedtime. Some people find that weird, they don't think the child should remember it. I think it would be great if my son remembers it, because then he will have something to balance out the media message about breasts being for sex. The more children who get to school age who remember being breastfed, the better.

––––––––––––––

Age 29 | One child, breastfeeding one-year-old

"Often people don't perceive you as a sexual person when you are in a wheelchair"

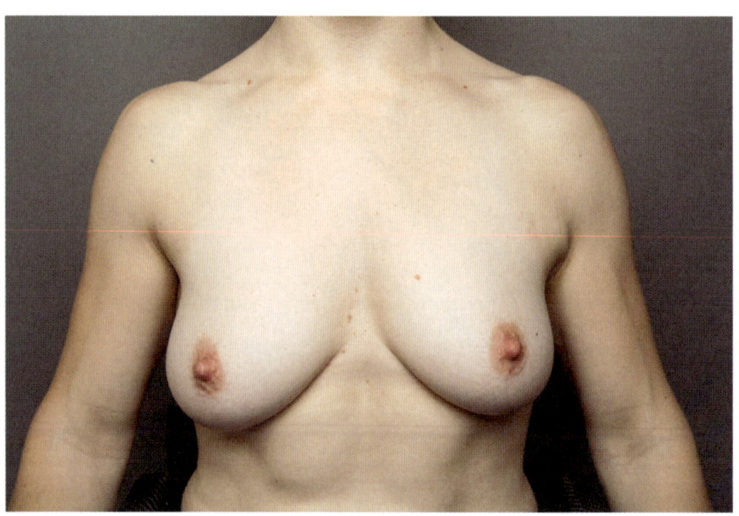

I think my breasts are one of my good features. They've always been relatively big. My friends were jealous of them when I was growing up. I was a small person and I suddenly grew these pert boobs. I can remember people accusing me of sticking my boobs out. I didn't mind, we had a laugh about it. I did ballet and horse riding, so as a result of that I had good posture.

I remember being at a swimming party when I was 13 and a friend's dad said, 'Oh, where have they come from?' Erm, that was embarrassing, but probably more so for my friend. I remember suddenly noticing attention from older men. Not inappropriate, but attention all the same. Your breasts make you suddenly grow into a woman. I was a D cup by the time I was about 14, and I was only about five feet tall!

I was short, my bottom was too big and quite muscular. I never felt like I had a great figure. But I did feel like I had great boobs. They were very high up when I was 18 and I had to shorten bra staps. I remember wishing they were a bit more pendulous. Now they are a bit more pendulous, thanks to gravity, I wonder what I was thinking!

When I was about 23 I lived in France and the women are very slim there. A woman I was working for told me I was too heavy to ride her horses. I became very conscious of what I was eating and I developed bulimia. I got fitter, I lost weight. I lost some of the fat from my breasts and they changed a bit.

In France there are lots of things in pharmacies about health and diets and losing weight. I'm not really sure they should sell slimming pills. The ads made me more conscious of weight even though I didn't take the pills. I also read women's health magazines and they talk about weight. I was just miserable.

When I was 26 I had a spinal cord injury as a result of an accident. Obviously it was really traumatic. I was told I would never walk again, never do sport, never dance.

I remember thinking in hospital, 'God it would have been awful if I had really great legs, at least I've got great boobs, at least I have them!' *(laughs)* But it wasn't till I'd been in hospital for four months that I felt like that. At least I had my arms, at least I had some muscles that worked.

Being in a wheelchair does affect your sense of femininity and how people perceive you, although I didn't think about sexuality for a while. Often people don't perceive you as a sexual person when you are in a wheelchair. A pair of jeans and top would look more sexy if I were able to stand up. Although because people are higher up they can look down my cleavage. You've got to be careful about not wearing low-cut tops.

Without movement, clothes don't drape as well as they used to. I found dressing to look good hard to start with. Although I can wear skinny jeans now because my legs are less muscular. *(laughs)* This long after the injury I am aware of what looks nice. In a way having bigger boobs helps because I look feminine despite being muscular. My breasts are important in making me look and feel feminine.

Six months after I broke my back I got together with my husband. I was intrigued to see how sex would be because I have limited sensation. I have normal sensation only to the hips. My friend took me out, 'We have to get you a vibrator, see how it is!' It's very different sexually to what it was, the sensation has changed. I have the same post-orgasm feeling, but it's not the same orgasm feeling. And I can't just move any way I want to move, I have to move my stupid legs out of the way. My breasts were quite sensitive before the accident, and important to me sexually. That hasn't changed.

The actor who played Superman had a spinal injury. His website talked about spinal injuries and sexuality, and about how it was harder for men to deal with, because men can't get an erection or ejaculate. An article about how it was worse for men! Someone with such a big name... I might complain, but I've got so many things I need to do.

I don't think of myself as being disabled. You don't often see women in wheelchairs in the press. I'd like to change that.

As a GB athlete I wear good sports bras. I do feel a bit unfeminine constantly wearing sports bras and tracksuits. Having smaller breasts is generally better for sports, but in my sport it doesn't matter, in fact it might add weight and that's good.

I much prefer sunbathing topless. Frankly, I don't find it comfortable wearing a bikini top. I sunbathed topless on honeymoon. It might bother my husband a bit more. I'm like, 'What the hell, they're only boobs aren't they?' You get hot and sweaty, and they have wires, and if it's supportive it pulls on the back of your neckm ... I'd much rather be topless.

They're only boobs at the end of the day. Society has made us believe that nipples can't ever be shown, although you can show plenty of cleavage. Nipples are an absolute no-no. British culture tells us we mustn't go there, but in France they sunbathe topless. In Austria they are very relaxed about nudity, they have naked saunas and stuff. The women just sit around with their legs spread! They have no qualms about anything. I quite like a sauna and it's much nicer to be naked.

I think breasts are very comforting. I remember my mum giving me a big cuddle and they were very comforting. They can also be very sexy. I think other women's breasts can be attractive and sexy. You could equally think a woman has great hair or great boobs!

I like thinking and talking about the body and body image. I think it's important to raise people's awareness. The way women's bodies are perceived is different to the way men's are perceived. That doesn't seem fair. Women's bodies are constantly criticised.

I wouldn't consider cosmetic surgery on them. I can't bear the thought of someone cutting me open and doing something to me. I can't understand why anyone would have an operation and have something put into their body. After my time in hospital I find it hard to understand choosing to go under the knife.

I agreed to do this before telling my husband. It's my body, I'll do what I want! But he did ask why I was putting my boobs in a book. To start off with he questioned it a bit. It wasn't an issue though. I'm not sure I could have done this if it wasn't anonymous though, because showing your breasts is seen as selling yourself. It can come back to haunt you in a negative way.

———————

Age 34 | No children

"My daughter can sit next to me to breastfeed because my breasts bend round the corner"

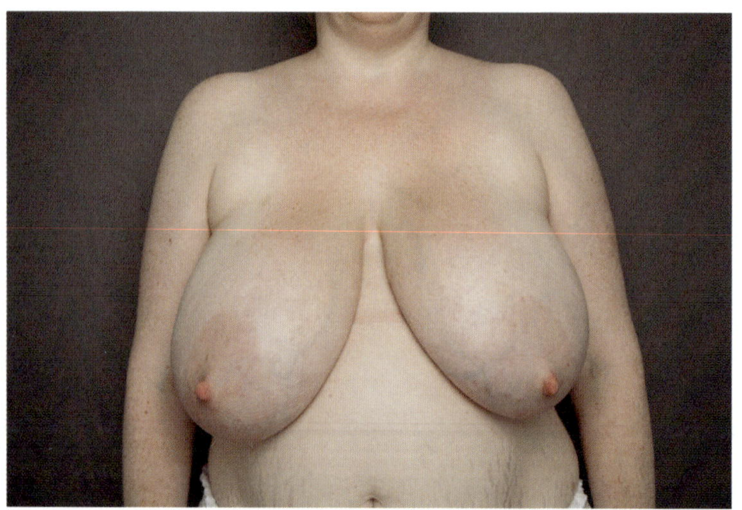

I'd describe my breasts as big! I've always been known for having big boobs. When I was 14 they went from nothing to big straight away. I was at a girl's school after 11 so I didn't get many comments. Before having a baby I was 36H and now I am a K.

I'm happy to have big ones. I've always been confident about them. I think they are ideal. At university people would say I could win a marathon because my breasts would finish before me. *(laughs)*

My mum's side of the family are pretty much flat-chested. My dad has a big build, so I think I have taken after him and it's come out in the boobs. My mum used to say I should share it around!

I wish I could get things to fit me nicely. After children I would consider having them reduced if they don't shrink down on their own, and it doesn't look like they will. I never used to be able to buy bras easily, but its better now and I can get quite nice ones in specialist places.

I was in my late teens before I went out with boys. They were always quite pleased with my breasts. My husband says he wasn't a boob man, he was more of a legs or bum man, but he must have changed his mind when he saw me! He converted. He's very pro-breast now. If I say they are too big or flopping about, he says they are lovely just as they are.

I used to work for the police and, looking back, some of the comments I used to get were sexual harassment. You know those frames of pins and you can do hand prints in them? Once they tried to get me to do a boob print. I didn't do it. The sexual harassment is done in a 'humorous' way, and we got on well, but it was a situation where I wouldn't have wanted to be on my own in a room with one of them, it was uncomfortable.

I'm planning on breastfeeding through the pregnancy. Apparently when the baby is born you switch back to colostrum, which might put her off. I'm hoping to tandem breastfeed. It can be quite helpful with jealousy issues. Breastfeeding has gone quite smoothly for me. My daughter can sit next to me to breastfeed because my breasts bend round the corner. Their size can be quite useful.

Friends have asked me if I'm going to stop breastfeeding soon, letting me know what they think. Every now and then my husband says, 'You won't breastfeed her when she's four will you?' But then he used to say, 'You won't breastfeed when she's two will you?' And she's nearly two now. I know someone who is breastfeeding a four-year-old. I don't really have a limit; perhaps five because of school. Although you could have bedtime feeds and no one would need to know. I'm assuming she will stop herself before that age.

———————

Age 38 | One child, breastfeeding 21-month-old, pregnant

"When I was thinner I always wanted bigger boobs, and now I've got them, not really"

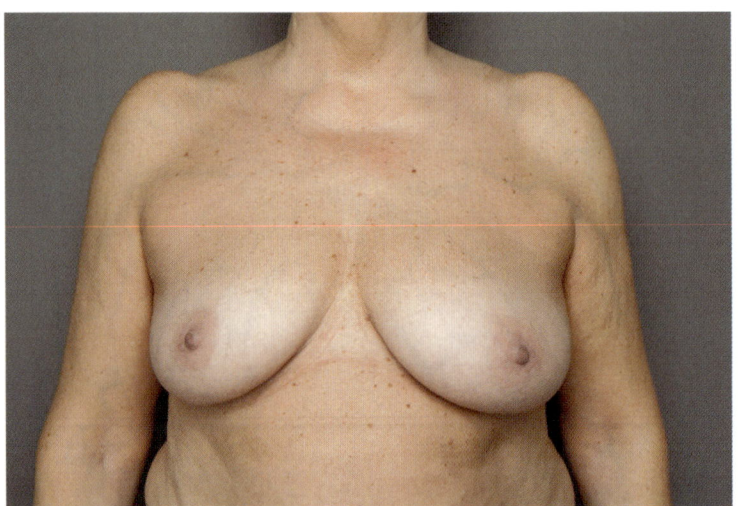

At the moment I'm feeling terribly overweight, so feel that my breasts are too big and they are attracting attention. When I was young I was very skinny and never had any breasts. Always wanted them, thought they would be a marvellous thing to have. I totally disagree with that now. They change the shape of your dresses. I think they make your look cluttered and, at my age, matronly.

I work with a mixed bunch of people, perhaps people I wouldn't normally associate with. Some men make comments or look at my chest. It could be called sexual harrassment actually. The other day, one young chap in his 30s said 'You've got a fine pair of buns.' To some people that might be very offensive. I just laughed it off, because it was an off-the-cuff remark. It didn't worry me because I'm fairly outgoing. Another chap the other day, said 'Are you still going to the gym?' I said, 'Yes, I am, why do you ask?' And he said, 'Because your buttons are bulging on your blouse.' Now, how come he noticed that?

I'm not being funny, but I am quite shocked, at my age. I'd understand if they saw a young thing, but for somebody of my age I think it's quite unusual. It's mainly in the workplace, although there have been comments from the odd acquaintance. One said how 'womanly' I look, which I find offensive actually, because his wife is the trophy stick-thin jobby. It makes you wonder whether men like it when they see somebody more rounded. It's difficult in a social situation.

I've always been able to wear simple shift dresses, but now they are much more difficult. I don't think the line of the clothes falls as well on the bigger-breasted person. I'm a 38C or D, but I was a 34A. I've put on a lot of weight, because I've developed a sweet tooth in recent years.

Breasts are important sexually, they make me feel more of a woman. My partner hasn't commented on my changing breasts. I've been with him 36 years or something, and he's 65, so he's of an older generation. I don't know how important my breasts are to him, to be honest. My breasts certainly play a part as an erogenous zone, I suppose more around the nipple area.

I always used to go topless. I'm a sun-worshipper and I always hated the lines. I don't go topless anymore, I've crossed that age barrier. There's something not so nice about being of that granny age, definitely. Because I've put on weight I wear a one-piece whereas I always wore bikinis before.

When I was thinner I always wanted bigger boobs, and now I've got them, not really.

—————

Age 58 | Two children

"Because I have rejected my breasts they aren't erogenous"

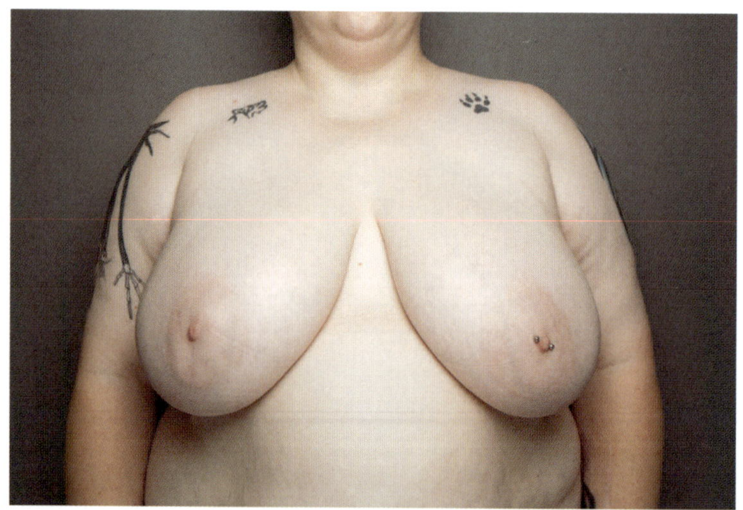

I absolutely hate my breasts. I would give them up tomorrow. I'm 40GG and I've been this size since I was 14. I had to give up running in my teens because it was so painful and I couldn't find a good enough sports bra. When you run they constantly jig, and because of the weight of them there would be a pounding pain in my shoulders and back, and shooting pains in my breasts. I gave up sport and got bigger and bigger. I went to the doctor when I was 15 and pretty much begged for a reduction, but they said no.

I have a lot of issues relating to my breasts. For one thing, I like wearing men's clothes and it's hard to find clothes that fit. I spend my whole time trying to cover up my breasts. I find men's clothes really comfortable. My therapist tried to explore this with me. Really, it's purely because they are more comfortable. Men's T-shirts are also funnier. I don't want to wear a sparkly girly T-shirt. Sports Direct is my Mecca. I should be their spokesperson, except I'd be the fattest spokesperson going. I don't want to be a man, but I don't feel comfortable in women's clothes. I remember looking like a meringue in bridesmaids' dresses, and feeling like I was on display, and they felt restrictive.

I suffered with eating disorders as a kid. I had a granddad who was particularly horrid. He told me if I lost weight I would be able to run faster. So I wouldn't eat; I was living off a sandwich and an apple a day. I did so much sport and a lot of running. It made me realise how quickly you can spiral out of control. I got very thin. I was a size six to eight but I still had these massive boobs. I have friends who have been in hospital with anorexia. I'm not blasé, but I refuse now to panic about my size.

It feels horrible to pin the eating disorder and body dysmorphia on my granddad, but it was his fault. He was a very hard man. 'You're fat. You're useless. You aren't going to get anywhere.' I think the media was an influence too. There should be honesty, not pressure to look perfect. And what is perfect? It changes. Magazines aimed at 15-year-old girls criticise women without their make up, or bingo wings, or cellulite. People are obsessed with size. Until it changes we are going to have a really sad world.

I see little girls in shorts and high heels. It makes me want to cry. I feel terrified for my niece. What happened to just being a kid?

My breasts represent something that should be very special and sacred and important, for mothering and breastfeeding. But they've been taken and destroyed. Now they represent everything that's wrong in the world. It's OK to have glamour models flaunting their breasts for men to look at, but people will still sit and stare at a mother breastfeeding. How can people be so twisted?

I've got borderline personality disorder. It can lead to erratic behaviour, self-harm, suicidal behaviour. These are self-harm scars. *(shows me)* I've been hospitalised. I've been through eight years of therapy.

I started harming when I was 12; that's when a lot of things happened to me. I realised I was gay. I found out I couldn't have children. I lost my best friend to leukaemia. My good granddad died. I managed to hide the self-harming until I was 22 when I had a massive breakdown.

I felt like I was lost when I found out I couldn't have children. When I was 11 my periods started. I had five, and then they stopped. The doctor said, 'You've got PCOS *(polycystic ovary syndrome)*, it's one of the worst cases that I've seen, there's no chance you will have children, there's nothing we can do except put you on the Pill to give you regular periods.' My world just ended. I think she has a lot to answer for, because I think I just gave up. I think in a way hating my breasts is related to rejecting some of these aspects of becoming a woman that were difficult when I was younger.

I'm the stereotypical 'butch' lesbian. Because I am obviously gay, some random men think it is absolutely fine to come up to me and go, 'Your tits are massive! Can I have a grope?' If they could hear themselves and hear what they've just said. Imagine if I asked to hold their penis. If it gets to the stage where I am going to get into an argument with someone, my friends will step in and help. I've literally been in the corner of a room and people have been groping me.

I went for a job interview and the man interviewing me knew my cousin, who's a man. He said, 'Oh, you look just like your cousin except with massive boobs.' Well, that was a job interview, it was meant to be professional, it was not OK to say that. Just because I dress asexually it doesn't mean people have a license to say what they want about my boobs.

I get 'Yes sir,' in shops. When I picked up my sister's kids from nursery there were lots of 'yummy mummies' there, and the looks I would get! It was like I was trying to steal their children, ridiculous. People don't like to admit they judge you on your looks, but they do.

If I could have my breasts removed, I would. Which is bad because my partner has had breast cancer three times and had a mastectomy.

She never removes her sports bra, not even when she goes to bed. I respect that, because I know how I feel about my clothing. If that's what she needs to make her feel comfortable that's fine. It hurts me that she can't see how beautiful she is. *(cries)* I'm getting all emotional now. I accept her as she is.

My breasts don't feature sexually in this relationship. I'm aware of not wanting to 'flaunt' them. I don't walk around with my boobs out. It's not me anyway, but it would feel like kicking someone in the teeth. I've got breasts that I hate and she has had to go through horrific times to do with her breasts, which she lost. It makes me feel guilty.

She had so much chemo it damaged her heart, and she has a pacemaker. So she can't have nipples tattooed on because you can't tattoo within six inches of a pacemaker. All the women in her family have had breast cancer. Her mum sadly passed away from it.

On our first date she explained to me what she had been through. I had to explain to her about my scars and my self-harm. It was so intense for a first date to explain all this. You have to tell the other one, because at some point you will see the scars. It's so hard.

Because I have rejected my breasts they aren't erogenous. My nipples are numb. I don't get any sensation from them. I got a nipple pierced, and everyone was asking if it hurt. I just didn't feel it at all.

My ex-girlfriend was obsessed with my breasts, to the extent that I asked her if she would leave me if I had to lose my breasts for any reason. She said she would. Then she said she was joking, but she wasn't, I knew she would. It was always my breasts with her.

My ex ended our relationship because she'd been seeing a man for about six months. I lived rough for a while. I thought I was indestructible, that I was brave enough to cope with anything, but I felt very vulnerable. I thought I could fight anyone, but when you wake up in a park at 6am in a park on your own it's terrifying. You think every little noise is a mass murderer trying to kill you. I was very lucky I didn't have any problems. Men and women can be attacked, but you feel more vulnerable as a woman. I get mistaken for being a man every day, but my breasts very much identify me as a woman.

____

Age 31 | No children

"There was no need for them to be that big"

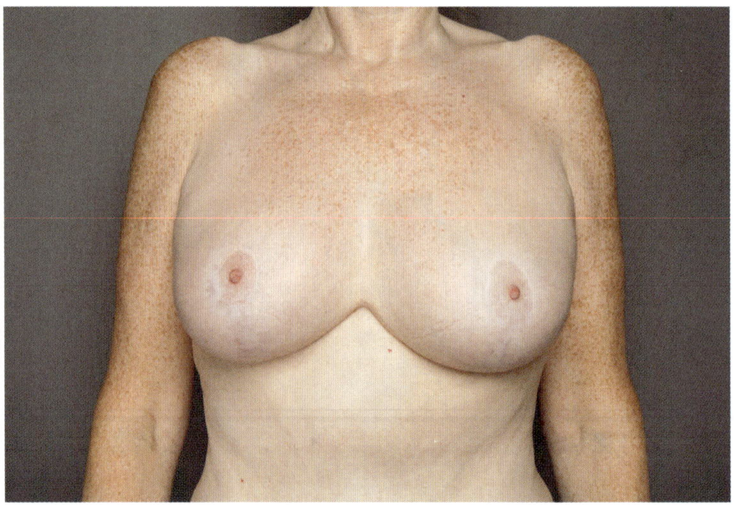

Since I've had the reduction getting into clothes is a lot better, which is really good. I wish they were smaller. I'm a 38D. I was a 38GG before, which was very big.

I had the reduction about five years ago, and it was the best thing I ever did in my life. When my breasts were too big, I couldn't get clothes that fitted me properly. If I bought anything to fit my bust it was huge at the bottom. I could never wear a bikini. The bottom would have been huge compared to the top, I'd have had to buy two! I wouldn't have worn a bikini anyway.

I wasn't big breasted when I was a teenager, I was in proportion. I had a very good figure. My breasts became bigger with each child and never went down, just got bigger and bigger. I always felt that men were just talking to my breasts, not to me. They were always in the way. My back was aching a bit too. There was no need for them to be that big. I hated it. I could never get any nice clothes at all.

I decided in the end to get rid of them because I felt I was into later life and desperately wanted to wear nice dresses. When you're so big you have to have out-size dresses. I couldn't really buy anything. I looked dowdy and bulky. It was about me as an older woman, thinking I wanted to wear nice clothes. I'm not bothered if I'm attractive to men, as long as I like the way I look. I love the way I can dress now. Absolutely love it! I've got two drawers full of bras. I just bought a bikini for the first time ever. I feel good about myself, and I didn't before. Confidence is brilliant.

My husband didn't want me to have it done at all. He liked them. I think he saw them as there for him. It didn't cause rows, because as far as I'm concerned it's none of his business. I do what I like, whether he likes it or not, and if he doesn't like it he can go elsewhere. I don't mean that in an awful way, but at my age I am not putting up with anyone telling me what to do.

My daughter's exactly the same but she's not had a reduction. She's so big she looks like she's going to fall over all the time. Her husband likes them.

Breasts in films and magazines are perfect compared to me and my friends! *(laughs)* They are wonderful. It gives an impression that all women's breasts are like that, and most women know that is not true. We're all different shapes, we've got one bigger than the other, and nipples are different. We sag as we get older. I just wish they would have a bit more decorum. You can't expect men to treat you one way if you are doing that. I think it demeans them. But their breasts are beautiful: they wouldn't be in the papers if they weren't.

When I had mine done I could have had implants done at the same time and pulled them up. But I wanted them to be natural. I was hoping for a smaller size. I would be able to get in Dior then! You have to be very small, virtually non-existent, to get into Dior. There are beautiful clothes, if you are talking Dior, Versace ... the most beautiful material, beautiful designs, but you have to be small. They don't make them for big people, that's the problem. I'd love to just get into one of them before I die. If it was up to me, I'd have them off! *(laughs)*

Along with the breast reduction I had liposuction too. I thought, 'in for a penny, in for a pound!' I had a tummy tuck and liposuction on my tummy. All three in one go. I wouldn't have the tummy tuck done again in a million years, that was very painful. It's the worst operation ever. You are doubly incontinent for a while because you can't get up. It's really difficult. Whereas I didn't feel a thing with my breasts.

You have to get to the best weight you can before you have a breast reduction done. And if you put on weight after, it will all come back. The surgeon said, 'You'll have gone through all this pain for nothing, so be aware of that'. And of course I wasn't … I've put weight on, and I really wish I'd been better.

The children were fine about the reduction, but more worried about the operation. My son was worried about me not coming out of it. It was all, 'Mum, I don't want to lose you! Please don't have it done'. He couldn't care less about what I look like. My daughter is the same, 'I don't know why you're bothering Mum, you look absolutely fine!' I won't have any more surgery done.

I didn't breastfeed. I couldn't bear the thought of doing it. No. I would never have breastfed in public, ever. I was very annoyed, because when I had my children they were trying to insist that I breastfeed. You stayed in hospital a lot longer in those days, at least seven days, sometimes 10. They were saying, 'You really must do this. This is good for the baby'. Making you feel guilty. Well, I wasn't going to feel guilty, because I was determined I wasn't going to do it.

It's extremely important to breastfeed children. But I just couldn't bear to do it myself. *(laughs)* All of the antibodies, everything in breastmilk, is so good for children. I just couldn't do it myself. I really don't know why, I don't know at all. To have something suckling my breast …

I've got no qualms about other people doing it, it's fine, absolutely fine. I would turn away, because I don't think it's my business.

I can't stand the sight of nipples. I have covers to cover my nipples, even with a bra. I can't bear to see nipples. It comes from my parents being prudish. My dad used to check me every time I went out as a teenager. I had to stand at the top of the stairs to see if he could see my pants. I used to wear mini-skirts, and he'd say, 'Right, back, you're not wearing that!' They were very, very prudish.

———————————

Age 62 | Three children

"Breasts are powerful, not submissive"

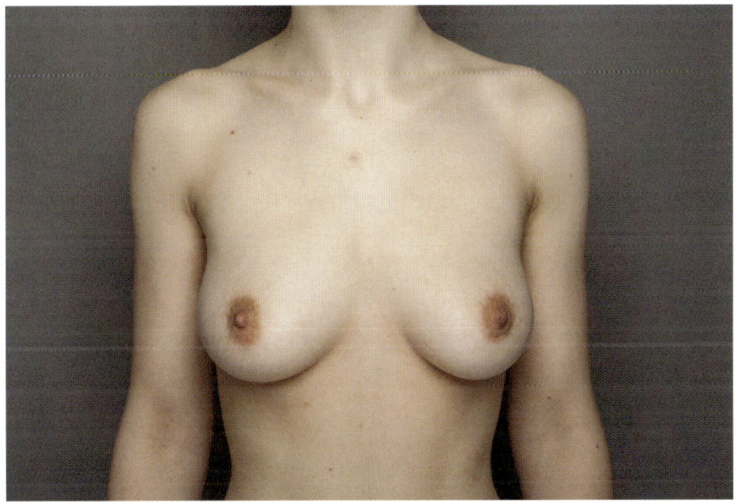

How I feel about my breasts has been very fluid.

I became interested in Femen (an international women's movement) when they were on the cover of the *Sunday Times*. The image was nothing like the typical image of a topless woman. It redefined what a woman could be. I thought, 'I will be involved with this.' I couldn't at the time, I was still too young. I thought I would finish university first, and I wanted to be sufficiently informed.

My work with Femen hasn't been as extensive as others, but in this country I'm probably one of the most active. That's illustrative of how comfortable we are in this country; people don't feel the need to do it. In Ukraine women did it even though it put them in danger. However, in a country which calls itself free, I spoke to a policeman about the actual laws: if I am standing there topless they can arrest me and it's down to the discretion of the individual officer. I think that's so fundamentally wrong. It's legal for men to be topless, but it's illegal for women. That's unfathomable, it's insane. Men have breast tissue too.

There are no matriarchal cultures today, despite the fact that we have a Queen. Not that she is going to be getting her breasts out any time soon. *(laughs)* I think everyone secretly thinks matriarchal culture would be better. Men keep making wars, maybe we'd have no wars if we had matriarchies.

I think that fear is at the core of not allowing women to be topless. Women are still blamed for men making advances on women. Part of me doesn't really understand why people are so threatened though. I didn't see many topless women when I was growing up, that's a given. But I saw my dad sitting topless in the garden throwing tennis balls for the dog. It doesn't even cross your mind to question it.

I think I started questioning things when I tried to set up a feminist society at school and I was knocked down. I started to read feminist writers. I'm interested in how women can be misogynists. Coming from an all-girl private school I can tell you it exists.

Femen are trying to get media attention, there is no shrouding that. That's what activism involves, getting people's attention. Being topless gets attention. The sex industry in Ukraine is shocking. The female body in Ukraine is utilised to make money, and they thought, 'Fuck that' and turned the whole thing on its head. I strongly believe that from the outset they have intended to change how the world looks at breasts. What's fantastic is that I think it's working. When I saw that first article I thought they were amazing, empowered and feminine. The more I look at pictures of Femen, the more normal it becomes. We are so easily programmed as a species.

When I was first presented with the idea of being topless, I felt threatened. My friends think I am insane. None of them are interested in Femen. The only person who stood outside the Tunisian embassy with me topless in the snow to support me was my boyfriend. He knew I was slightly terrified about doing it on my own. When the police saw we were taking our tops off and had slogans written on us, a riot van arrived with about 15 policemen. Then they realised we weren't the 'real' Femen – we didn't want to climb up the walls and scream – our aim was just to stand there and protest.

A police officer said, 'I'm really sorry, I will have to arrest you if you take off your bra, there's no way round it'. If I had been arrested I wouldn't have got the pictures taken, so I kept my bra on so the slogans could be seen.

I didn't want to get arrested; I was still at university. I'm a London kid. I wanted to do this because it mattered, but if you get arrested and get a criminal record here, it's hard to bounce back from that. You might find it difficult to get a job. We've got it too good to put ourselves out there. People in the UK don't want to go about Femen in quite the same way. We'll have to find a slightly different way of doing it. Politically we don't have the same reasons and it just won't work. We haven't all been topless at the same time yet. I don't know what will happen with Femen in the UK. I don't know if there are enough people ready to embrace it fully.

There were protests at Tunisian embassies all over the world. It was very well orchestrated everywhere except in London. Women did topless photos in support of Amina after she was arrested. There was such strength in it. It's dangerous for Muslim women anywhere in the world to take part in that.

I had a topless photo on Facebook, but I'd painted over my breasts and nipples with blue and yellow, the Femen thing. It was removed, which was absurd.

I haven't told my father about my involvement with Femen. I think he would have a reaction. It comes down to a sense of ownership. Do I own my own body? If I do, I can do what I like and not feel ashamed. I've been having an identity crisis. I have to hide everything from my father. I'm not sure what to do. I want to be honest about who I am. Life is fluid and you are influenced by every moment you experience. In light of that you change every second.

Since Femen has started, since seeing these strong women emerge, my view of my breasts has changed completely. I wouldn't have taken part in *Bare Reality* two years ago. When you contacted Femen UK I couldn't think of any other members who would do it and I was very interested. It seemed like an important project.

I can't wait to read the rest of *Bare Reality*. I'm fascinated to know how different women feel about their breasts. It will be interesting to see what men think. Men are terrified of the desexualisation of breasts. Men who whistle at women in the streets and objectify them will probably be really uncomfortable about this project. My boyfriend is such a good guy, he identifies as a feminist. He knows I am doing this and he's really excited about it. Why do men respond so differently to things?

I see my breasts as something that can change the world. Breasts are powerful, not submissive. They have more significance than they have ever had. The illegality of our breasts makes the difference between men and women more extreme.

———————————

Age 20 | No children

"Because I'm pregnant they're not as I've always known them"

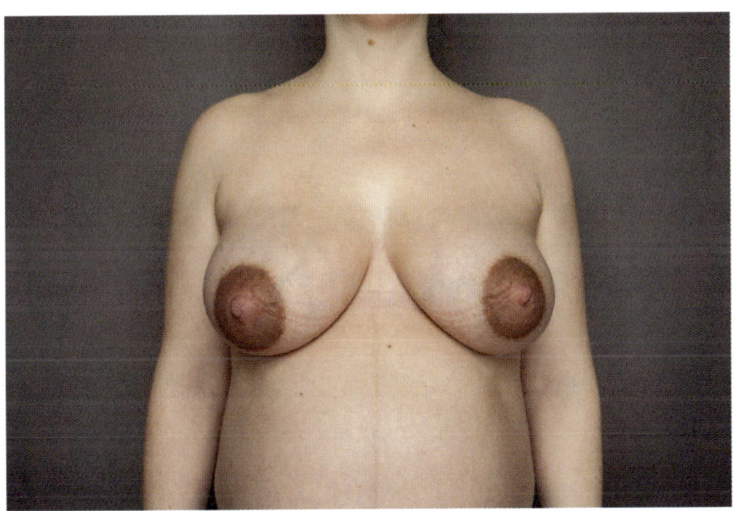

I've got slightly mixed feelings about my breasts. Because I'm pregnant they're not as I've always known them. The areolae are big and incredibly dark – that looks quite strange – and they're much fuller, much bigger. They were always fairly large anyway, larger than perhaps I would have liked. They feel quite big at the minute! *(laughs)* I am sure there are lots of people who would like that, but I'm not necessarily one of them. I was a 32DD before pregnancy. My ideal size would probably be a 32C.

There a few reasons why I don't like having big breasts. When you are large it can make you look a dress size bigger than you are. It limits what you can wear and feel comfortable in. I've found bra shopping isn't very enjoyable. You see all these lovely pretty bras, all displayed in a small size, then you pick up the bra in your size and it looks like a hideous boulder holder! It doesn't even look like the same bra! Bras look like hammocks, massive granny bras.

For reasons I've never been able to figure out, even larger cup sizes are so massively padded. My boobs are big enough already, why would I want to make them look bigger than they are? I don't like the padding. I don't want or need them to look bigger than they are, and it can give you an odd shape as well.

There's a specific type of bra I like, underwired, balconette-style, lacy, so it doesn't look like you have so much material. I look everywhere to find the right bras, all the big department stores.

I try and disguise my big boobs with the clothes and types of bras I wear. Some bras make you look bigger and give you a cleavage. I don't particularly like a cleavage looking like a bum. I don't like that look at all, I'd rather I was just supported in a bra, rather than being squashed together. I hate that look.

I was chuffed when I got my first bra, I was desperate for those sort of things to start happening. Maybe I wanted to feel grown-up. I didn't have really big boobs at school, they didn't get larger till I was about 17. They suddenly grew quite quickly, and I got stretch marks that I felt self-conscious about.

I used to feel very self-conscious about my breasts, and in my early 20s I had to learn how to dress myself. There are some people who have larger breasts and don't think twice about it, whereas I didn't want to draw attention to having a larger pair of boobs. So it comes down to the type of bra you wear, the types of clothes you wear. There will be some tops I think will look nice, but no, it looks matronly because of the size of my boobs. You have to think about what you're wearing. If you wear something low, and you've got an ample chest, whether you want it to or not it suddenly looks tarty, in my opinion.

I used to go topless sunbathing when I was younger, early to mid-20s, on beach and girly holidays. But I always felt a bit self-conscious. I wasn't 100 per cent comfortable. But I wanted an even tan! Lots of other people were topless, it was just what you did. If there was no one else going topless I wouldn't, and I would go topless on the beach, but not by the pool. I think topless sunbathing is declining. It was a 'thing' for a while, there was a stage when shops by the beach would just sell bikini bottoms.

It seems like we have one extreme or another in magazines or on TV.

You don't see many women with what I'd call average-sized boobs. They are either flat-chested, and you can see the breastbone, and the definition, a more fashion look, aimed more at women. And you've got the other extreme, where women have obviously fake, round, full boobs, a very sexual look, aimed more at men. I don't think there's much in between. I think the majority of women aspire to be thin and the majority of men like women who are fuller-figured.

Partners have made it clear they like that I've got fuller breasts. I'm quite curvy: large breasts, small waist, large hips. I think it's probably the combination.

When I was first pregnant they were too sore and sensitive. Then they became sensitive in a more erogenous way. My partner thinks all the changes from pregnancy are great, which sometimes I struggle to believe! My body is changing so much, really quickly as well. All for great reasons, obviously. If you've had the same physique for ages, and then it changes, it can alter how you feel about your body. And when you're with your partner, how you feel about your body is part of things. We've had quite a few conversations about things, and he does still find me attractive. He thinks it's great. We're not having sex as frequently but that's more me than my partner, due to feeling tired and achy, and I don't feel in the mood as frequently as I used to. In the first trimester I felt too nervous about it, and in the second I got more libido back. It's not the same, because you can't do the same things as you would normally, but breasts are still part of my sex life.

From what I've heard my boobs will get even larger after the birth. Which I'm not necessarily looking forward to! *(laughs)* Oh, crikey! I haven't got any control about what happens to them. Whatever happens, happens. It's part of life, you're going to get grey hairs, put on weight, lose muscle tone. Changes happen for a reason and they happen gradually, you have to accept it.

I'm planning on breastfeeding, but it will be decided as and when. The plan is that I will breastfeed and also express, as my partner also wants to be involved in the feeding. But we will see. He's totally on board with breastfeeding.

I'm not entirely sure about breastfeeding in public. I've never minded other people breastfeeding around me, I don't have an issue with it. I just don't know if I would feel comfortable with it in public. I'm not going to know until I'm in that situation. I'll probably be fine, but who knows. I can just go into a different room.

———————

Age 32 | Pregnant for the first time

"The female body is beautiful"

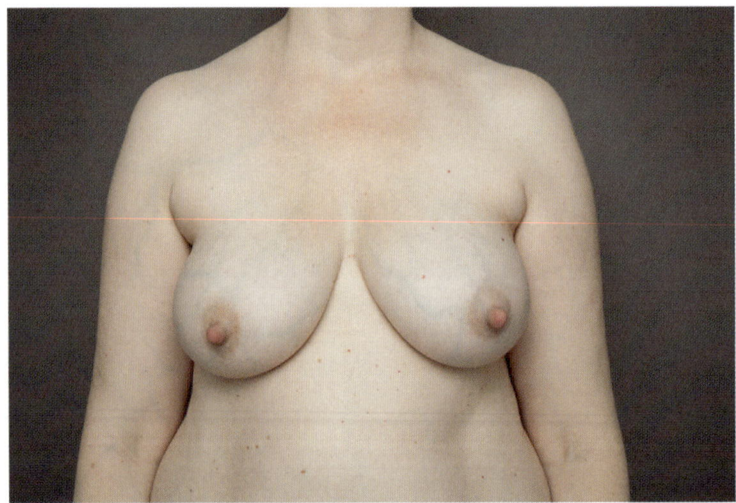

I like my breasts. If I dress properly my figure looks good. I haven't got dressed up for such a long time though.

Becoming a mother changes your relationship with your body. I had the birth I wanted to have and that was empowering. I feel like I've become a woman and accomplished something. I am here because a woman gave birth to me, I have given birth, and the line continues. I laboured at home, but wanted the back-up of hospital for my first birth, so I went in quite late on. They thought I wasn't in labour, but I gave birth an hour later! I'd done hypnobirthing and I was in myself, and in control. I was calm and collected. So I think they thought if I wasn't screaming I couldn't be in labour. I was sceptical about hypnobirthing, but it was brilliant.

My parents took me on naturist holidays from the age of eight. It helped me realise that everyone's bodies are all different: there is no ideal body. You don't look at the bodies, but you can't help taking them in. You never see that stick-thin model type.

I never felt that anyone was really looking at me on naturist holidays. There were a lot of Germans and as a nation they have a very different attitude to the human body. It was about human relationships, not bodies. We stopped going when I was about 14. Towards the end I did feel a bit self-conscious and wore a long T-shirt, but it was more about my family seeing me naked, not strangers.

I remember my mum getting dressed once and watching how she did her bra up. It intrigued me. It was before I hit puberty and she said, 'I don't think you're going to be small-breasted'.

I'm a voluntary breastfeeding peer supporter with the local NHS Trust. I was interested because I started out breastfeeding pretty naively. I thought it's just what women do. He fed well, and I had good support at the beginning, till he hit four months when he got distracted. It went wrong and I needed support. I was lucky enough to find it, and I had the reassurance and comfort to get through it. Having come through that, I was so grateful to have access to that support, that I wanted to be able to offer it to someone else who needed help.

My son is 18 months now. I thought I would breastfeed for a year, but having gone through the 'Troubles', as we call them in this house, from four months to nine months, I thought, 'Why would I give up now?'

I was ill last week and my period started again. My supply took a big hit. Bless him, he was so upset. He doesn't talk much yet, but he does baby sign language, and while he was latched on he kept signing, 'More milk, more milk'. It was only like that for a couple of days and then my supply went up again. Breastfeeding is a huge parenting tool for me. When he bumps his head, or he gets upset, or comes over shy, he has this base he can come back to for comfort. It's nutrition and antibodies and comfort.

Someone asked me why I was going to breastfeed and it really threw me. Why wouldn't I? I'm part of the human race, and that involves procreating and feeding and raising a child. My time on this planet is short, and I will use my body to keep the race alive. I know if I didn't, we wouldn't crumble away.

Men used to be attracted to my breasts and I could dress my figure to get attention. I knew they were a decent size and men would look at them. I don't want to sound arrogant, it's more that I was confident in them. I could put them in different tops and they would do a job in attracting a mate! *(laughs)* Although it's probably not right to derive confidence from your body, and you don't want a mate to be attracted to you for a body part, it's natural in the first stages. I was more confident that dressing a certain way would attract people, not my 'sparkling personality'.

I love breasts, I think they are fabulous. The female body is beautiful, more beautiful than the male. Women are more graceful and elegant even without clothes on. My husband has a fabulous body, and I love his body, but I think women are prettier to look at.

———————

Age 37 | One child, breastfeeding 18-month-old

"I stopped wearing bras when I started to think about the politics of body image"

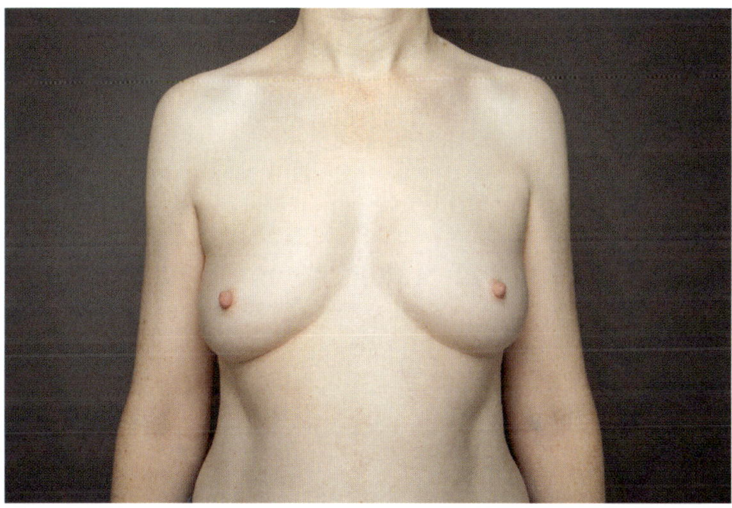

I'd describe my breasts as small. I was very self-conscious at school when all the other girls started to wear bras and I didn't need one. Flat-chested comments were made at school. The word 'small' has stayed with me all my life. Growing up you become more comfortable in yourself generally, you move away from that peer pressure.

I have a strong memory of doing an Outward Bound thing at school. I remember two girls were holding up their tops and comparing their breasts. I was fascinated, probably in a bit of a sexual way. The fact that the memory sticks with me means that breasts were becoming intriguing and important for me, without identifying what was behind it. It was a confused feeling.

In my late teens I became a feminist and started to think about the politics of body image. I stopped wearing bras, because I didn't need them anyway. That was quite liberating. I didn't want to be forced into bras. But it was also sexuality. There is something quite sexy about seeing the outline of a breast without a bra, and that was part of my emerging sexuality.

I wear a very thin T-shirt bra when I go to work, because of the nipple thing. I'm in a senior position, and have to speak at conferences. I don't want my nipples to stand out. People think that's inappropriate. It's interesting, because they're just your nipples really!

As a woman you have to work harder to be taken seriously. I don't want people to look at my chest, I want them to look at my face. You make compromises. I also dress more femininely at work. I think you have to, to be heard. That's not comfortable with my politics at all. As a lesbian, I'm not interested in being attractive to men, but you have to fit into a box. If I wore jeans, with my nipples poking out, no one would listen to me. It's like men having to wear ties.

My partner really likes my breasts. I don't get very aroused through my breasts, they're not a big deal for me. They are for her though – that's always a balancing act! I really love her breasts. Breasts are quite often involved. I tend to rely on my girlfriend to check my breasts for lumps. It's more fun that way! *(laughs)*

My experience of lesbians is that they're not looking for breasts that pop out of the newspaper at you. They've seen more women and more women's breasts and have a less stereotypical view. But it's difficult to generalise.

On a political level I don't agree with breast enhancement surgery. It's trying to fit in to a stereotype, that bigger, rounder look. Some of the women you see in the media have had ridiculous enhancements. I don't think they look feminine or beautiful. The cosmetic surgery industry is awful; it's all about women fitting into a comic-book stereotype, and it's a huge money-making exercise.

You couldn't take your top off in public, people would stare at you, and it's part of the inherent sexism in society. But why shouldn't you do that? One rule for men and another rule for women. I've gone topless on holiday with women, but I wouldn't in a mixed group, that would make me uncomfortable.

I went shopping the other week and I could hardly find a bra that wasn't underwired or push-up. The marketing of bras has become more sexualised. The marketing for Playtex bras used to be about 'Cross Your Heart', a safe feeling. They were bigger, more encompassing bras, they kept you all tucked in: completely different to Wonderbra, which is a very sexualised look.

The other thing that drives me mad is lingerie for young girls. That's really changed in the last few years. You see lingerie in the shops for tiny girls, who clearly don't need bras. Both the knickers and the bras are adult, frilly and pornographic!

I've been having this conversation with a few women recently. When we were younger there was a strong feminist movement and things got better, but it feels like things are going backwards at a rapid pace. You wouldn't have seen the same sexualisation of women 10 or 15 years ago. It's dispiriting. We let our guard down.

———————————

Age 45 | No children

"My boobs disappeared, my periods stopped, my hips shrunk"

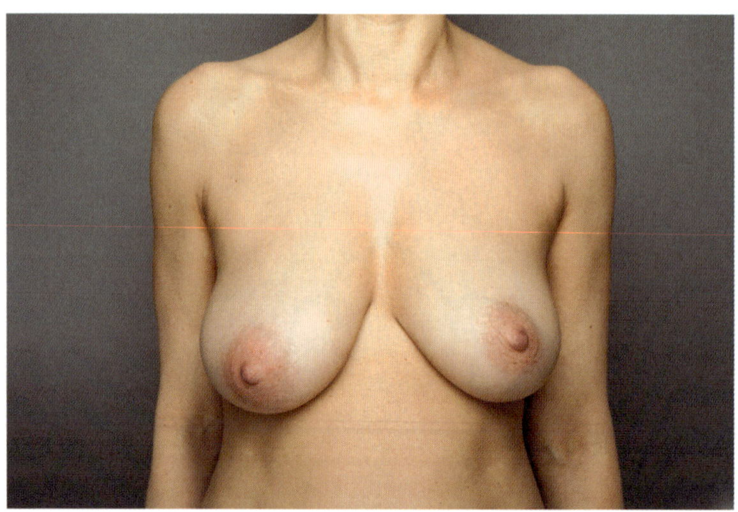

I don't think I have any strong feelings about my breasts. If anything they annoy me. They have caused me problems over the years. I've had lots of cysts which have needed investigating, a lot of tests and mammograms, and quite honestly it's been a pain. It's never been anything sinister, but every time there is that concern.

My doctor checks them for me on a regular basis. My breasts are so cysty and lumpy that I have no idea what I am touching. Is it something potentially suspicious or a normal lumpy bumpy bit? So these days, rather than get stressed out, my doctor does it all for me. We have a good relationship! *(laughs)* My doctor is a woman but I don't think I would mind if it was a man. I think I will always avoid doing my own examinations.

I'm a stylist. You do have to take breast size into consideration when you dress someone. I suppose I prefer the look of dressed smaller-breasted women. If you are not careful you can look top heavy very easily. I have to be very careful of what I am putting on up here or I could look like I am going to topple over. So it's easier to dress women with smaller breasts.

In my line of work I don't think I have come across any woman who has said she likes her breasts. I can't think of anyone who's said, 'I love my boobs'. The well-endowed ladies think they are a pain and want to minimise them and cover them up. They can feel like they are a pair of walking boobs.

I'm a 32D and a dress size eight to 10. I've not wanted attention from men, and I would prefer to have smaller boobs. But hey, this is what I've got. After my degree I worked in a nice bar in Berkshire. I had a great time there, but really, the entire time men would just talk to my boobs. I found it very uncomfortable and annoying.

I feel like I should love my boobs because I have a physique some women would want, but I don't and it sits uncomfortably with me. I think that's more to do with my issues and inhibitions about my body.

By the time I was 15 I had stopped eating. I developed anorexia. Though I had started to develop boobs at that age, they shrank, I stopped developing.

As a teenager, life felt very out of control, and in my head it made sense that if I stopped eating people would start to notice and be concerned about me and help me. I remember it now clear as crystal. I didn't know it would become a way of life, I just wanted my parents to notice. There are very few things you have control over, but you have 100 per cent control about what you put in your body.

When you stop eating your body becomes more childlike again. My boobs disappeared, my periods stopped, my hips shrunk. I was happy about that even though I hadn't set out to achieve that. I wanted to retreat and make myself as fragile as possible so no one would expect me to deal with the difficult things in my life. I always felt safe while I was anorexic. It's like a shield – while you have that, no one can get in. It is hugely scary for a recovering anorexic to let that barrier down.

I was 33 when I had my first baby. I was a bit concerned about how I would react to my body being so out of control with a baby bump. It didn't bother me nearly as much as I thought it would. Yes, I did put on weight, and I didn't like it, but I can't imagine there are many pregnant women who do. 'I love the fact that my arse is big!' *(laughs)*

I didn't breastfeed, and I didn't try. I think it's to do with some ingrained body attitude. I didn't come across too much controversy, just the occasional comment, because I was so definite about it. I've never regretted it, it was the right decision for me.

I didn't want the whole responsibility of breastfeeding. It's my husband's child as well, 'You can flipping well get up and feed him in the night!' I thought I would be tied to the baby the whole time. It was me being a little bit selfish I suppose. But if I had made myself do it, or someone had made me try to do it, I would have resented it and then I would have resented my baby. I loved him and I didn't want to resent him.

Both children were emergency caesarians in the end. I was pretty ill after each birth, and you need to recover. Bottle-feeding did mean my husband could get up in the night sometimes and feed them. After nights of being in hospital and not sleeping at all, that worked for us as a family.

I've never been a Mother Earth type. I worried during my first pregnancy that I had made a mistake, that the baby wouldn't like me, that I wouldn't like the baby, that it would be horrendous. Maybe a lot of other women feel the same way. Thankfully, when I had the baby there was a rush of maternal something and I thought he was the cutest thing I had ever seen and I loved him instantly.

It's depressing that model agencies sign up anorexic models. I make the distinction between fashion and style. I am in style, not in fashion. Fashion is very transient, vacuous and materialistic. Styling, what I do, is about nurturing the person, hopefully making them feel better about themselves. It's about improving people's lives. Fashion uses women and perpetuates unhealthy ideals of what women should look like and be like. It's not just about body image, it's also about how young you are, how much money you have. And what about this gap between the thighs that a lot of children aspire to? They are just clothes hangers, there is no body underneath the clothes.

I feel worried about my son and my daughter. My son is very body-conscious already. He's very sporty, and wants to be an athlete. I do worry that it is something to do with me, but he picked up at a very young age the difference between healthy and unhealthy diet, and how much sugar you can have.

Because of my history with anorexia my antennae go off with anything to do with my children's bodies. I don't want to be so aware of it that I create problems. I will not have scales in the house.

Photoshopping makes me so cross, I hate it. It objectifies women's bodies. Leave our bodies alone. What is wrong with the female body just the way it is? I know it is done to men's bodies as well, but they aren't used to sell everything like women's bodies are. It is irresponsible and dangerous. It should be illegal. Those who do it should really question why they are doing it. It should not happen. It's total disrespect. We are supposed to be living in an era of equality, but clearly we are not, because you just have to look at the manipulation of women's bodies in the media.

———————

Age 41 | Two children

"In our culture you have to hide when you breastfeed"

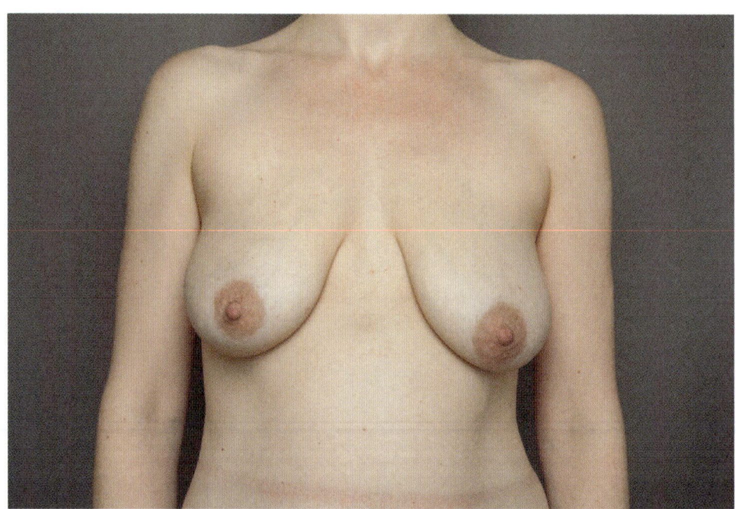

I've never felt particularly sexual about my breasts. In fact, if anything, I've preferred to minimise their obviousness. Since having children I would say they're not as attractive as they were, but I feel more confident about them, even though they're a bit saggy.

I think a lot of that is because I struggled to feed my first child. I felt that they had sort of let me down. Having not even particularly liked them very much before then, I was almost embarrassed about them. I thought, 'Oh no, I've failed!' Now, having successfully fed three children, how they look is less of an issue. They've done what they're supposed to do.

I've no idea why they didn't feel like part of my sexual identity before. I just didn't like being a very womanly, overtly feminine shape. I don't know why, it's odd.

I went through a phase of not wearing bras in my 20s. They make you look a bit bigger, and I didn't want to look bigger. I used to wear a supportive stretchy vest top under my clothes. I didn't strap myself down, but it was along those lines. It was about diminishing, rather than emphasising, what was there. I always wear a bra now. If I didn't I'd feel floppy.

I remember starting to get comments about my breasts when I was in my late teens and they were quite full. I didn't like it, and it was part of the reason I quite liked wearing modest things. Interestingly, my gay friend used to draw caricatures of me which were quite busty, and I remember thinking, 'I don't like that'.

I was a probably a D before, but I'm a C now. I haven't lost a lot of weight, I've always been pretty much the same weight, but it's probably getting older, having three children, a bit less connective tissue – I don't know. Also, I've changed how I exercise over the years. I do more running and things like that. Now parts of my breasts are around my belt line!

I've never particularly enjoyed my breasts being played with sexually. They've never been a big part of any sexual experience. Sometimes I enjoy it, but if anything I tolerate it. Sometimes it makes you want to go, 'Just get off!'

Breasts are presented sexually, but most women I have spoken to say that breast fondling isn't a big part of their sexual experience. That's the complete opposite of how they are presented, as the iconic sexual fondle toy. Are we all just existing in a myth bubble when it comes to breasts?

I think my breasts are quite important to my husband. He does quite like them and he plays with them. But he likes them as part of a general feminine shape. I don't think they do it for him in isolation.

In our culture you have to hide when you breastfeed. I remember when I had my first baby and I was like, 'I don't care, I'm going to do it, I'm going to breastfeed', not in an obvious way, but I certainly wasn't going to hide. But you're made to feel very uncomfortable. People look, and they don't like it.

My father-in-law made a comment about going to a coffee shop and there being women with their buggies, breastfeeding. And I thought, 'Like me, do you mean? Because I had to stop and feed a baby, because I was looking after your grandchild? The generation which is going to keep you in your nursing home! Right, that's fine!'

It's so odd that the only use they have, their primary reason for being, is the one which makes us feel the most uncomfortable.

I would say the people who disapprove are elderly or middle-aged, men and women. It's very odd, you do get 'tutted'. It's quite difficult to breastfeed my baby, even though I've got my black breastfeeding 'burqa', which is a breastfeeding cover. You just tie it around your neck and it's like a big scarf really and it goes over the baby so you can breastfeed discreetly. But now she doesn't understand why that's there, so she grabs it out of the way. She can't look around. Eating is a social thing. While she's eating she likes to chat to the people next to us! I think the 'burqa' makes people more comfortable and that makes me more comfortable.

It does make me cross. I find it extremely hypocritical considering you can walk past shelves of … it doesn't matter what the magazine is, it could be the *TV Times*, and it's still like this. *(thrusts breasts out)*You can sit there reading *The Sun*. Most pictures with women advertising something involve quite a lot of cleavage, which seems to be tolerated beautifully! But as soon as breasts are given any airplay for feeding the baby it seems to make people feel uncomfortable. I don't know whether it's about power. Breastfeeding stops fertility doesn't it, so perhaps it's linked primarily back to that.

Younger people are interested, especially children. They are accepting of it. They'll come over and have a look. I remember when one of my sons came over and said, 'Is it really real milk?' I squirted him with it! It's probably going to scar him for life. *(laughs)* 'Yes, it's real milk!'

I love breastfeeding. It feels perfect. I remember my mum saying to me she enjoyed breastfeeding. After she had the baby she thought there had to be something else, and breastfeeding was that. That's how it felt to me. It felt right. Blissful really. I love that blissed out feeling, it's lovely.

When women have breast implants they are often quite thin. And if you are thin you generally don't have a lot of breast. Breast is fat tissue at the end of the day. So, sickening as it is, probably a child's body with a great big pair of breasts is exactly the image to have.

I'm more of a feminist since I've had children. I always believed in equality, but not in such an obvious way. I've matured. Producing, feeding and looking after children is so massively undervalued by society. I just didn't know that before. And you want to make the world a better place for children, you don't want to send them out into that.

———

Age 35 | Three children, breastfeeding 10-month-old

"It broke my heart when my daughter told me she had breast cancer"

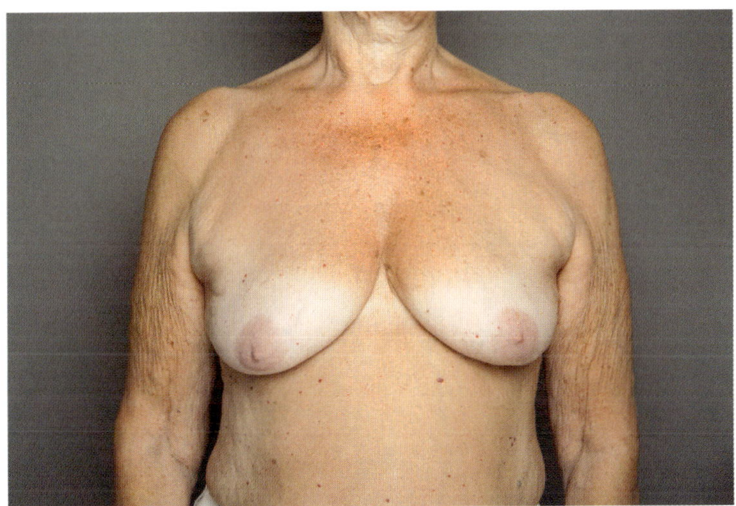

I'm quite happy with my breasts now, but of course when I was younger I wasn't. They were never big enough, but there was nothing I could do about it. The advantage was I played a lot of sport: tennis, badminton, hockey, you name it, I did it. Big breasts are not advantageous to sports.

What's changed? Confidence and age. I'm so used to walking around nude at home. It's nice and warm in Spain where I live. Maybe walking around naked at home affects self-confidence. My husband is not so much for nudity, but I don't like clothes on. I like to feel free. I'm not a naturist, I just like being naked at home. I sleep 'in the nud'.

I've just celebrated 55 years of marriage. It's wonderful! We've grown so comfortable with each other, and there's nothing to hide. I think my confidence comes from my relationship with my husband. I always know that if there is a problem, my husband is there in the background for me to fall back on.

When I grew up I had no confidence. I grew up in the 1930s, everything was hidden. I had two brothers; we never saw each other naked. My mother died when I was two, of tuberculosis. My father married again when I was six. They kept themselves very separated from us. I never saw my step-mother's breasts. You didn't speak about sex or anything like that. It was a funny world.

In these modern times, young people are proud of their bodies and I think it's great, but I tell you what I don't like: pregnant girls with tops that show their tummies sticking out. There are a lot of things I am happy to go along with – I like crop tops – but it's my background you see, the modesty coming in. I like to see a nice young body, but not when women are pregnant.

Nowadays, I think it's great to be emancipated and have no hang-ups and live the life you want to live. You can have sex with whoever you like. I didn't have sex until I was married and I had my 25th birthday on honeymoon. That was to do with contraception: you were terrified of being pregnant. That would have been dreadful in society.

Breastfeeding in public is OK, but I would like it to be more discreet. Sometimes you have to breastfeed, the baby needs feeding. The first time I saw my daughter breastfeeding I thought it was beautiful, quite extraordinary. *(cries)* It was so emotional. I watched my daughter-in-law breastfeed but it didn't have the same emotional impact, maybe because she wasn't my daughter.

I couldn't breastfeed my daughter because I had tuberculosis. When my son was born I was dying to feed him but I don't think I had the right care. My breasts went absolutely rock solid. Oh, the pain. I was brought up to be stoic, but I cried sometimes. The nipples were breaking away. The nurse said 'You can't breastfeed', but I have a feeling she wasn't the right sort of nurse. I only breastfed for two days.

It broke my heart when my daughter told me she had breast cancer. She's had it twice and had to have a mastectomy. It was dreadful. To think of your daughter going through that. The second time round she didn't have to have a mastectomy but she had to have this horrible chemotherapy. She has the hormonal kind of cancer.

I hope everything will be alright for her. We are going for another MRI and brain scan today. I am very worried about it. She doesn't seem too worried. I am concerned. She is such a kind, nice, caring person. Some people are too good, and these horrid things happen to them.

I had a lumpectomy. So many women get cancer and breast cancer. It's scary. When I told people I'd had a lumpectomy lots of women told me they'd had one too. Initially when I was told I had breast cancer I thought I was going to die. They only had to take a little lump out. They said I might have a funny-shaped breast, but I said, 'I don't care at my age, what the heck'. My husband was so supportive, he really is a good man.

My breasts used to be erogenous but we don't have sex anymore at our age. We gave up about five or six years ago. We used to have such fun, it was great. We'd have a laugh and roll around. It took me a while to get used to sex, because of all my inhibitions. I was a virgin when we married when I was 25, and I don't think my husband had many sexual experiences. I don't think he was a virgin exactly, but it might have only been a one-off against a wall or something! *(laughs)* He'll still come round the back of me and put his arms around me and put his hands on my breasts.

I think we stopped because I slowly lost the urge. I don't know why. If you don't use it you lose it. I'm not sure now whether if I got the urge, if I could urge my husband. I'm not sure how it works with the male.

I live in Spain and go topless on the small beaches, if other people are. But I am careful because the sun is hot, and my breasts see less sun and they can burn more easily. Most sunbathing is in the complex where we live, and I wouldn't go topless there, because the other people are my neighbours. Surprisingly enough, the young girls wear a thong and bare breasts. My husband will go, 'Look at that!' and I go, 'Yeah, I know, it's lovely!' But older women also walk around topless on the beach. They were all brought up in the Franco era, and I think there is a rebellion against those times when everything was modest. I think there are fewer inhibitions now.

I don't know what young men feel about young girls walking around with bare breasts. Do they have emotional or physical reactions, or are they used to seeing it? Maybe it's only within the confines of the bedroom and a relationship that it becomes erotic.

We're aged from 50 to 100 at the retirement complex we live in, but I am the eldest, I suppose, who does aqua aerobics and Pilates. In the changing room we are all shapes and sizes. Some look good and some don't particularly. I am happy with myself and I don't think about other people. We've been doing it for five or six years and it has taken some of the women all this time to walk around totally in the nud. There is one lady, a little tubby sweetie, and she goes into the changing cubicle.

My grandchildren were talking about body hair. I asked them, 'Do you take off your pubic hair?' They said, 'Of course we do Gran!' It turns out they wax it. My granddaughters do each other. They said they just don't like hair. I think it's great being hairless; it's very clean and I am fussy about hygiene. I'd do it myself, but I would look very odd, wouldn't I? This is obviously a fashion among young girls. I guess they all discuss it; they don't seem to have any inhibitions. I wouldn't mind shaving or using cream. You get less hair though as you get older.

My husband is very hairy, bless him. I don't like it but I've never said anything about it. Why should I not say something to him? Maybe I will. We ought to be totally open with each other. 'Shall we transplant it from there to his head?' That would be wonderful. You never know, that might do something for him! He's got quite a good body for his age – he's two years older than me, and he works out – it's just this hair. 'Can we have a cutting session darling?' *(laughs)*

––––––––––––––

Age 79 | Two children

"I might be ambivalent about my breasts as a self-defence mechanism"

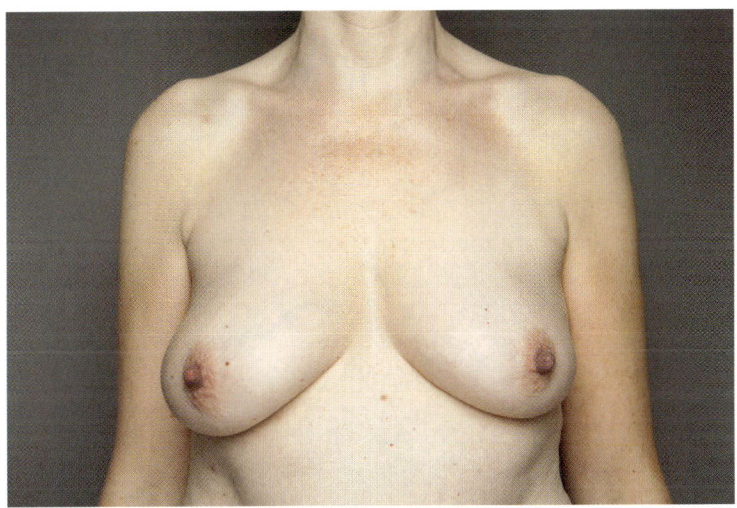

I don't think about my breasts. They don't make me powerful or feminine. I didn't feel a burning need to breastfeed and I didn't breastfeed for that long. If I got breast cancer I would be more concerned about losing my hair, which is more important to my femininity than my breasts.

I feel differently about my breasts than I do about the rest of my body. I've got nice legs, I quite like my face, I've got nice eyes, I like my hair. I like myself. I've had low self-esteem about doing things, but not about my body. This is going to sound big-headed but if I walk into a room, I generally look around and think, 'You are one of the most beautiful women here'. I think I look quite good. I might feel differently about my breasts if they were huge and attracted attention from men, but they never have. I don't dress in tight clothes, or very low-cut tops. I wouldn't feel comfortable. They're not for the world at large. I'm quite straight-laced.

I don't remember my mum talking to me about growing up. I think I went to get my first bra with a friend's mum. My mum had me quite late in life so she had quite old-fashioned views. When I started my periods she said I couldn't use tampons because that would mean I would lose my virginity. She got me the belt and the Dr White's stuff. When I talked to my friends I realised they weren't using stuff like that, they had moved on. But my mum said no. She also said I mustn't wear red trousers, because it would give out the message I was a tart. It's only in the last couple of years that I have bought red trousers. She had a big influence on me.

My parents were very traditional. My dad got in at 5pm, his slippers were waiting for him, we had dinner at 5.30pm. I never saw my dad naked. I accidentally walked in to the bathroom once when my mum was in there and she just closed the door on me. I've seen her naked more in the last few years because she's elderly and I've had to clean her.

My mother is a manic depressive. My brother died when I was 13. She plummeted into the blackest of depressions. My mum just wasn't able to care for me, she was completely lost. So just as I was going through puberty, I had to live in various other places because it was affecting my exams and stuff. I left home when I was 18, but I kind of lost her when I was 13.

I might be ambivalent about my breasts as a self-defence mechanism. I have a lot of self-defence mechanisms, and what I call my 'walls', based upon a very important time in my life when I didn't get from my mum what I could see what my friends were getting. There was no birds and bees talk, no body awareness talk, no periods talk, nothing. Friends' mums were quite matter-of-fact with me, because they weren't my mum. Maybe that's why I am very matter-of-fact, I wasn't taught any other way. My breasts probably do mean a lot to me. You could go on ad infinitum talking about various issues, but you can't keep going on forever. I'm not unhappy, I'm a happy person and I move on. I do think there is a connection with my breasts though.

For a woman of nearly 88, my mum has a fantastic pair of boobs. I don't like seeing her naked though. She always took very good care of herself; her skin is great and she doesn't have a single grey hair. She always had a bra on and nice clothes, but she's spent so long in hospital and care homes that she's got into the habit of not wearing a bra. That's fine in hospital, but I don't like it when she's at home in trousers and a jumper and her breasts are down by her waist. I don't know why I don't like it, but I think it's because she's lost her self-respect. I've got her dressed and said to her, 'Can you go and put a bra on please? I'm taking you somewhere, I don't want you walking around like that. It's obvious you haven't got a bra on'. She forgets because when she is at home no one sees her. The only people who see her are me and her carers.

I was never scared of getting old till I had to do all this for my mum. To see the degeneration of the body of a person who was so lively and vivacious. OK, she was traditional, but she did so much. To be reduced to this person whose world is so insular scares me. Not wearing a bra represents losing self-respect.

My first child was born through IVF, after five years of trying. Right from the start I wanted a caesarean. I'd lost faith in the ability of my body to do anything naturally when it came to pregnancy and birth. I couldn't get pregnant naturally, so I thought I wouldn't be able to give birth naturally. They wouldn't agree to a caesarean. I didn't like it but I understood. As it turned out my blood stopped clotting and I was admitted to hospital a month early, and given a caesarean under general anaesthetic. So I never saw her being born, and I was drugged up to the eyeballs. I wasn't really aware of her till she was about two or three days old. There are photographs of me breastfeeding her and I am completely out of it.

I had a visit from the midwife, who said she was latching on fine and everything. The next day I didn't think anything had changed, but when she came back she said, 'Oh for heaven's sake, you're going to get really sore nipples, the baby's not latched on properly'. She literally yanked the baby off and it really hurt. I remember plain as day thinking, 'Hah! I've got it all wrong'. I was absolutely devastated. From then on, it all went wrong. She wouldn't put on weight and was crying and crying.

I belonged to the NCT and went to the breastfeeding counsellor. We talked over what had happened and they said I'd had a major crisis of confidence. They recommended a breastfeeding weekend, where we stayed in bed from Thursday till Monday. I didn't wash, I wasn't allowed to get up, my husband brought me my dinners. That didn't work. When she was six weeks old I was on the phone to my mum and said I couldn't cope anymore. My mum said she was hungry. A midwife came out, weighed her and asked how I felt about bottle-feeding. She recommended a mixture, keeping my 'best' feeds and all the other feeds being a bottle. The idea was that if I was more rested I might have more milk. We did breast and bottle for six months. When I started bottles I was able to start enjoying her. With my second baby I breastfed him for the first four weeks to give him some valuable antibodies, but my mindset was already there, I knew I wouldn't carry on.

I don't like my breasts being touched sexually. Not at all. My husband is very grabby with my breasts and he cannot see anything wrong with that. I didn't like it with previous partners either. I find him quite crude about breasts, he's always been like that, and we've been together 23 years. It has caused problems. I can be washing up and he will come up and go 'Phwoar!' *(indicates his hands grabbing her breasts from behind)* Sometimes I swing round and say, 'Why have you done that, what are you hoping to achieve? Do you think I'm going to say, "Take me, you sexy beast?" Get off.' It has caused problems and it will continue to cause problems.

He thinks I should like it and he doesn't understand why I don't. He thinks they are an erogenous zone for all women. I like my neck being stroked and kissed, I like my back being stroked. That's what to do if you want to put me in the mood. He does do that and he can see I am getting in the mood. A woman would see it's working and carry on doing that. But he sees I am getting in the mood and ruins it by going from my back straight to my breasts, and wham, it's over for me. It's disrespectful.

———————

Age 48 | Two children

"I wanted to design them, to make them more important to me"

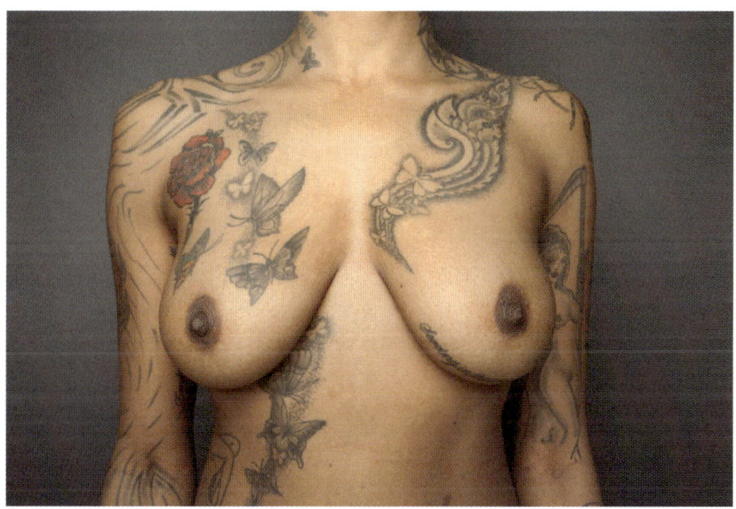

I don't really think about my breasts, to be honest. They're just there, they're just a part of you. I probably got them tattooed purposefully because I don't think about them a lot. I wanted to design them, to make them more important to me.

If I had to lose a breast, honestly, I'd prefer it to be the one with fewer tattoos! I'm not good at pain, so I wouldn't want to have to go through the tattoos again, and one of them has all the butterflies and stuff.

What do my tattoos mean to me? I like butterflies and ladybirds, they go all the way down to my ankle. A lot of women have butterflies, it's quite a feminine tattoo, but normally above the butt, wrists and ankles. I haven't seen anyone who's got them from the top to the bottom of their body.

I wish all my tattoos had meaning, but no, I had money and free time and wanted to get more body art. I had about three months of constantly healing. They're just like jewellery that you don't change.

I get more comments from men about tattoos, there's a little bit of fascination. 'Where do they go, do they go all the way round?' But I think if you mark up your skin you have to accept you will get questions about it, and not be precious.

I've had wolf whistles and men looking at my boobs. But unless I am going to wear a jumper or a big coat, it's part and parcel of having breasts. I know it's not perfect, and in an ideal world it wouldn't happen, we shouldn't have to be prepared for comments. But it's easier for me to get my head around, because it's not always men. I get comments from women as well. It's not as bad – I don't think women are objectifying me – but you can't help but look at them! They're there.

I've got polycystic ovaries, so I take medication, and that affects my size; not my whole body, just my breasts. The bigger I get, the better. I'm never going to be a curvy woman, so my breasts are my curves. I think my breasts are quite small at the moment. I could get my mum's bras over my head and still have space, it would be like a bonnet. She has bad back pain and multiple sclerosis and has had several reductions.

Wearing pretty underwear is important to me. One, because people can't see it, it's like a secretive thing. Two, it makes me feel good. It's the closest thing to my skin. You can be having a crap day, and look like a mess if you've been running around the office, but you kind of know that your underwear is really nice. A feel-good factor. When I was younger, I couldn't leave the house if my bra was white and my bottoms were black. It felt wrong!

Sex is wrong if there's no breast manipulation. Not wrong, but... no, I'm going to stick with wrong! It's important. Sensations, and the act in itself.

Looks-wise, I couldn't necessarily date a woman who was flat-chested. At the same time, I couldn't necessarily date a woman who was considerably larger than me. I'd feel like I could get lost!

My partner has breast implants. In clothes, breast jobs look amazing: they're pert, you can go without a bra, it's like they are exactly as they're meant to be. But if you're lying down without a bra, the tits don't go how everyone expects, they just sit there. And even with a really good job, there's scarring.

I think sometimes women worry too much about glamour modelling objectifying women. I sit on the fence about it. They're just breasts. To me the model is no different to Naomi Campbell or any other high-class runway model, because technically she's still a piece of meat. Her body is her asset, whether it has clothes on or not. If a girl has a great set of tits and she's comfortable with it, doesn't feel used, and isn't coerced, and she's paid a decent wage for doing suggestive poses, I wouldn't be against it.

I also feel men should take responsibility. If you're a grown man you should be able to look at a pair of tits and not objectify women. We shouldn't make excuses for men.

Unless you're Beyoncé, black women aren't packaged as that kind of sexy. Although they are packaged as sexual beings, it's not seen as a sophisticated form of attractiveness. It's a much lower level, open-access sexuality, not what you take home to mum, something dark and sexual. I know black boys who have said black women are ugly; it's quite sad, it's self-hatred, and it causes problems.

———————

Age 32 | No children

"They started to show naked boobs after the Second World War"

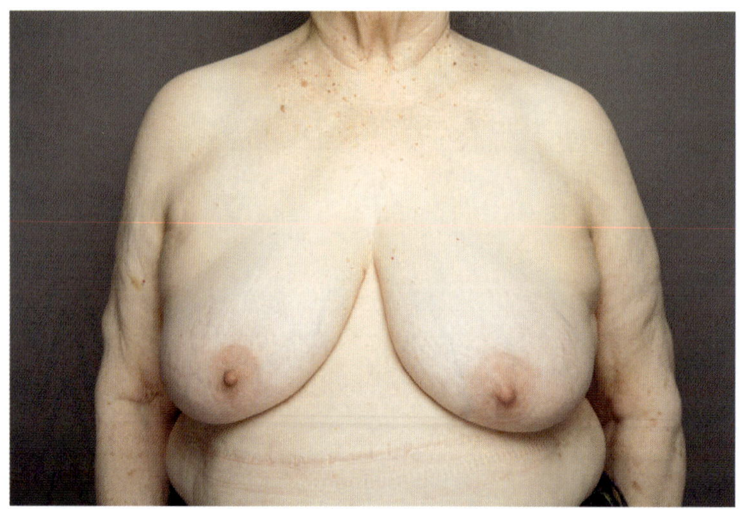

My breasts are just there and not perfect, shall we say. They are 40D, ordinary, a bit droopy.

They are part and parcel of being a woman. It's lovely if they bring pleasure to you and your husband, but they are for babies when all is said and done.

When I was young you didn't show your breasts, no low-cut dresses or short skirts. You had to be demure, or you were considered a 'fast' young lady. The bras I used to go for were for comfort and keeping a natural shape. I didn't want my nipples to be seen, so I liked bras that disguised them. If my nipples can be seen it makes my body open to the public, rather than being private. Nipples are for a baby.

My mother used to wear corsets, but I don't remember if she wore a bra. I never saw her getting changed. My mum got my first bra for me when I was in my teens.

I had three children. Breastfeeding was just normal then. When you were 'confined' you were expected to breastfeed. The nurse put the child to my breast and showed me how. It was difficult with the first child, due to being an inexperienced mum. I didn't know how to hold baby in the right position. I was sore to start with because baby had to suck for some time. When the milk became abundant my breasts became hard and that was a problem. I leaked milk and had to pad my bras. Nursing bras had a flap on them in the middle, but they weren't very good, they were horrible.

Talking about being confined takes me back. You had the midwife with you, and the doctor would come at the crucial moment when the baby came. With my first baby I stayed in hospital for nine days. I wasn't allowed to get out of bed for about five days. When I got out of bed I couldn't walk properly because my legs were so stiff. I had to have a bed pan and that was awful. I had my next two babies at home so that I could go to the loo! *(laughs)* To have a homebirth was considered unusual, you were supposed to go into hospital. I think it's much nicer for mum and baby to be at home. Although I do feel sometimes that the mums get up and start active life too soon. They don't realise that their body has to recover from the birth. Getting up too soon can lead to a prolapse.

I was in a big ward with about 20 women. The babies were kept together in a nursery, and a couple of nurses looked after them. They were brought to the mums for a feed every three hours. The idea at that time was that mums had to have rest, because they would have sleepless nights when they got home. They were thinking of the mum. They thought the babies would cause us trouble when we got home, they didn't realise the babies would also be a pleasure. I didn't like the arrangements, that's why I had my other babies at home.

We had to lie on our tummies at certain times of the day, with a pillow underneath, to reduce the size of our stomachs. At another time of the day we had to do exercises in bed. I remember distinctly that one woman had only just finished breastfeeding her baby and hadn't closed her nightie and we had to do a side-to-side movement with our arms outstretched and there was this woman with boobs swinging around. *(giggling)* We had some laughs. But I didn't want to go back into hospital after that.

Breastfeeding in public was taboo, it wasn't considered nice. You arranged your day so you wouldn't do it in public. You wouldn't do it in a crowded room of your own family either. People didn't want to see it in those days either. I think breastfeeding is natural, and good luck to mums who aren't embarrassed. After all, the child is more important. It's also good for mum if the baby doesn't keep crying.

When my granddaughter was breastfeeding her little girl on demand it looked so natural. Both seemed to do well on it. Not only that, the little girl has never needed a dummy. I'm glad it's changed now, for mum and child.

Breasts are part and parcel of sexual attraction. They are important to me. When a man fondles your breasts it does arouse you. It did me, anyway. They are one of the erogenous zones.

When my husband became infirm in his 70s we stopped having sexual relations, because he was afraid of the activity. I was in my late 50s. It was quite young for me to have to subdue my urges. He was my best friend. My love for him was such that I wanted him to have as good a life as possible considering his infirmity.

Some young women go too far now, they show too much of their body. They've got no surprises to present to a future husband, and I think that is such a pity. A gift is far more precious when you have to unwrap it. Life has changed so much. I can't imagine everyone is as promiscuous as it's made out. But there are young girls who have babies, and they shouldn't; they are far too young to have that responsibility. There are young girls with more than one child before they are 18, and I feel that is sad. They are not mature enough in themselves. They suffer, and the child suffers. They aren't wise enough to know who the right partner is, and they give in to their sexual urge. There is more to a long relationship than the sexual urge, and I know that from my second husband. A deep friendship and companionship is very necessary in a long-term relationship. I have to say relationship because people aren't always married now. But in God's eyes, they must still be married.

You have to work at a relationship sometimes. You have to talk things through and come to an agreement, and then problems can be solved.

The media changed after the Second World War. They started to show naked boobs. It was probably a reaction to men and women not being together. There was a fashion of a sort for some clubs to employ topless waitresses. I can remember seeing a photograph in the paper, discreetly done, not like it is now with full nudity, there was a sort of netting draped over the woman. But of course it was all there! It didn't last very long, and it was only certain areas of the country where this happened. Now these clubs are everywhere, although now it's full nudity. You only used to get that in the Folies Bergère.

I don't like the nudity in the papers, it makes me turn away. I don't think children should be able to see it, it gives them the wrong idea about people. It only serves the people who publish it and make money. I think they've got a lot to answer for the harm that has been done to boys and girls. It's so sad. If I see the word 'Sun' on a paper, I avoid it! If I speak up I am a prude or 'old-fashioned' and it is said in a derogatory way.

In general I don't think men have the same respect for women as they used to. They respect some women more than others. When you look at it, they respect the ones who are more demure, as I would call it.

Life has changed so much in my lifetime. I think times will turn, for the simple reason that life goes in cycles. But there is a lot of good now.

———————

Age 81 | Three children

"Every young person strives to be like the images in the magazines"

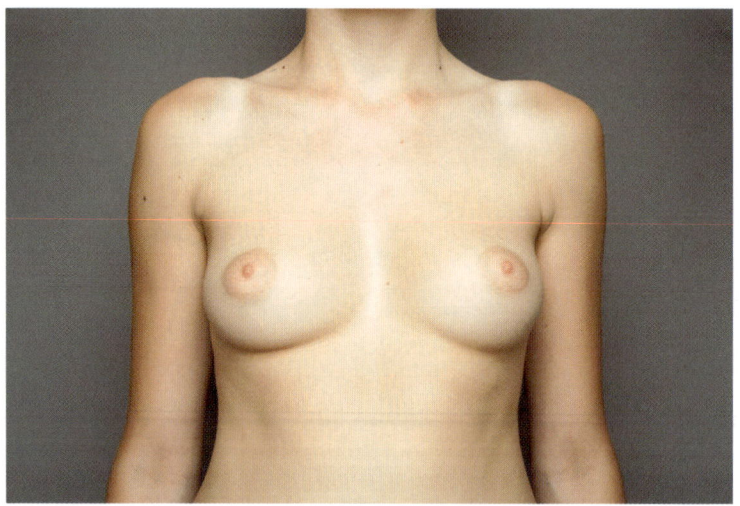

I like them, I wouldn't change them. They are nice and pert, but I haven't had children yet.

I like it when they're brown. When we go to France I sunbathe topless all the time. I wouldn't do it on the beach in England. Actually, let's be honest, I would. I just haven't done it before. I sunbathe in the garden topless. I don't mind if anyone sees but I'm not blatant about it. If it was acceptable I would do it anywhere. I've never done it with young guys around, but I have in front of my dad's friends. I don't care.

I don't get attention for my boobs, they aren't big enough. It's about the full package, you know? Girls with big boobs do get unwanted attention. I'm probably a small 34C. My sister is big – she has amazing breasts – but she hates the attention.

I don't know what it is with men and breasts. I've Googled, 'Why do men like breasts?' What answer did it come up with? Pert breasts show your youth, something like that. The younger the better, the more fertile you look.

Your boobs and fanny are private, and men are not allowed to see them, which means they want to see them. But tribes get them out all the time. I reckon if we had our boobs out all the time there would be less of a thing about them.

I used to be a model. My boobs were smaller then and I was thinner. I was a small B then, and size six to eight. I gradually got fatter, now I am a 10. I was never one of those skinny ones, not a supermodel. I wasn't tall enough, or confident enough, to do castings for catwalk. I did magazines and hair. The clothes are definitely not designed for boobs. Clothes are designed for skinny women because that's what people think looks good. They want a coat-hanger walking down the catwalk.

I got spotted when I was 16 in Covent Garden, twice in a row, both within about 10 minutes: once by a top hairdresser, and once by a high-end agency. It was weird because I'd been looking at magazines, thinking I could do it. Not because I was up myself, but I thought I looked like them. I don't look like them anymore! *(laughs)*

I did bits and bobs to start with, mainly hair stuff. When I got to 18 I decided not to go to uni and really try it. I did it till I was just over 20. Now I'm 22. Your career is mainly over by the time you are 25. Obviously male models can do so much longer because they get more beautiful as they get older. Thirty is perfect for male models, that's when they earn money.

I wasn't 100 per cent into it. I didn't like the lifestyle. Casting after casting and constant rejection. You have to beg for your money, agencies don't just give you your money. None of the models I know live in big houses, they aren't doing amazingly well. And to be a model you have to travel, and I didn't want to leave my boyfriend and dog.

Once I went to Majorca and there was the hottest male model ever. Most male models are dicks, really up themselves. They're good-looking but their personalities are awful. Nothing happened though, because I had a boyfriend. They were the best photos I've done.

I had a test shoot with a photographer early on. I was wearing clothes, and he kept saying, 'That doesn't work, take it off,' until I was basically naked. Well, I was completely naked. I was 18, but I was still quite naive and innocent. He was probably late 30s. I didn't realise, I thought, 'Ooh, is the bra not working? OK, I'll take it off.' Afterwards I thought it wasn't right. I told the agency and they said, 'You shouldn't have done that.' I look back, and I think I was stupid. I've heard lots of rumours about particular photographers who are known as perverts.

None of the models I knew had an eating disorder. Well, they had an eating disorder to an extent. I was very rigid about what I ate, I always knew my calories. I thought I ate whatever I liked, but I didn't. I felt really guilty about eating anything bad. I really restricted my eating, and that was the same with all the girls. You ate as little as you could, just not quite to the extent of being anorexic. I ate breakfast, would try and skip lunch, until I got so hungry I would eat again. I would say now I am at my natural weight, and I do eat what I want. I should probably eat less, because I eat a lot of chocolates, biscuits, crap like that, and drink alcohol. I'm lucky with my metabolic rate. I'm only 22. After 25 it goes! Hopefully by then I will be healthier.

I think my boyfriend likes my breasts. I like them being touched and stuff, but I don't need them to be touched.

I do snapchat. Basically, you take pictures and send it to someone and they can only see it for however many seconds you say, and then it's gone, unless they screen grab it. Some girls' pictures have ended up on Lad Bible. Lad Bible is funny, but it is sexist. My sister sends me naked pictures of herself, she finds it hilarious! Not in a sexy, weird way, she'll send an awful angle of herself, it's so funny. I would only send naked snapchat pictures to my boyfriend or my sister. You shouldn't send a naked picture to someone unless you 100 per cent trust them.

Women are sexualised in the media – that is all they are. Every young person strives to be like the images in the magazines; they want the flat stomach, the big boobs, the skinniness, they want to be tall, they want to be perfect. It's shoved in their faces constantly.

———————

Age 22 | No children

"If I'd had big breasts I would have been a different person"

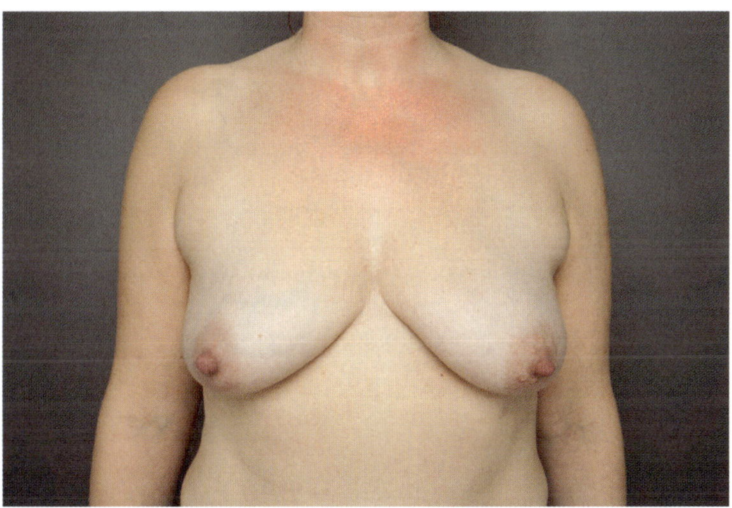

My breasts aren't central to my being. The only time I really noticed them was when I was pregnant and they were big. I didn't like them big. They've always been relatively small and so they've been easy to handle.

My husband loves them! He likes them when they're little, he liked them when they were enormous, he loves them now. He thinks they're just wonderful. When I said I was doing this he asked if he could photograph them, and I said 'No!' (laughs) He'd be on them all day if he could. My husband is generally keen full stop, he just loves everything. It's very nice after all these years. If I had cancer and lost them it wouldn't make any difference to him. He likes my breasts, but they're not me. He loves me, not them. They're an added bonus.

Most of the time they're not particularly important to me sexually. I have to be seriously in the mood. Most of the time I don't like being faffed with, but every now and then I absolutely love it, and then he thinks it's Christmas. When they are erogenous, they seriously are, but when they're not, they're not.

Breasts are meant to be seen as sexual. It's to do with abundance, you know. If you've got large abundant breasts which are full and perky, it shows that you're young and at your sexual peak. When you're old and saggy it's obvious you are not at your reproductive peak. I think it's in-built for blokes. Some are more fixated than others – maybe they missed out when they were young or something.

I breastfed quite happily. The only reason I gave up was because I wanted a drink on my birthday. It was inconvenient at times. If I heard a baby cry, milk would come through my bra like a fountain. I heard this baby gurgle, which made me think about my baby. Bear in mind I had maternity pads on both breasts. Next thing I know, I can feel dripping on my shoes; the milk had come through my maternity pads, bra and top and was literally dripping on to my shoes. The milk patches were huge. My little girl loved watching me squirt milk across the bath!

Feeding was easy and I really enjoyed it. Both babies latched on beautifully. I breastfed everywhere, I never felt uncomfortable, I didn't give a monkey's! I didn't hoike my breasts out in front of some grandpa, I'd put a shawl over the baby, and I had special pop-down bras. I think I had a special shirt if I remember right.

If I won the lottery tomorrow I wouldn't mind stopping them going south, although I wouldn't have them made any bigger. I think you can have something attached to the nipple and sort of drawn up. I wouldn't mind them looking like they used to, but I'd have to have money to burn before I even thought about it.

I don't understand why anyone would want to make their breasts any bigger than they are. The only time I had big breasts, when I was breastfeeding, it was a nightmare. I didn't like the look of them, they were uncomfortable, my shoulders killed me, I had to wear a bra in bed. Oh, it was awful. I don't understand these women who've got perfectly normal, healthy breasts having them sliced open and foreign stuff shoved in there. If my daughter wanted it I'd have her committed! I think there's something wrong in their heads. They are unhappy and they think having their breasts enlarged will cure the unhappiness. But the problems are still there: what you think about yourself is still there, all you are is poorer.

There are probably pictures of my breasts knocking around somewhere. Somebody stole one of mine. I had a top on in it, but only just. I was wearing a bra, pants and suspenders, and drinking a yard, standing on a table! *(laughs)* One of the guys at college went through my blooming photo album and nicked it.

Every Fresher's Week, we had a thing called the 'Pornographers' Ball', or the 'Dirty Disco', and we had to wear really slutty clothes. I wore lace camis, string vests, all sorts of things. There were hardly any women at college, so the men would wear whatever they could nick out of my wardrobe! I did get my boobs out at some point, to get a reaction probably! It was a long time ago. Because my breasts were so small, they never bothered me; nudity never bothered me. So it was for a laugh really, to give them a bit of a thrill. Nobody was nagging me to. They were gobsmacked. Most of these guys came from private boys' schools and the only women they'd ever seen were their mums and sisters, so yeah, you could hear their jaws hitting the floor. Which was part of the fun in a way. They'd never come anywhere near, they were so scared. In a way it was quite funny, because it gave you a bit of power. They were completely out of their comfort zone. They were quite scared of me, because I was quite sexually confident and they were not.

It's not just women who are sexualised these days, men are too. They've got to look smart, have beautiful bodies, chiselled features. I think society in general is just more sexualised. It worries me sometimes – where is it going to go?

I suspect if I'd had big breasts I would have been a different person. I used to say, 'I'm really glad I haven't got big boobs because they'd get in the way of my badminton swing'. Because I have small breasts they've never defined me. If you've got big breasts that's what people see. Men just spend their entire time with their eyes glued to them. I must admit my eyes are glued to women with big breasts!

I've always been confident with men, talked to them like people, looked them in the eye. I think that's because I've always been dealt with like a person. If I'd had enormous boobs then it probably wouldn't be the same.

If I want a man to find me attractive I want him to find who I am attractive, not two pieces of flesh stuck to my front.

Age 47 | Two children

"Boys like big-breasted girls because of what they see in the media"

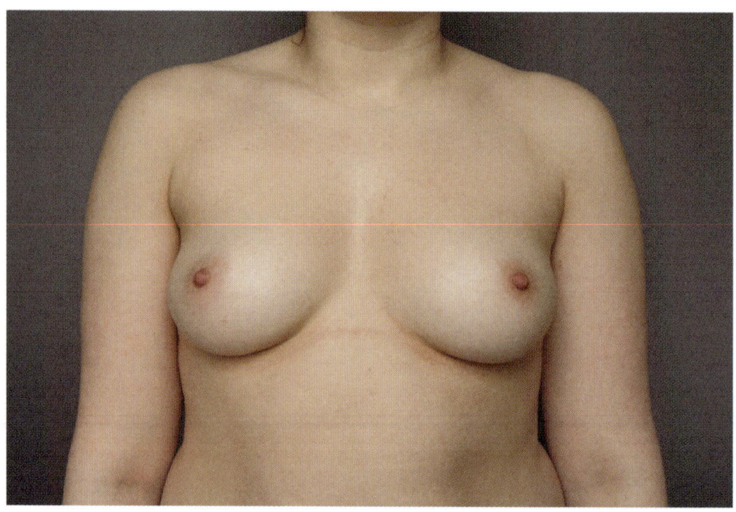

I don't dislike my breasts. I've definitely come to like them more since going to college and university. At secondary school I didn't like my boobs and was very self-conscious. Boys were interested in girls with massive boobs, and I was, like, 'Oh, OK, mine are just normal size!' When I was at school, I thought wearing padded bras would get male attention.

Boys like big-breasted girls because of what they see in the media. My boy mates read lads' mags and car magazines: it's like boob central. They've made banter comments about my boobs: 'Oh, your boobs are looking big today!' I think men and boys think they have a right to comment on what the female body should be like. Obviously everyone's entitled to their opinions, but they are built on Page 3, lads' mags, car magazines. When they see bodies like that, rather than real women, they expect everyone to look like that. It puts pressure on my generation, but it depends on how strong the individual is.

Guys almost expect girls to try and make themselves look like girls on TV and in celebrity culture and stuff. Unless they are really stupid they must know not every girl is perfectly rounded and pushed together, with cleavage.

How women look in porn affects what men expect; not just boobs but the body in general. I don't watch it personally, but I've seen some. It's not just their boobs that aren't natural, you get other things like anal bleaching. A lot of my male friends look at porn. They are quite open about it. Men think sex is some massive extravagant event; they expect a certain level of 'dirty', rough and ready sex, rather than love-making. I think they know the boobs in porn aren't real, but they don't care, they like it. An exaggerated woman's body gives them a better show.

My boyfriend at the moment likes my breasts. He likes natural-looking girls. He'll say stuff like, 'Your body is nice how it is, it's in proportion'. Sometimes I like him giving them attention more than other times, I guess it depends what sort of mood I'm in. But it makes me feel good knowing he likes them, so that makes them important to me. They are an erogenous zone; coupled with other stuff, they help.

One boy I was with said very openly that they weren't big enough for him, blah blah blah. We broke up shortly after he said that. We'd been together five months. I said, 'If you don't like me like this, then you're never going to like me.'

I do dance at uni and no one wears a bra under a leotard. Bras restrict your movement. Dancers have boobs, but they are toned and flatter, rather than big and bouncy. I've got used to that being the norm, so I'm more comfortable with my boobs. I think dance gives me and my friends body confidence, and confidence in general.

The people that I work with in a clothes shop are very negative about their own bodies, but I don't really know why, because I think they have lovely figures.

You have the 'magic' bra, the 'push-up', the 'boost', with an inch of padding. They always use these positive words. They encourage you to make your boobs bigger, not accept what you've got. You can buy into changing your bum as well as your boobs – you can get padded knickers now. It's all about making your body like J-Lo, or Beyoncé. 'Buy this bra and make your boobs look two sizes bigger!' At the end of the day, you're going to take it off! I think it would be embarrassing to take it off with a guy. I don't know how savvy they are, they probably think what you see is what you get.

I don't think I would ever have implants, because it's quite major, invasive surgery. I don't think I could put myself through that. Now I'm fine with my breasts, but if after breastfeeding they go a bit further south, then ... it's hard to say. If your breasts change from having children, it sort of tells a story, like stretch marks. I find it sad when people are ashamed of stretch marks, because that's your baby, those are your baby marks.

I never used to check my breasts, maybe once in a while if I saw an advert on TV or went to the health centre and saw a poster. But ever since my auntie died from breast cancer, I've started checking them more regularly, maybe once a month. I am worried about it. If I had to have a lumpectomy or a mastectomy, so be it. Just get it out of me.

I don't sunbathe topless. I'm not afraid or ashamed to get them out, I'm more afraid there are pervy men around, that they'll see me in a more sexual way than I want to be seen. If I was going to sunbathe topless it would just be to not have tan lines, it wouldn't be so people would look at my boobs.

At university a lot of the theme nights encourage girls to portray themselves in a slutty way, like 'Golf Pros and Tennis Hoes'. At a popular night called 'Carnage' you have to buy a T-shirt. There are different themes like the beach, or 'Playboy', and they want you to wear the T-shirt and not much else. Universities all over England do the same thing; a company puts on these events. Even the nights at our union are called 'Flirt'.

A little while ago there was a thing on Twitter (they have hashtags and trends) and it said 'Big boobs don't count if you're fat'. I thought that was really shallow. And it wasn't just boys writing these status things, it would be girls as well. You see more criticisms than compliments. You don't get compliments very often.

———————

Age 20 | No children

"Girls send pictures of their breasts to boys"

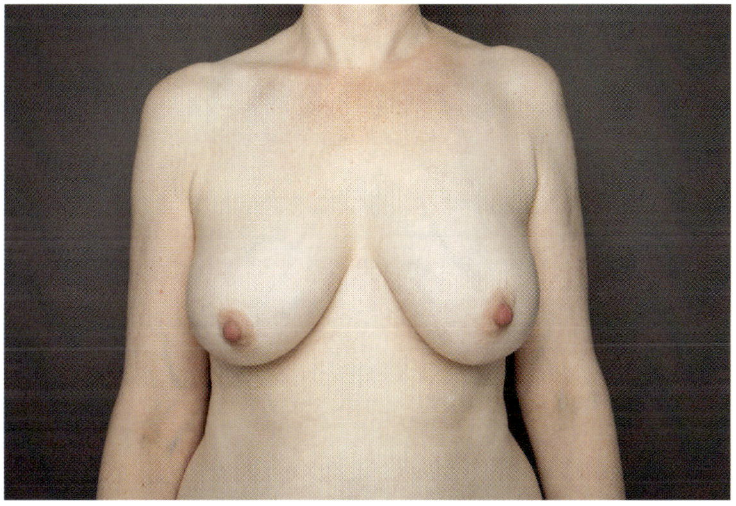

I feel OK about my breasts. I don't feel too self-conscious about them. They are quite pale and they have blue veins. No one has said anything negative about my pale blue breasts! I think partners have liked them.

When I was 16 I was a bit radical, starting to feel political, and didn't wear a bra. I wasn't trying to be flirtatious, it was more, 'No one can tell me to cover up and tell me what to wear. I can do this if I like.' I got attention for being attention-seeking, but it felt uncomfortable and unwanted.

I started wearing a bra again in my mid-20s. I got a bit bigger and also it was about going to work and feeling like I had to dress differently. If you don't wear a bra to work you will be taken less seriously, rightly or wrongly.

Bras are all a bit balcony-style now. I don't like the feeling of being pushed up. I wouldn't choose those sorts of bras, but lots of people are choosing them. I think it's to conform to a look, size and shape. Society's ideal breasts are large, pushed-up, lots of cleavage, Page 3-style breasts.

In my job I meet a lot of young women who get pregnant. The young ones are less likely to breastfeed than the older ones. I think younger women are more self-conscious about doing it in public. They are more aware of a sexual aspect of their breasts, and so they feel uncomfortable. All my friends have breastfed. I'm not self-conscious about talking to women while they breastfeed.

Page 3 should definitely go. It objectifies women. It's such an outdated thing, it's horrendous. I can't believe it really. And what was on the top shelf has moved down now.

The Internet and social media have changed what people think is acceptable to have in the public domain. We have the scandal of children accessing the worst pornography on the Internet. People are becoming more immune to it, and the threshold for what people find tolerable is shifting. The ISPs could give us better protection, but they don't, they choose not to.

I've been doing some work around children at risk of sexual exploitation. When you talk to young people individually, they are horrified about what goes on around them. There is some insidious, horrible stuff going on in playgrounds. Their sexual activities are recorded, sent round to each other, uploaded on Facebook and YouTube. Young people are 'sexting'; girls send pictures of their breasts to boys. There is bullying going on around these sorts of things.

There is peer pressure. People want to belong to the group, but that means they have to buy into a horrible culture. I work with lots of people who self-harm and this will be one of the reasons why. A picture of breasts, for example, can go round a school.

Young women are used and 'sold' across gangs. For instance, there are initiation ceremonies where they go along a line of young men and give each one a blow job. I know young girls who have done this. They are just 14 or 15. They're used as 'honey traps', entrapping a member of another gang so they can be ambushed. They are raped as a weapon in gang culture. All this sexualised stuff in magazines has shifted what is tolerable, and the world is becoming a more scary place for young women.

Age 47 | No children

"I'm completely ambivalent about my breasts"

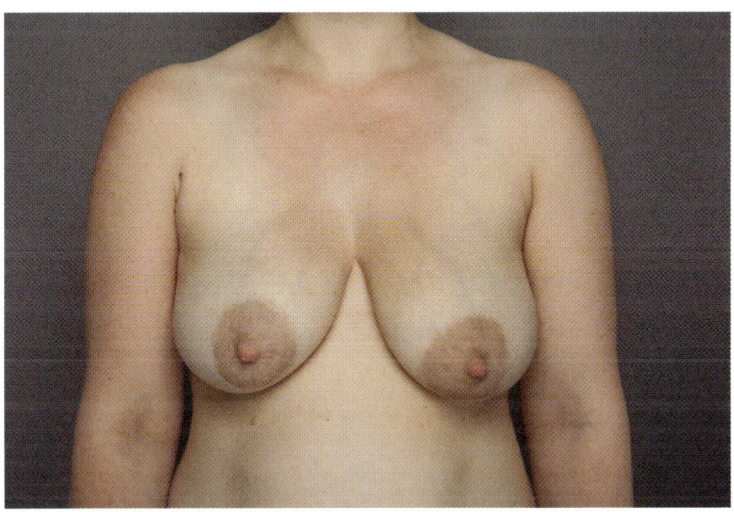

I've always been completely ambivalent about my breasts. If I had to describe my breasts I'd say, 'Well, they're boobs aren't they …' I'm happy with them on a functional level, but they don't even register on an aesthetic level. I don't show them off.

They've worked brilliantly feeding children for the last three years. I'll feed my children whenever I need to and I'm not bothered about getting them out in public. Sometimes people have come over and I think, 'Oh, here we go', and I'm more than ready for criticism, but they've always been supportive or ignored it. I've never encountered any negativity, but I know people who have. When you're breastfeeding all people can see is the baby's head anyway.

When my baby arrived I thought my toddler would want to feed again, but he didn't. He never showed any interest until she was 10-months-old, and then he asked to feed again. I think his jealousy kicked in because she was more mobile. I've let him try. I was always prepared to feed them both.

There are more acrobatics when you feed a toddler. There's a lot of stretching and pulling, but you're more accustomed to it by then.

Breastfeeding rates in this country are pretty poor. It does take work, some women don't stick with it. People think it will be easy and natural, but it involves learning new skills. I think there should be more learning during pregnancy. At antenatal sessions they pass a doll around, and you think, 'Right, I'm holding a doll against my chest, how is that of any relevance at all?' Learning that it might hurt for the first week or 10 days would help, as your nipples get used to it.

For me, their whole purpose has been breastfeeding. It is a nice thing for me to do, as well as for my children. Some women find the let-down toe-curling, but I like it. Maybe that's just me though – I also like the feel of hot wax!

Sometimes I have felt my boobs are too large to dress properly. I would love to wear sweet little dresses. I find breasts cumbersome more than anything; like when you have to hold them down when you're running for a bus. I've never found a bra to fit me nicely, but then I haven't been to a fitting for years. I used to wear bikini tops instead. I was happy to stuff them in, then put some clothes on.

I've had a few people talk at my breasts. I'm like, 'Hello, I'm up here!' Someone came to the door asking for charity donations and looked at my boobs.

My breasts have never done anything for me sexually. They are important to my husband as part of the overall package. He would spend more time on them if he could, but I find it quite annoying. I'm not a very sexual person, whereas he is. I think he would like to bring it out of me, I'm sure he thinks there is more to be discovered. But it doesn't feel like my body is for that at the moment, I can't get back to where we were before children. It's probably hormonal, and not enough sleep. But I think there is only so much I can blame on hormones. I think it's also where my head is at, and our relationship. From talking to women I gather sex drive improves as children get older.

———————

Age 38 | Two children, breastfeeding 14-month-old

"I've never worn a bra"

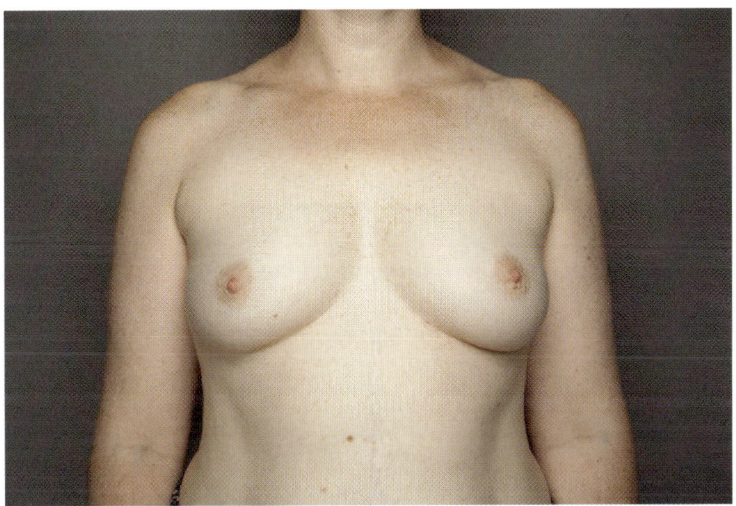

I've always felt pretty good about my breasts because they are small and manageable. I find them easy.

I've never worn a bra. When I was about 12 my mum bought me a starter bra. It felt ridiculous. I've never needed to contain or support them. I've lived quite an alternative lifestyle and known women who are happy to live differently. I haven't felt a need to cover them. If I was wearing something thinner then in some situations I might wear a vest so you can't see the nipple.

Where I live there are quite a lot of Muslims and religious people and I'm conscious of not being perceived in a sexual way. I am happy to be topless in an appropriate situation. I used to go to a lot of rainbow gatherings. They are very earthy get-togethers, normally very remote, and it's about having a connection with the earth. People swim naked or sit around topless. Not everyone, it's choice. There's no sense of the male gaze, or voyeurs, it's very comfortable.

I have a daughter. Her attachment to my boobs is interesting. I breastfed till she was three and she is four now. When she goes to bed she has her hands on my boobs. If she's hurt she wants her hand down my top. I don't mind her hand there, but I don't like her fiddling with my nipples. They are such a source of comfort for her. She breastfeeds her dolls and animals and has a very wholesome attitude to boobs. I'll be interested to see how that develops.

Just being naked around your kids helps. They need to feel comfortable and relaxed in their bodies. I want to take her to a Rainbow Gathering to help her be comfortable.

We went looking for swimming costumes and they were really skimpy. Why would you put a four-year-old in a frilly little bikini, what's the message? Girls' clothing is very sexualised now. It makes me want to run to the hills. I talk with friends about creating some kind of lifestyle, being closer to the land. I've decided not to apply to school for my daughter, which opens up a whole new world. I've made contact with other home educating families and hanging out with the kids is great, they have such a wonderful energy and they are kids for longer.

I had a Catholic upbringing. We had catechism classes every Saturday till the priest was removed because he'd been molesting … I went to a Catholic girls' school; it wasn't a great experience. I became veggie at 12 and vegan at 15 and I was an atheist, so I didn't really fit in. So I left. *(laughs)*

We don't have Barbies, but my daughter has seen them and thinks they are a complete delight. Unfortunately I also had a reaction: 'Bloody Disney princess crap'. She latched on to that and she's really into Barbie now. I should probably buy her one but I can't bring myself to yet. My partner says we should let her, it's her choice, but it's everywhere, so what does choice mean?

Breasts were a good part of sex, but now I can't bear them touched. But then we don't have sex much. I don't call him my partner any more. We've had a rocky road. We have sex occasionally but I don't want breasts involved. He also associates breasts with breastfeeding and I think he's traumatised by the birth. Poor him eh? *(laughs)*

I had this fantasy I would have a home birth, and with hips like mine it would be no problem. Breastfeeding was going to be a breeze. I had to go to hospital, I had forceps, I was in there for three days and she wouldn't breastfeed initially. There was a lot of pressure in the hospital to give her formula but I persevered. I had thrush in my breasts for six months. I would dread the next feed, it was excruciating. That was hard. I tried researching it, going to the doctor, homeopaths. After six months, breastfeeding was good. I think because it had been so sore, after that it felt like bliss.

I had post-traumatic stress after the birth, but I didn't tell anyone. Everyone's like, 'But at least the baby's OK!' And you're like, 'Yes, of course, I'm grateful'. It was a tough time.

Breastfeeding was blissful and I didn't want to give up. I think of myself as strong in my mind, but I definitely felt pressure from my daughter's dad to give up. I think he felt it went on too long and it was blocking his connection to her because he couldn't put her to bed. I'm happy we got to three, but I didn't continue as long as I could have.

You have to be careful talking about breastfeeding, because so many women don't, and there is guilt around it.

———————————

Age 40 | One child

"They are my assets and I have been blessed with them"

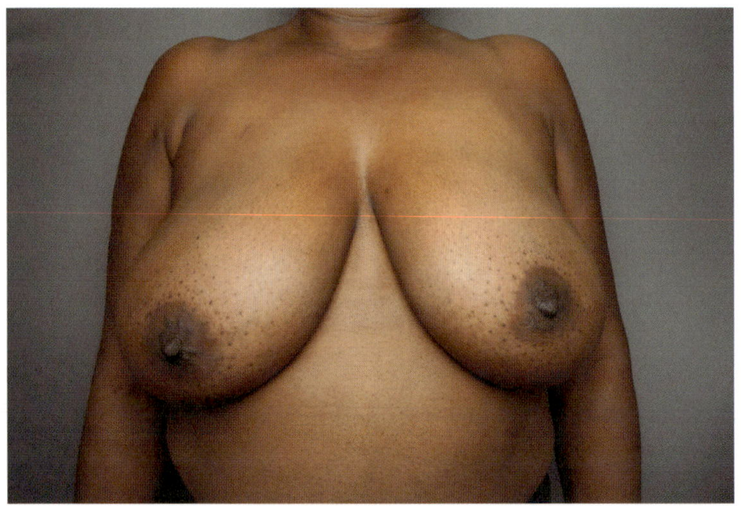

I love my breasts. I think they are fantastic. They are part of me and I wouldn't want them any other way.

My mum and my family encouraged me to be positive and confident. I can't hide, I am 6ft tall. I was the only black face at the school, the only black in the village – like the only gay in the village! *(laughs)* I was the tallest and I was the naughtiest too. At school I was a 38DD, and it never bothered me because I have been taught to carry it off. A lot of tall women are hunched over and you can see they don't even love themselves.

My mum always said I need to look after myself, in terms of health and looks. When she was younger her mum said to her, 'No matter what, even when you have children, you have to look after yourself'. That's the mantra I have lived by.

A lot of women don't understand how to dress. We're ladies, it's important for us, for our own self-esteem. We have to know how to take care of ourselves. Don't let anybody put you down, because you are what you are.

I wear my heels on purpose. I'll give you an example. I'm an advisor to the Metropolitan Police. Years ago, when I first started, I was scared, kind of shy. I hadn't been exposed to that level of leadership and those kinds of people. You know they say 'fake it till you make it'? Well I did. I wore my bright red trouser suit and my heels that make me 6ft 5in tall. I walked in there, having kittens, but all they saw was this tall black lady in a power suit! It can help being a tall woman, because they have to look me in the eye, or look up to me.

Dressing your breasts in meetings can be more complicated. I am a 38GG or a 40G, depending where I buy my bras. They are slightly above average, as I call them. *(laughs)* As a stylist I know about dressing for my shape. It depends what meetings I go to. I went to a football club recently and I asked my friend who I was going with, 'Tell me about who we're meeting with. Shall I have legs or my tits out?' I was only joking. I dress with discretion, nothing popping out. When I walk into a room, people will stare anyway.

If breasts are big and look droopy, people are drawn to look. But if you dress right – for me that means a V-neck – people are drawn to all of you. Some people's eyes are at my boob height. Dressing starts with foundation garments, it starts with your bra.

I get men looking at my breasts all the time because the majority of men are short. I just brush it off. If the man is jolly and makes some normal conversation it's OK. If the focus is on my breasts then I will pass a comment back. I would stop the conversation and look down the front of his trousers. Or I would say, 'Do you have a good view?'

I took part in this project because I like inspiring, positive messages. Women should love themselves. Even if they have small breasts they should love them. I love my breasts. They are my assets and I have been blessed with them.

———————

Age 45 | No children

"Mine are very large and I've only got little legs, I'm like Humpty Dumpty!"

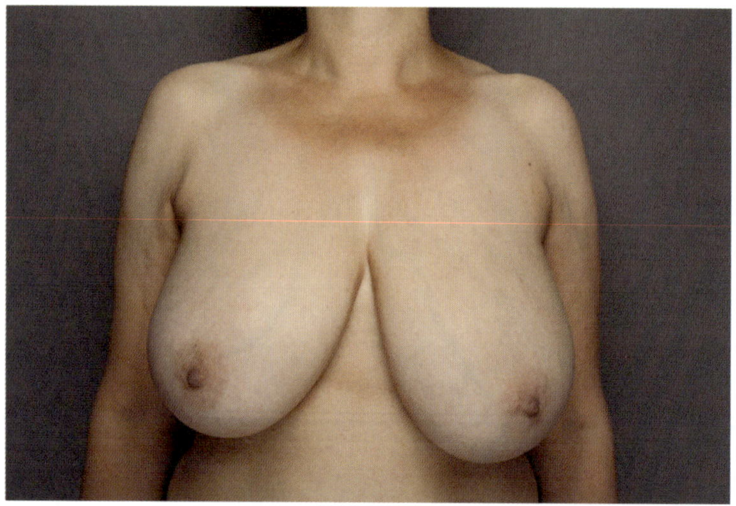

Mine are very large and I've only got little legs, I'm like Humpty Dumpty! I would have preferred my boobs to be smaller but they haven't adversely affected my life.

I developed early, I was big even by the age of 12. I wore bras before my friends. As a teenager I couldn't wear tops that other girls wore. I always had to wear a bra, and back then bra straps could not be shown. I think it's liberating that women can wear strappy tops with bra straps showing now.

I wore big tops to cover my boobs because I did find chaps were looking. When I was 13 I was already a C cup, and I hated the comments. I would get comments when I was swimming and I was too young to handle it. 'Nice knockers!' and 'Phwoar!', grunts and noises. I wasn't ready for it. I would have looked like a child if I hadn't had boobs, but they projected me into womanhood. So I would wear big tops, and they made me look big all over.

When we went bra shopping my mum would launch at us with bras and shove them against our fully-clad bosoms in the middle of a department store. That was the extent of our bra fitting.

I grew up playing sport so I needed firm bras. My breasts didn't get in the way of the sport but I would have liked them to be smaller because of bouncing around. They didn't have good sports bras then, you had to tighten the straps to the maximum.

I went to a naturist beach by mistake once. I was with people from work. We didn't have swimming costumes because we'd just finished a meeting, and this fellow we were with said he knew a good beach, so we thought, 'Alright then'. There were three girls and two blokes, we were sitting there having cans of drink and a bite to eat. This fellow who had suggested it just stood up on the beach and pulled down his trousers and his underpants. We hadn't taken in that it was a nudist beach. I was sitting down when he did it so I was eye-level to his tackle. I said 'What are you doing?' And he said, 'I'm going for a swim, it is a nudist beach.' Really he was giving us a flash.

Once when I was breastfeeding, someone said, 'Your boob is bigger than the baby's head.' I can remember that upset me a bit. They thought it was funny. Of course, my breasts were even bigger when I was breastfeeding. When you're doing something like that you don't really want people to comment at all.

Breast cancer is so high profile, there are races, breast cancer awareness. It's a good thing, but it's very high profile, you are aware. You enter a 'worry stage' with your breasts around menopause. I went through menopause early. I have been for a mammogram but I missed the last one. My friend with breast cancer was furious with me for missing it. I was told mammograms are painful, but it was just weird. I think it is better for larger-breasted women.

I feel that my attitude to breasts has changed with age. I went from being a bit embarrassed by them and shy, to finding them a nuisance with the sport and bras that didn't fit, then there was breastfeeding, now they are just part of me, then you enter the worry stage. What comes after the worry stage? Then you die! *(laughs)*

Age 55 | Two children

"Eating wasn't for me anymore"

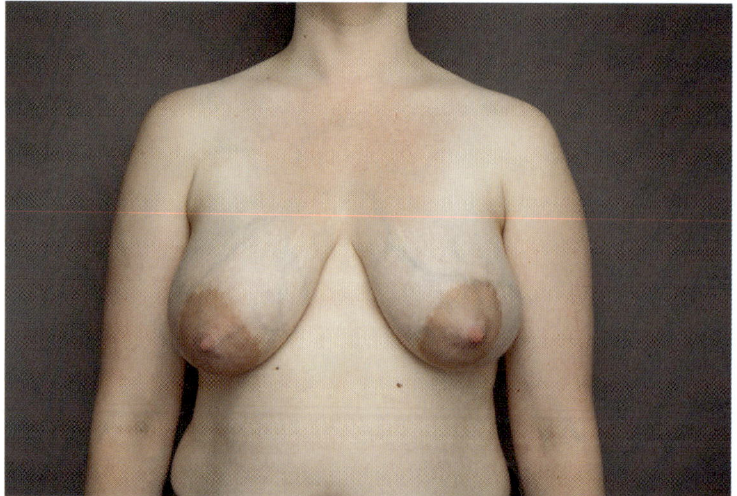

I've never been happy with my breasts. When I was about 14 I developed purple and blue stretchmarks on them. I wouldn't wear low-cut tops or bikinis. I hid them away.

I was also never happy with anyone touching them, including boyfriends. As soon as their hands went down, I'd say, 'No, no, you can't touch them'. They've always been very sensitive. I've never liked the feeling of anyone touching them; it's almost painful, especially when I have my period.

I have very big areolae and I'm self-conscious about them. You get lovely, perky, perfect pictures of breasts in magazines and on TV. I've seen small ones and big ones on the beach in Holland, but I'm still prudish about my own breasts. I think in general Dutch people are more open about everything. It's normal to walk around naked on beaches, to see your parents naked, but I'm prudish.

I've always been very insecure about my whole body. I suffered from anorexia between the ages of 18 and 21. I wanted control, but I liked being skinny too. My whole life was one big horrible mess and I had no control over anything, but I could say no to food. I went down to 47 kilos. I had no face, boobs, or upper arms, but I still had this! *(indicates hips)* That's my build.

My mum had body image problems, she was always on diets. My sister teased me about being fat. My mum was always saying, 'Don't eat that, you'll get fat.' When I got anorexia she said, 'You're losing too much weight,' and I said, 'Well, isn't that what you've always wanted?' I was angry at her.

I have become more happy with my body as I've aged. I'm not 16 anymore, I don't have to prance around on a beach going, 'Look how skinny I am!' I don't care, my partner doesn't care, no one cares.

I like that I am more relaxed about my body now. I've gained respect for my breasts since feeding my baby. I've stepped away from looking at them just sexually. I had a lot of trouble with the idea of feeding in public because of seeing breasts sexually.

The thought of a child sucking my breasts panicked me, because they are sensitive and I also thought it would be kind of gross. I wanted to do it for health reasons for my baby so I had to get over it. As soon as she nursed for the first time I realised it was completely fine. The sensitivity has never been an issue. In fact, they are less sensitive now.

I want to be a good role model for my daughter. Girls have more and more trouble with their body image because of the media. I sign any petition I can about not Photoshopping. You are so judged as a girl on your appearance. Everything is airbrushed. People should be educated about what women and men look like. I'm worried about my daughter growing up with all this.

I'm a mum now. This body has made a child. I have more stretchmarks now and I don't care. I'm proud of myself. I had issues and I didn't look forward to breastfeeding, but I do it and I do it in public.

———————

Age 31 | One child

"I was so determined to breastfeed my second baby"

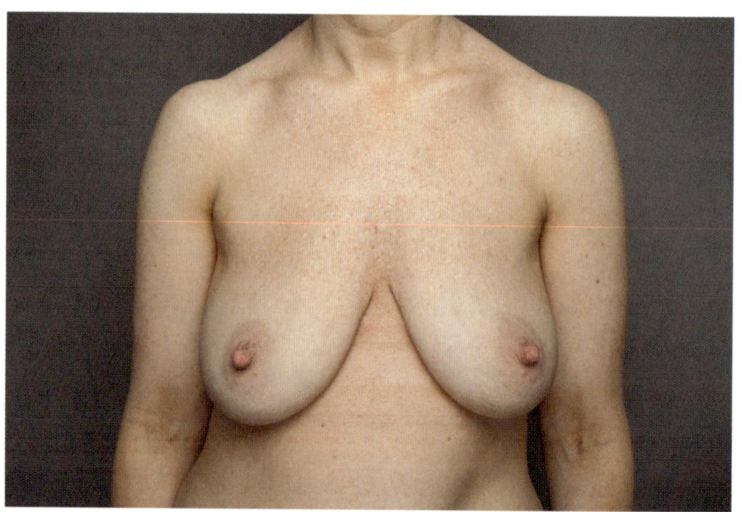

I like my breasts now although they've headed south after having kids. My breasts were one of the best things about me. A boyfriend thanked my mother because my breasts were so wonderful! *(laughs)*

I had a caesarean, but my breasts were the biggest change to my body after my first son. After the baby is born you think everything will spring back quickly, but it doesn't. After my second baby I put on about 20 kilos.

I don't think women know how much they will change. I had morning sickness and was very sick the first 16 weeks, I wanted to step in front of a train and kill myself, and there was no help. I ate lots of bread and carbohydrates. I'd have to get up and eat bread and cereal to get back to sleep. I put on a lot of weight.

I had trouble breastfeeding my first baby and I stopped breastfeeding after about seven weeks. He had a bad latch and I had cracked and bleeding nipples. I told health visitors I needed help, but I was just told it was OK, babies can take a certain amount of blood. There was no help with positioning. I knew nothing about correct attachment or anything I could do to help myself. I had mastitis and thrush in my breasts.

I was so determined to breastfeed my second baby. *(starts to cry)* I knew where to get support second time round and it was much easier. I had read more, and had friends who had breastfed through problems. The more I breastfed my second baby, the more I loved my breasts. Also, I saw them more, I was getting them out every day, so I got used to them.

Now I love them. They have served the purpose of breastfeeding. They look nicer to me than they used to. I am more confident about them, and I have special memories of them. I appreciate what I've got now.

I was in Australia for 6 weeks after my second baby. When I was over there my mum and my best friend, well, my ex-best friend, were telling me I should be putting him on to formula, when he was six months. He's two now, and he's still breastfeeding. *(breastfeeding during interview)* I was getting pressure to stop, 'You're supposed to be going out drinking with your friends, and you're supposed to be going away for weekends with your husband.' I didn't want to leave my children, but even if I wanted to do those things, I didn't have to stop breastfeeding.

After my experience in Australia I was quite upset for about six months. I thought it was so awful that women are treated like this. I looked into breastfeeding and I found out about breastfeeding counsellors. I was really interested because I love being around other mothers and children. I'm a breastfeeding counsellor now with the Association of Breastfeeding Mothers

I want to help create a community where women help each other with breastfeeding. Once I am qualified I can give more advice. I want to do something more with my time while I am at home with the kids.

I haven't asked my husband if he minds me still breastfeeding. He sees it all the time so it's normal for him. He's a bit old-fashioned, so it's more that he's been forced into the lifestyle, he goes along with it.

I don't have much of a sex life. It's not a breastfeeding thing, it's work stress. I sat him down for a chat and said, 'We're a married couple, we should be having sex.' I put on my sexy underwear and I said, 'Right, we're going upstairs to have sex.' 'But I've just eaten dinner!' 'I don't care, we're going to have sex, now.' I was really scared, but afterwards I thought I shouldn't be scared, we should be doing this much more often. But then nothing else has happened.

The other week there was a nude scene on TV, and my husband said, 'Mmm, she's got breasts like you.' They were nice breasts!

———————

Age 38 | Two children, breastfeeding 27-month-old

"Breasts are an integral part of my identity as a woman"

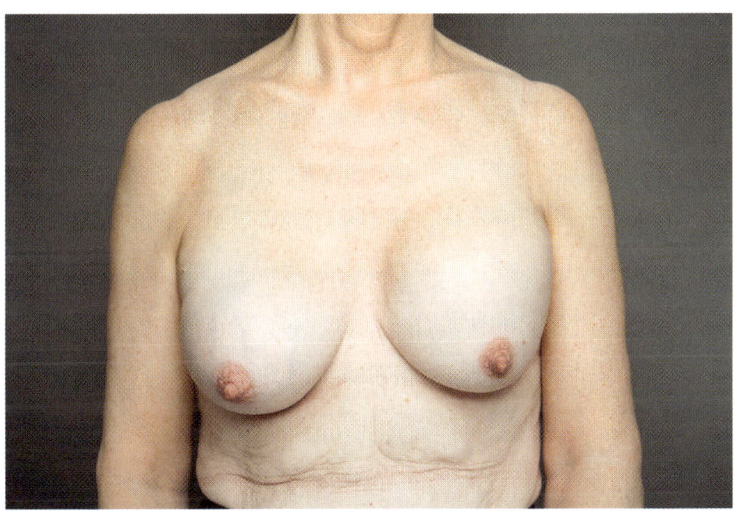

I knew from the age of five that I identified as female. I regarded my male genitalia with absolute horror. I wondered what this bit of skin was. I hoped it might fall off. *(laughs)* As I got older I realised I was stuck in a body I detested.

I was dreading puberty because it meant becoming more masculine. I'd read a story about school boys in Italy who were castrated to retain their soprano voices, and they didn't grow facial hair or develop typical male bodies. So, at the age of 10 I planned to run away to Italy. I saw it as the only way out. But I realised I would probably be caught, in shame, and my father's reaction would have been … After the Christine Jorgensen story broke, my father's opinion was that freaks like that should be locked up and the key thrown away. I knew I had to hide how I felt about myself, for fear of losing his love, and also fear of being incarcerated.

I did once tell my mother how I felt. I was standing in one of those old-fashioned deep sinks while she was washing us. I told her I was a girl and I shouldn't have a penis. All I got was a smack on my wet backside and I was told, 'Don't be so silly, and for God's sake don't let your father hear you talk like that'.

I hated what happened to my body when I went through puberty. Once I got to grammar school I knew that I'd have to pull myself together, otherwise the verbal abuse I'd had at primary school would probably turn into physical abuse. I resolved to fit in, but I found myself attracted to boys, which back in those days was a complete no-no. I felt like a freak.

After my father died I found the courage to go to my doctor. He referred me to the local hospital's psychiatric unit. The psychiatrist tried to persuade me to undergo electro-convulsive shock therapy, which I refused. He then suggested to me that if I was put on a course of testosterone it would make a man of me. I bloody hated that idea. I discovered quite by chance that one of the hospitals in Manchester had opened one of the first gender identity clinics. My psychiatrist was glad to get rid of me to be honest *(laughs)* and he referred me. I was 27.

The clinic diagnosed me with gender dysphoria. After six months of hormones, my body started changing and I grew breasts. I loved the fact that my body was becoming as I knew in my core it should be.

I told my mother when I was referred to the clinic. I was nervous because of the earlier rejection, but I had two choices: either tell her, or just disappear and never contact her again. I couldn't be that cruel, I had to give her the choice to accept it or not see me again. The only way I could actually tell her was in the third person as though it had happened to a friend of mine. About two-thirds of the way through the story my throat was tight like a vice was round it, and tears were pricking, and my mum said, 'And that little boy was you, wasn't it? I'll always love you and we'll get you through this together'. From then on, we were so much closer. She was marvellous, she supported me until the day she died.

There is so much more help now. But even in this day and age, so many transsexuals think of suicide, and many of those actually try to commit suicide. The suicide rate is appalling. I've seriously attempted suicide twice.

I always detested what was between my legs. My ultimate goal was surgery to remove it. I had the penectomy, vaginoplasty and labiaplasty. It's the most painful operation you can imagine. I came around in recovery and thought, 'Fabulous! It's gone!' It was such a wonderful feeling to know that I didn't have that thing between my legs.

They create a clitoris which is very sensitive. It's great, it works, I have orgasms. *(laughs)* I have full sexual intercourse and it all works. The act of penetration isn't just physical, it also happens in my head. It looks as though I was born with it, even though they do far, far better ones now. It passes. It must do! Of course I don't lubricate like other women, although by this age other women don't in the same way either. I've finally caught up with where I would have been! *(laughs)*

The hormone therapy developed my breasts, but they stopped growing when I reached an A cup. Because I had been through male puberty my back was larger than a typical female, and an A cup on a large frame is very small. So I opted to have breast augmentation about a year after the penectomy. I had implants which took me to a B cup. Because of the tightness of the skin that was as large as I could go.

Mentally I felt fabulous. They looked how I had imagined myself from when I was seven or eight years old. I had the body I dreamed of for all those years. It was like all my Christmases had come at once.

Men noticed me a lot more, they became more attentive. If I was out with friends a man might come across and ask to buy me a drink. I had offers of dates from strangers. It was very flattering. I was finally myself and getting attention from men. I had wolf whistles, comments like, 'She's good-looking'. It made me feel good about myself.

A few years ago I had a rupture so they had to take out the implant. Because of modern techniques I could go up to a D cup. I was 64, but that was when I noticed men talking to my chest. It was a most unusual experience: instead of looking at my face when they were talking to me, they were looking at my chest. There was an initial feeling of 'Yes!' and then I felt slighted. He wasn't interested in talking to me, he was only interested in eyeing up my chest, and it was as though I was irrelevant as a person.

Without a doubt the lower surgery is what made me feel most like a woman, but the breast surgery was the icing on the cake.

I've had about 10 partners. Not everyone has known I am a trans woman. No one who hasn't already known has guessed. I was going out with a man from a group of friends from my church. It became more serious and he moved in with me. All was well. I thought he knew, although

I'd never told him. I thought it was my business, it was so personal. It became more difficult to tell him. He made a reference to getting married and having children, and I thought, 'Oh hell, I've got to tell him'. So I sat him down and brought the subject up. He went bananas. He called me a freak, he punched me, he broke my nose, broke a number of ribs. I was black and blue. That was the first time I had suffered from male physical violence. It put me off men for a number of years. I was asexual for a time. I felt I couldn't have a relationship with a guy because I didn't know when the next punch was going to come.

Breasts are an integral part of my identity as a woman and of my sexuality. I have a very high level of sexual pleasure from my breasts, they are very, very erogenous. They are the outward sign of my femaleness and I love the fact that when I am in bed with a guy he will be attracted to them. That in itself makes me feel more feminine. I get this sort of hotline between my breasts and my vagina, and my whole body starts to glow and the desire increases. Whereas, if he was solely interested in my vagina I don't think I would be turned on to the same extent. Breasts are an essential part of my foreplay.

When I finally got my breasts it was like winning the lottery. I was so pleased. I've got the complete picture now. I'm so proud of them. I love them.

———————————

Age 68 | No children

"I want to raise awareness of breast cancer in a positive way"

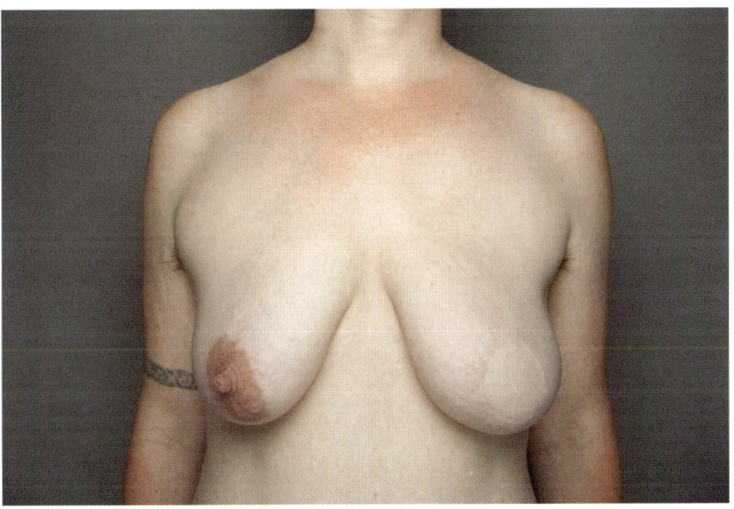

My whole life I thought I had wee saggy boobs and big nipples and was self-conscious about them. I love my breasts now and am trying to get in touch with them and all the pleasure they have given me. I've breastfed two children. I don't want to be hard on them anymore.

None of my partners ever had a problem with my boobs, it was just me who had a problem with them. I've always been down on them, although I loved them when I was pregnant and breastfeeding.

About a month after I'd stopped breastfeeding my younger son I felt a lump. I thought it was probably hormonal but I went to the doctor. I was diagnosed with oestrogen-sensitive breast cancer. I've always had funny hormones; I have polycystic ovaries.

From that moment I thought, 'Right, I'm going to start loving myself.' I was 41.

I'd also split up with my partner for a wee while and was going through a bit of heartbreak. I think emotional stuff may have triggered cancer as well. For the first time in many years I felt like I hated myself. I might even have had post-natal depression. I wondered if hating myself was the trigger for the cancer. It could be one of the problems, but there's also the hormones.

When the cancer was discovered it was at an early stage and I didn't need chemotherapy, just a mastectomy. I take Tamoxifen. I'm lucky I didn't need the really horrible stuff. I had the mastectomy and reconstruction all at once so it was a nightmare of an operation. I don't know if I would have gone for a reconstruction if I'd had to have it later.

When the plastic surgeon first saw me, he said, 'Oh, you've got droopy boobs, but I can fix that. We'll make your new one up here and then you'll come back later and we'll fix the other one. You'll have a great set of boobs.' I told him, 'Make it as droopy as the other one.'

He was a lovely guy, but yeah, 'droopy'. He thought I could get a free boob job out of it. I didn't think of it as insensitive, he was looking at me and being honest and he didn't say it in a horrible way. I didn't take it badly, but it made me realise I wanted it as natural as possible.

The nurse who did a mammogram after the operation told me it was one of the best reconstructions she's ever seen. It's just like the other one. It helps that I have big nipples; the scar was literally just around the nipple line.

I had a tummy tuck as well, they took the skin and fat from my tummy. I didn't want an implant, I wanted it as natural as possible. I'm numb on my tummy now. And look at my belly button. They had to pull the skin down and give me a new bellybutton, which is bizarre. I had two butterfly tattoos there, and now I just have the wing of one butterfly. I wasn't expecting that. Amazingly, the tummy was the worst thing. You look a bit like Frankenstein, covered in bruises, padded, drips, horrific-looking.

I had lots of friends and family who totally supported me. I lived at my mum's house afterwards for a while. A friend came up for a week to help with my son and give my mum a break. It's quite an amazing experience to realise how much you are loved. (*starts to cry*) It's funny, I think I am over it, and then I get all emotional.

I can feel my boob on the skin outside but not the inside. With my tummy it's the opposite; I can feel the inside but I'm numb on the outside. I can get an itch on the inside of my tummy and I can't scratch it.

I recovered well from the operation. I got really healthy before, lots of juicing, vitamin C.

Although I am still pretty healthy it's chocolate and crisps again. I limit myself to two cups of caffeine a day. I inject mistletoe, I don't know if you've heard about that? It's a herbal treatment that's been used in Germany for years. It stimulates your immune system. My homeopath prescribed it, and I get the needles from the NHS. It's quite an expensive treatment and I am very lucky the prescriptions are funded in Scotland, where I'm from. But you know what people in this country are like about alternative health, they don't believe it.

I don't take the same levels of Tamoxifen anymore. I had headaches, mood swings, I was a total monster. It makes you feel pre-menstrual all the time. Every doctor I've spoken to has said it varies from woman to woman, and it's not like taking it will stop me getting breast cancer again.

I have thought maybe I should have my ovaries out. It's like choosing to have mastectomies before you even have breast cancer. It's difficult, it's every woman's decision. I have thought about it, but it's not routinely what they do anyway.

Straight away my partner didn't have a problem with the scars. He kisses them. My breasts have always been great sexually.

I was a bit nervous standing having my photo taken for this project, but I shouldn't be really, because another thing that's come out of all this is that I've become a life model. I work with one artist. He doesn't add a nipple. We talk about my scars sometimes. I see him every six months or so and he has commented that they are fading. It's a way of embracing my nakedness.

I need checks every year because I'm more at risk. I'll have a mammogram every year, but some people think mammograms put you at risk. I've only had one so far.

Although friends have moaned in the past about stretch marks, or saggy boobs, or hairy nipples, they are now more appreciative of their bodies since I have been through this. If we could all just be more appreciative of the good stuff that our bodies do ... I've been doing lots of things recently to show my boobs and my body how much I love them. I hope I won't get sick again.

I never got down about it or let myself go into that negative fear. It's like giving birth: if you go into the negative fear place there is more pain. I don't think 'bad luck' and I never did. There was only one moment I panicked, and it was literally only one moment, and I thought, 'No, that's not how I'm going to handle this. It's a lesson I've got to learn and it's something that will make me stronger.' Obviously, no one wants to get cancer, but you have to get on with it.

As soon as I heard about this project I knew I wanted to get involved. I want to raise awareness of breast cancer in a positive way. When you are told they are going to remove a breast, it feels like the worst thing you can have done as a woman. It's not the worst thing that can happen. Breasts are just a body part. I know of someone who died because they refused to have a mastectomy. You can get through it.

Age 43 | Two children

"Conversations with my mum about weight started at a very young age"

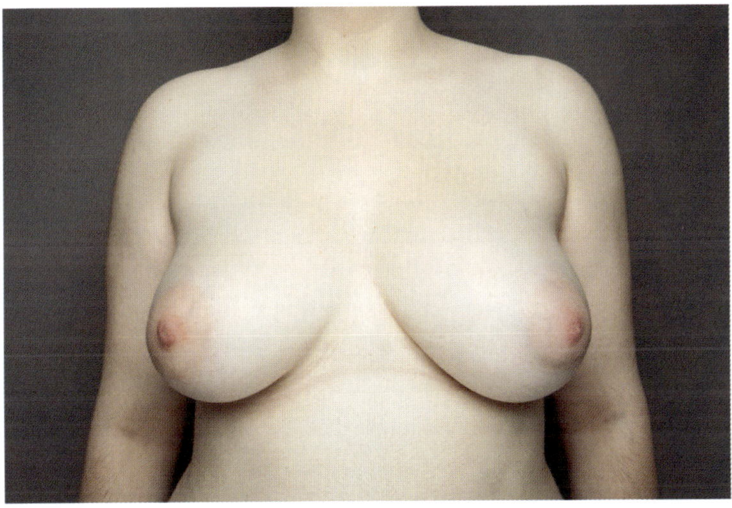

What do I think of my breasts? That is a big question. I like them, they're quite big, not too saggy. They're not the best pair I have ever seen, or the worst, compared to my friends and pictures in magazines. Even if you try not to compare yourself to people in magazines it's hard not to.

My dad is Turkish and Muslim, my mum is Jewish. I identify as an atheist but I have this weird ethnic mix. If I am around my muslim grandparents I do think about what I am wearing, I will cover up out of respect, I worry about adhering to their culture.

I find what you are supposed to wear to school and work more of a concern, you know, not wearing your skirt too short. I used to work in a gift shop and a shoe shop. They had different expectations of how you had to dress. In the gift shop it was very much high necked tops, whereas in the shoe shop you had to appeal to young women, wearing revealing clothes was almost encouraged. I'm not afraid to wear low cut tops in the office now. I'm still trying to figure out what's appropriate for work.

Conversations with my mum about weight started at a young very age. 'Should you be eating that?' and 'You could be so beautiful'. She does think I am beautiful but she has implied I would look so much better if I lost weight. It doesn't make me feel great. We've had some of our biggest arguments about it. She says she has struggled with her weight and how she looks all her life, and she doesn't want me to go through what she has. That's her angle, it's not a fat shaming exercise, she doesn't want me to suffer like her. But it really hurts to have that conversation with my mum. If she thinks I have potential she will push me, and I respect that. She doesn't expect me to be a size six, eight or 10, she just thinks if I looked after my weight more I would look better than I do now. If I was a size 12 I would be really hungry.

I'm wearing a 'No More Page 3' T-shirt, which is funny because this interview is the opposite! I think what Page 3 does is very damaging to young women. It's like, 'This is the benchmark, this is what men find attractive. I don't look look like this, therefore I can't be attractive to men'. I think Page 3 affected me, and it affects all women, and men too. It impacts on every single person who's ever come into contact with it. It affects our perception of beauty, it makes young women think they are valued for their sexuality, and not for their thoughts and actions.

Breasts are great, they are all great. What is so great about this project is highlighting how fabulous they all are. All bodies look completely different, and that should be celebrated, rather than us all conforming to one image.

I went to a girls school and I come from a family of women. I didn't have much exposure to men. I did notice men in the street would look at me differently when my breasts grew. I didn't feel like a sexual person until university. Well, I did feel sexual, but I didn't have an outlet for that till university. Freshers was when I found myself in situations I never thought I would be in. I took a gap year before uni and that's when I lost my virginity. At uni I found myself having more casual sex than I ever thought I would. 'This is attention from guys, this is new!' It was almost like I felt grateful that people found me attractive. With the benefit of hindsight that's a ridiculous attitude.

I was part of a sports club in my first year which was very centred around lad culture and drinking and there was a lot of pressure to conform. I ended up sleeping with half of them. Wahey! *(Ironic laugh)* I did 'topless après'. It's when you get really drunk at the top of a mountain and take your top off. That was potentially really silly, and I didn't want to do it, but I did it anyway because other people were doing it. Lads and girls egging me on. All the girls did it. Ridiculous. I pandered to this stuff.

I haven't had a boyfriend. I go through stages of thinking that's really abnormal. I do want one. But actually I wouldn't have achieved the things I have achieved if I'd had a relationship.

My breasts aren't that important in sex. They're fine, but I don't like people being too aggressive with them. It's nice to be touched there, but I don't like biting. I've had lots of comments for my breasts, like, 'Oh my god, they're really amazing!' That sounds really arrogant. *(laughs)*

I was kissing a male friend of mine who I have slept with a couple of times at the end of a night recently, and he was like, 'Oh can we, can we?' And I said no, I just wanted to go home, I said, 'I know it's happened before, but I don't want to'. He basically dragged me. I don't know whether to say this or not ... He basically forced me to give him head. It was pretty horrendous. That was a guy I thought I had a good relationship with. It's not great. It's pretty shit.

Halfway through I managed to stop him. We were both horrendously drunk, which doesn't help. He says he doesn't remember it. I managed to run home. He followed me home, and my housemates literally had to kick him out of the house.

It still upsets me. I feel sad and angry. I never say I was a rape victim. I think a lot of young women accept that sort of behaviour, because our attitudes to consent are blurred. Just because you have slept with someone before doesn't mean you are asking for it. I always ask female friends to let me know they have got home safely, because part of me worries something is going to happen to them. It shouldn't be like that.

I wrote to him. I told him what happened was not OK and it's really upset me, and he doesn't get to treat me, or women that way. He said he was really sorry and he didn't realise, and he felt sick at the thought. I should have called him out on his drinking. I will never look at him in the same way again, but he's still part of my friendship group. It comes back to feeling so grateful that someone finds you attractive that you find yourself in a situation you don't want to be in. So, maybe it is my fault. I don't look like the women I see in magazines, I don't like women in the media, I don't look like a Page 3 model.

I have had sex since, but it makes me feel sick thinking about it. It's too early to know how I feel about sex now. I think it's good to talk about it. It's affected me more profoundly than I thought it could. It's a bit shit. Sorry.

———————————

Age 21 | No children

"They were like balloons after a party"

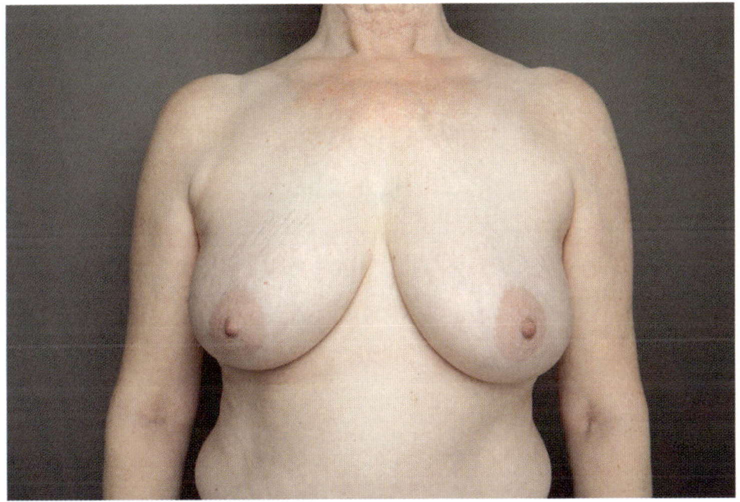

I think my breasts are quite reasonable. They are probably one of the parts of me I don't mind compared to other bits. I didn't like them when I was younger because I was very flat and had a pigeon chest.

I was dead ashamed of not having any bosoms when I was coming up to 16. I remember being in a pub with a friend who was quite bosomy and incredibly confident. She pulled back the top of my sweater and said '28AA' and laughed. I was consumed with embarrassment. I felt unfeminine. I would have liked bigger bosoms.

Then when I was 16 I went on the Pill and they were marvellous! I was delighted with them, I couldn't stop looking at them! I'm not sure if people's reactions to me changed. I am quite vague and very short-sighted; I've never worn my glasses out of vanity, so I might have been lusted at but I wouldn't know. I couldn't see much past the end of my nose! *(laughs)*

I remember my first pretty bra. It was very slighted padded, white with tiny rosebuds. It was ever so pretty. When I put it on and then put a jumper over the top, I could see the beginning of a womanly shape, and I was absolutely thrilled. Mum was born in 1918 and was quite unusual for her generation. We had a very comfortable, open family. I can picture my mum's bosoms now. Not dissimilar to mine, but she had much more pronounced nipples. I had a sense that she thought they were quite nice.

It never occurred to me not to breastfeed my children really. Breastfeeding had been out of fashion but was coming back in. It seemed like if you were on your own in the wild and gave birth, it would be the next obvious thing to do. It's like the last process of giving birth, kind of a conclusion. It felt absolutely right.

I do have to tell you this. In the maternity hospital where I had my first baby, the Sister was appalled that we wouldn't sit with the curtains around our beds when we breastfed. She would shout, 'You can't sit there in full public view, feeding your babies. We have men come in here!' That's the absolute truth. And the other thing was that we had to sit on hard chairs, we couldn't sit on the beds and feed our babies. She claimed that was to do with the healing of your fundus, but it wasn't. It was … well, I don't know!

I was 18 and not married. Only husbands were allowed to visit. If that Sister I was telling you about was on duty, he wouldn't have been allowed to visit or attend the birth. They were very sniffy about it. It was only the 1970s!

I'm fascinated by the way breastfeeding is approached now. It's been totally different for my daughters having babies. I remember a midwife, or a specific breastfeeding advisor, showing my daughter how to hold her baby in the most uncomfortable way imaginable. And when my daughter said, 'Oh, that's quite difficult', she said, 'When you're breastfeeding you develop muscles you never knew you had'. How would we have evolved as a species if it's that hard? Something's gone wrong when you've got books and DVDs about breastfeeding. Stick on the TV, sit on the sofa and put your feet up, get a nice cup of tea and whack the baby on. Nobody told me what to do. There's the baby's mouth, there's my nipple – as far as I'm concerned those need to come together, and that's it.

I knew lots of people who gave up. But they didn't like it, they found it a bit yucky. People now can be just slightly revolted, slightly horrified. It's bodily fluid. I think also people feel much more obliged to try. The whole of motherhood you're plied with, 'You should be this and that, put your child's interests first regardless'. There's nothing more evil than a mother who's not fantastic! I think if your heart's not in it then it isn't for you.

Pregnancy and breastfeeding significantly affected my breasts. They got much bigger and I absolutely loved them! They were fabulous, they were majestic, gargantuan. I had massive amounts of milk. They were stretch-marked, although I think that was mainly from going on the Pill, but I wasn't too bothered about that. But when I finished breastfeeding that was a real shock. Blimey, they just went. They were like balloons after a party. There was no substance and I was very taken aback. They weren't saggy, just much smaller – like someone had sucked the air out of them.

On our honeymoon my husband couldn't go anywhere near them because they would have spouted milk everywhere! *(laughs)* We had sex on honeymoon, but no touching of breasts. There was leakage anyway, but it could have been significantly worse. He became used to it. We would both wake up, and I'd say, 'Oh no mate, bed's soaked!' He came from an all-women family, although he would never have seen his mum's breasts in his life. He didn't even know about periods till we got married I think. Leaking milk didn't seem to bother him, but I don't know if I gave him the option to offer his opinion. When I got into the bath he'd bring me a cup of tea and we'd both laugh because they would literally pour!

I can remember going to Boots for breast pads and just looking at them and laughing. They were going to be hopeless. I used to cut big, old-fashioned sanitary towels in half, and they would get soaked. I think I drank too much water. If I heard a baby crying, it was 'Woah, here we go.' A door squeaking could make me leak.

I'm not like some of these women who apparently only have to have their nipples tweaked and they have an orgasm. Lucky them! I think it's a fantastic fantasy for blokes, isn't it: twiddle, twiddle, like a radio. I knew a hairdresser who said there was a woman who would have an orgasm when she was having her hair rinsed. It just goes to show how different we are, doesn't it?

The whole maintenance of women's looks has changed significantly and I think breast augmentation is part of that. If there is a way to make money out of how women look, it will be capitalised on. I think it's a lot to do with the fact that we live in a more visual age, the media is 24-hour. The way women look has been airbrushed and enhanced a million miles away from reality. Cindy Crawford said, 'I wish I looked like Cindy Crawford'.

Women are turned into things and bits of things. Girls think that's how they have to look to be acceptable. It's beginning to happen to men too, but women have always been under that sort of pressure. I think it's less to do with gender politics and more to do with capitalism. Women have to invest: it's money, it's revenue. The amount women spend on body maintenance! Regular bits of nipping, tucking, plumping, waxing, lasering, things being injected here, there and everywhere, dyes, tattoos, plucking and those awful trouty mouths.

Breasts are associated with women's sexuality, but I do think they have been sexualised by the media. There is a discomfort that they are sexual objects on the one hand and for feeding babies on the other. I think that disturbs people who think of them sexually. It's quite complex, that.

Breastfeeding is very pleasant, but it's entirely different. There is no connection from your nipple to the bits down below, as there is in sexual contact. It's the most warm thing. It's sensual. I can understand this being something that troubles people. It could be they only feel nice sexually because they are supposed to feel sensual for breastfeeding. If you think of the whole skin-to-skin contact with your baby, it is sensual. I stick my nose into my grandchildren's skin. It's not sexual, but there is a sensuality. I think it troubles us as a society.

I remember as a youngster feeling regretful that I didn't have enough. In my day the idea was (it's so funny when you think about it) that you don't need more than a handful. Well, whose hand? Oh, your boyfriend's hand. Well, that seems reasonable! *(laughs)* It's the whole ownership thing.

———————

Age 54 | Three children

"Stretchmarks aren't pretty but you can feel proud of them"

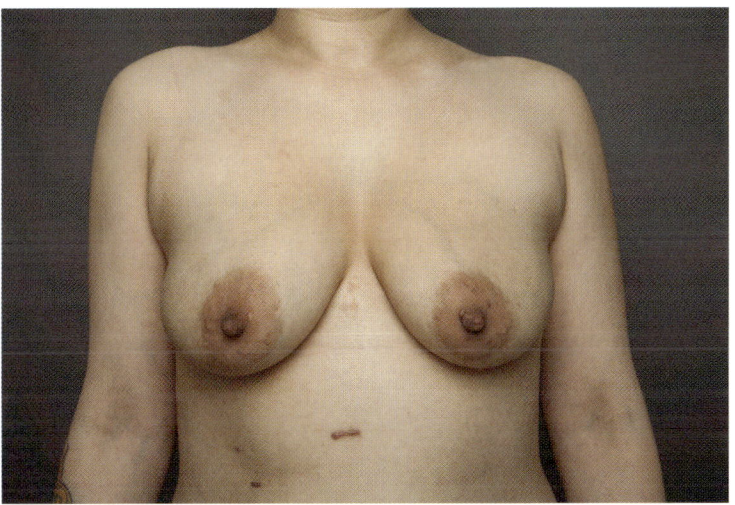

My breasts are alright. I don't put as much aesthetic importance on them as I used to. I do on my skin though. I was reluctant to do this project because of my scars.

I teach hypnobirthing and BabyCalm. I work with pregnant mums, mums and dads, babies and toddlers. Particularly in mothering, there is a misplaced sense of authority in the doctor-patient relationship. That can be good for people who are happy to have someone make decisions for them. For those of us who aren't, it can create tension and poor decision-making. I had a laparoscopy recently and I could relate to the experiences of some clients who have had the decisions and rights of their own bodies taken away.

I think I had qualms about this project for aesthetic reasons, but also I felt weakened by that procedure. A laparoscopy isn't a natural process. Scars aren't stretch marks. I wouldn't mind if you wanted to take photographs of what has happened to my belly, it's more about the physical story of the procedure. Stretch marks aren't pretty but you can accept them and feel proud of them.

My husband finds my breasts sexually attractive, but I think that's comical. I have my pop-psych ideas about breastfeeding. Where breastfeeding is not the norm, boobs are sexualised. My husband wasn't breastfed – he is definitely a boob man! It's not very feminist of me, but my husband's acceptance of my breasts helps me. You do want some kind of validation.

How breasts feel sexually matters more now. There was a time when I would recoil from them being touched sexually. That sounds terrible. That was from breastfeeding. Some women recoil from breastfeeding because they see their breasts as for their husbands. I was surprised that I felt completely the opposite. At one point I had to say something. I didn't want him to think I was rejecting him.

My daughter has always had a shallow latch, so breastfeeding has never been pleasurable apart from the oxytocin in the early days, where it was 'brain bubbles'. I've always had feeding aversion. I carried on because I was determined to let her self-wean. That's because I was forced to wean my son. I had a very misguided midwife. I know now she just didn't have enough training, and I don't think she even had any children. She said he was starving and I had to give him formula when he was just a couple of days old. It turned out I was over-producing. He had lost less than half a per cent weight more than the guidelines. She never asked me how the birth had gone. He had been taken away from me for a night in hospital and he hadn't been fed, which would have been part of the problem. She badgered me for a week and called me into her clinic. She persuaded us to mix breast and bottle, without warning us of the dangers of mixed feeding.

I prepared for the birth, but didn't prepare for breastfeeding at all. I didn't know there was opposition to it, or that some midwives would have such minimal training. I'm still angry. I'm angry that I didn't take the research I put into birth into breastfeeding, but I didn't know I needed to prepare for negativity. I thought breastfeeding was the normal thing for babies. I was nonchalant about it.

I know I need therapy for the anger I feel about it. But maybe it is useful the anger is there, because it might help stop it happening again. That midwife is now the senior midwife in charge of a midwife-led unit.

Birth can rob us of power. No matter what happens women often blame themselves, but they should be angry at the people who guided them into motherhood. Even if it isn't their fault, women still internalise it as 'I'm less of a women, I'm less of a mother.'

———————

Age 31 | Two children, breastfeeding three-year-old

"Sport has changed my body image"

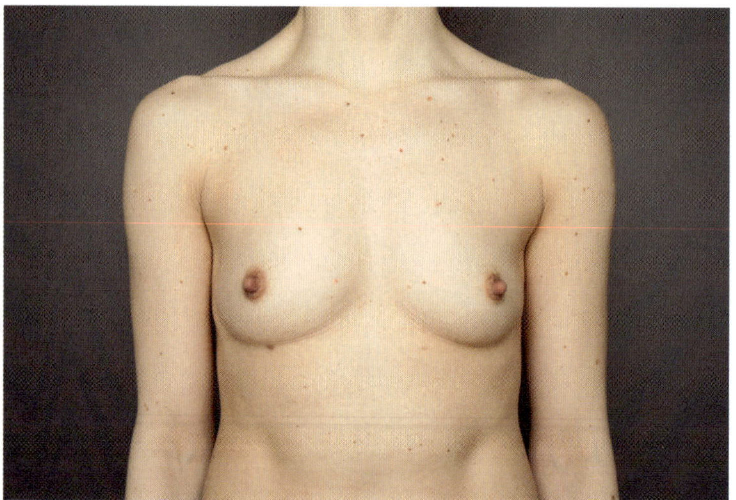

My breasts are small, but because of the sport I do, they would be in the way if they were big. They're just there. I like them. I remember trying my mum's bra on when I was a little girl and sticking oranges in it! My mum and all my aunties and my nan have good size boobs, big knockers basically.

There was a point when I really didn't like them. A few years ago I considered breast enhancement surgery. But if they were any bigger now they would be in the way, cost a lot of money, and what for? I've changed quite a lot in my outlook.

I considered a boob job not long after I got divorced. My confidence wasn't brilliant, but I was back out in the dating game. I wasn't myself then, it was a car-crash time. The ideal woman is presented as being size eight with big boobs. Maybe because I've got a boyish figure I thought I would stand out more with bigger boobs.

It wouldn't have solved my problems. I know that now, and I think I knew it then. I felt like a failure. I couldn't get why he'd been unfaithful and left me, so I thought, 'What can I fix?' Ah, I've just thought, the woman he left me for had fake boobs! I've never considered that before. Maybe that played into my psyche.

I really wouldn't like it if my daughter wanted implants. I want her to be happy with her body image. Ultimately it would be her choice and I hope it would be an informed one. I've got strong feminist opinions. I want my daughter to feel as valued as any man is on this planet. My mum did a good job with me, but society wasn't as sexualised as it is now.

I do triathlon: everything is about reducing drag and resistance. Especially in the pool, the smaller your protrusions – the smaller your boobs – the quicker you go. I wear a lot of compression gear, everything is about minimising. My wetsuit straps everything in. I want the least amount of resistance possible.

Most female triathletes have quite small busts. Because of the amount you have to train, it all turns to muscle. If I'd had big breasts I don't know if I'd have become a triathlete. Maybe I'd have seen myself completely differently. I've always seen myself as quite boyish.

Sport has changed my body image because the body has become functional. The more functional it is, the better in this game. It's changed all my attitudes, that someone can find you attractive for what you can do, and not for how you look.

In the sporting world, women are judged more on performance than what they look like. If you go and do as your coach tells you, and you're consistent, and you train hard, and you perform, then that's how you're judged. Even if you don't perform well, if you tried your best, then you're admired for that. There isn't a double standard, I've never come across sexism in the sport.

———————————

Age 39 | One child

"I'm planning to have breast implants"

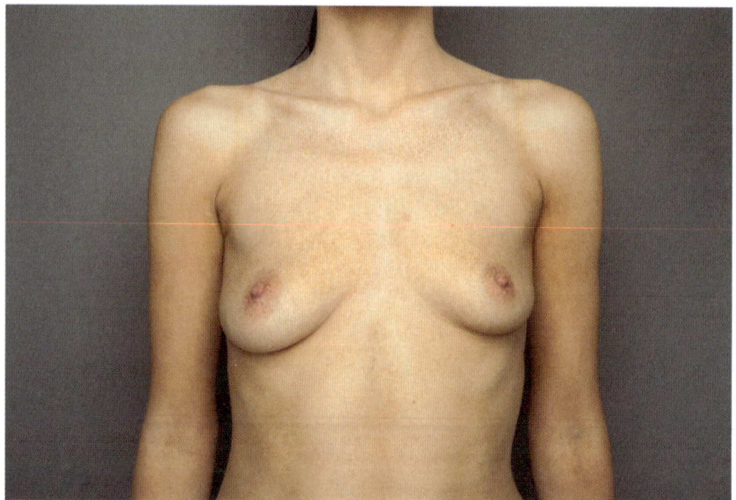

I would describe my breasts as saggy, skinny and horrible. I'm planning to have breast implants in a few days time. I'm very excited about it. I'm going to go from 32B to 32DD. Maybe I should go for something a bit bigger. Girls I know who have had implants say you always wish you had gone for bigger ones.

The surgeon is at one of the top London clinics and I know a few girls who have been there. So it should be safe. It would be cheaper in Poland where I am from, but if something goes wrong I can't go back there. I prefer to pay a bit more money and be sure they are going to look after me.

The clinic told me implants won't affect breastfeeding at all. I haven't really thought about breastfeeding, but I think it would be nice. Someone told me it develops a very nice connection.

I found a job in a gentleman's club so I could pay to have my breasts done. I realised there was massive potential to earn money. I'm hoping to pay for it within a year if I work hard. Since I started working in the club, I am surrounded by beautiful big breasts. My problem has become bigger: I am even more conscious about my breasts.

When I was new in the job, I would leave my bra on until the last seconds of the dance because I was self-conscious. I get lots of compliments for different parts of my body, but not my breasts. But they could pay me thousands of compliments and it wouldn't mean anything to me because I think my boobs are horrible.

I've started talking about my operation in the club with the customers. I tell them they will see the before and after! They say it's not a turn-on when the girls have implants. No one has said, 'Good for you, if that's going to make you happy, then do it'. Some guys have tried to discourage me.

They haven't put me off because I am not doing this for men, or customers, I am doing it for my own confidence. I talked to a guy for about 20 minutes and he didn't buy a dance. Then he had a dance from a girl with bigger boobs.

When I took my bra off once, one customer said, 'Oh, your breasts look bigger in a bra. You tricked me. I want a refund.' He's a regular, so I'm waiting till I see him with my new coconuts. The club could sack me if I refused him another dance.

One of the dancers told me to be very close to the customer when I take my bra off, because if I am close my breasts will look bigger. If I stand at a distance they can judge me. Also I can play with my breasts to hide them. She said once you've danced for a guy for two minutes he's already turned on, he won't register if one is bigger. Plus he's probably drunk.

I get comments in the club like, 'Have you studied anything?' They make out you don't do anything except undress, they don't realise you have a life outside of the club. Maybe they are just trying to make conversation, but I think they think I am just stupid.

I was once grabbed by a guy during a dance. Towards the end I had my back to him and he licked me in the, you know … intimately. I stopped immediately. He started apologising to me, but I couldn't even look at him. It was disgusting.

They forget where they are and get confused between a strip club and brothel. I've been offered money to do things. I had a guy who said he would take me out for a nice dinner date and he would pay me £300, but if I was interested in more money he would take me home for £1,000. He grabbed my hand, tried to give me notes and pay for my number. They aren't supposed to touch us or proposition us, but they don't care.

If there's something about myself I don't like, I change it. For example, when I put on weight I wasn't happy with myself, so I went on a diet and I lost 10 kilos. I totally hated a mole on my back. My mum called it a beauty spot, but how can you call it beauty? So I went to a surgeon and had it removed. After my breasts, hopefully nothing else will bother me. I don't think so. I am 90 per cent happy with how I look, it's just my breasts. When they are done it will be 100 per cent probably. Not probably, definitely. I'm pretty sure. Unless I put on weight. Breasts will be the last thing. It's interfering with nature. I don't like my nose though.

My bum used to bother me: in my head it was big. I met this guy who was fascinated with my bum. After four years of being with him I liked my bum, I thought it was one of my best assets. Although I was comfortable with him I didn't want him to see my breasts or touch them, even with the light out. They are unnaturally soft, there is nothing inside them.

I wouldn't mind them being small if they were full and the same size. There is hanging skin. It probably sounds like I am all complexes, but there are parts of my body I am happy with. I feel sexy when I am all done out, spray tan, hair done.

I'm an occupational therapist. I work in an old people's home as an activity coordinator. It's such an extreme: during the day I entertain the elderly and during the evening I entertain dirty men. *(laughs)*

I'm nervous about people's reaction to my new breasts at my day job. I'm going to hide them under baggy clothes. Whatever they say, I will deny it. 'I've bought this amazing bra, and I've put on a bit of weight.' Simple.

I'm scared of my parents finding out. My dad sees me as the 'sensible one', and if I tell him that I've spent nearly £5,000 on breasts ...They don't know I work in a strip club. My dad would disown me. Working in a strip club to pay for a boob job ...

I am also nervous about the anaesthetic. I've never had one. I might die, I might have complications. What if I wake up and I can't remember English, and I can only speak Polish? The anaesthetic might kill some brain cells!

I trust the clinic. The surgeon spent only five minutes with me. At first I thought it was because he does so many operations every day, but the consultant explained to me that he saw my boobs and thought, 'Great, this will be so easy'. My boss at the club also said not to worry, she said she could see that the results will be good.

Barbie is perfect. I've got a vision of a perfect woman: big breasts, nice bum, small hips, small waist, long legs, long hair. Men normally go for women with big breasts. I am doing this partially for men as well. I'm not saying I want to look exactly like Barbie, I know she's not proportional, but I want to make myself as attractive as possible. I've got so much more confidence when I'm pampered.

continued on the following page

"I look in the mirror and it's not me"

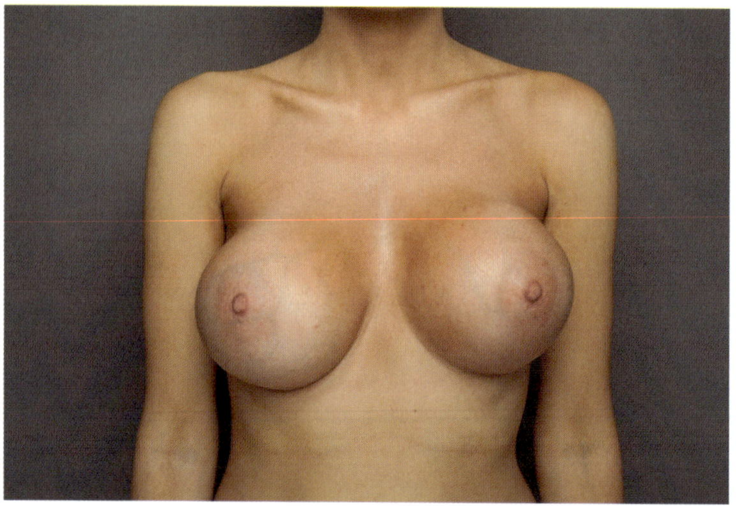

continued from previous page

It was like a luxury hotel, amazing. A friend came with me and we were taking loads of funny pictures. I was posing, I was so happy, no stress at all.

After the operation I didn't feel pain, but felt very heavy. The hell started after 24 hours. I felt like I'd been run over by a train and had broken ribs and spine. I had to keep the dressing on for a week.

When I went to the clinic a week later they took the bandages off. I really wish someone had been with me. I started laughing when I looked in the mirror. It felt like I was screaming inside. I thought, 'What the fuck have I done?' They were massive, hilarious. I looked like an inflatable doll.

Do you remember one was higher? Well, they are like that now, but the problem is magnified because they are bigger. I have a huge boob almost on my shoulder and a huge boob almost on my tummy. The nurse ticked the box to say the client is happy because I was laughing, and I had to say, 'No, hang on a minute. I am laughing because they look ridiculous. I am not happy.' She said I would calm down and be happy with the results. I had a feeling she was thinking, 'Oh shit'.

They printed out before and after pictures. Before the operation I remember thinking 'Whatever happens it can't be worse than this.' But actually I thought my new boobs were 10,000 times worse. I went to the toilet and took a photo and sent it to a few friends. I was standing in London, tears pouring down my face, people looking at me. I even sent the photo to my ex-boyfriend. He told me off and said, 'They look very, very fake. Now you look like a porn star.'

To be honest with you I thought I would kill myself. I couldn't see any other option. They couldn't take the implants out, they said I would be saggy and stretched.

My sister said she started laughing when she saw the photos, but I was crying. I said, 'No guy will want me now. I don't accept myself either. This is it, I don't know if I am going to survive the next 24 hours.' She said, 'Don't be stupid, some people are disabled, they've got no arms and legs. You've got DD breasts and you want to kill yourself. Are you crazy?' She kept calling to check up on me. I felt depressed for a week after the operation.

There was an accumulation of liquid. The surgeon had to use a huge needle, squeeze my boob like a spot and drain the fluid. After that things got better.

After all that, I kind of like them. From the side, they look glued on to me, very fake, but I like them from the front. I have a nice camera and sometimes I like to do a sexy shoot of myself. Depending on the light, one boob is high and one is low. That's why I'm scared of you taking a picture.

I have lost sensitivity. You could bite, and I would feel nothing. The surgeon said it might come back after a year, or maybe never. I'd rather they look good than feel good. You know where you get hair around the nipples? It used to be horrible when I plucked them, but not now.

I was self-conscious the first weekend back in the club. But last weekend I had loads of compliments. 'Oh my God, they are so full!' Guys don't see the scars. Also, one of the girls said, 'The boobs changed the game. I went to talk to some guys and they said they are waiting for the Polish girl with the big boobs.' *(laughs)* I am definitely getting more dances. I know this is because of the boobs.

I used to be told I had a beautiful smile, beautiful hair, beautiful eyes, beautiful bum, but never beautiful boobs. Now I don't hear about my eyes, smile, bum and hair, I hear only about my boobs. Which is worrying actually. You can't please me! Maybe when I get bored of my boobs I will miss the other compliments, but I am enjoying it at the moment. I flash them at any opportunity. The guys in the club who give me compliments only look at my boobs.

The girls in the club have these glass platform stripper shoes and I think I will treat myself to some. Before I wouldn't have dared to wear stripper shoes with those flat socks dangling from my chest! I thought people would think, 'How dare she wear stripper shoes when she has those fried eggs!'

To start with I wore very baggy clothes in my day job. But baggy clothes are not me. I can't pretend all my life to be something else. So I wore a tight shirt. Nobody said anything, but one woman started talking about boobs and asking me questions. She is gossiper number one at work. I'll just tell people I am on the Pill. What are they going to do, feel them? You can feel them now! *(I feel her breast; it's very firm, but not as firm as I was expecting.)*

I have to be careful with the photos on Facebook, because my parents don't know. They will be worried. I will deny it to my parents. My mum criticises my clothes in photos. She said, 'You look like a slut in this dress'. Now you can understand why I am afraid to tell her. They would disown me.

There are days when I look in the mirror and it's not me. It doesn't match my personality to have such big ones. My sister said I should have gone for a full C. She said it will be even harder now to find a normal guy to appreciate me for who I am rather than what's on my chest.

I told the surgeon I am not happy about one being higher, and that they are two different shapes. I was told the operation would reduce that. He said it's too early to tell; they will take any action required to make me happy, but they have to wait at least six months.

When I show you my boobs, I would like you to tell me, hand on heart, how badly lopsided they are. Try to take the best shot possible! *(laughs)* Are you ready for this?

(She asks me to show her the photograph on the camera back.) This one is much higher. Oh my God. And my tan. And my shoulders look so skinny, like I came out of a concentration camp. When I look in the mirror, I don't see this. But I can see an improvement.

———————————

Age 27 | No children

"I never even give it a thought now"

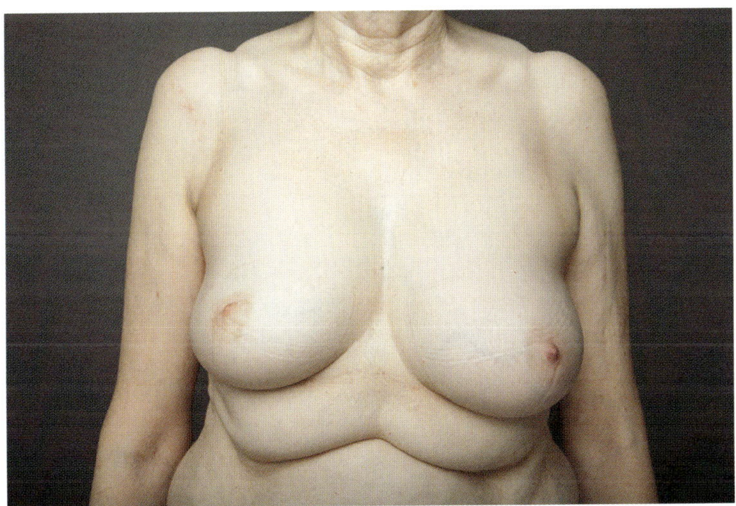

The lumpectomies haven't changed how I think about my breasts. I think if I'd been younger they might have done. I very rarely think about my breasts at all, they're just part of me. They're alright.

The first lump was found when I had a routine mammogram. The second time they found a lump it was at another routine check up. I had surgery both times, and radiotherapy the second time. For five weeks I had daily doses and they also took out the lymph nodes and the sentinel node under the arm to make sure it hadn't spread. The operations weren't too bad at all really. It was a bit painful, not excruciating, but uncomfortable for a few days. And then when the stitches came out it was sore for a while, but it wasn't terrible.

The service was excellent. They don't waste any time at all, which was really good. Because I was only in overnight they wanted me up and out. I was being sick in the waiting room while I was waiting for my daughter to come and pick me up, which wasn't pleasant. It was a short stay, I was only in one night. I thought that was harsh. The first time I had cancer I was at work and had private medical cover and I was in there for three nights. I don't think it needs three nights, but two nights would be better. But these days, they want you out, don't they?

After the radiotherapy, this one *(her right breast)* used to go bright red if it was very hot or very cold, which looked very strange! If the weather turned really cold, like it is right now, it would turn the colour of this cushion! *(bright red)* It surprised me when I took my clothes off. Apparently that can go on for years.

Initially I was aware of the scar and the difference in size, but I never even give it a thought now. It only shows when I wear one particular T-shirt; the stripe goes at an angle, instead of straight across. I still wear it because I really like it!

I would feel uncomfortable if I was topless. I wouldn't want to get my body out in public because it's … *(laughs)* I certainly wouldn't want to do that!

My husband was always happy with my breasts until I'd had the children. After breastfeeding I lost a lot of weight, not intentionally, it just all sort of fell off and they went all small and saggy. He didn't like that at all, and he made comments, like 'Your breasts have gone, you've lost them.' It made me feel quite bad about myself actually.

I think it's such a shame when people aren't happy with what they've got, especially when so many people would give anything to live a normal life when they've got some kind of disability. For people to worry about what they look like all the time and how other people see them is sad. I could understand if someone had huge breasts that gave them back ache and problems and they wanted a reduction. You get people with sores under their breasts because they're so huge. But if it's to make them look sexy or whatever, I just think it's sad.

If my daughter wanted breast surgery I would be upset and I would try to tell her there was nothing wrong with her as she is. I wouldn't like her to have surgery unnecessarily; it's invasive, it can go wrong and anaesthetics are always dangerous. I'd hate her to feel pressurised by society to look different.

Age 67 | Three children

"I regret not using my womanly wiles"

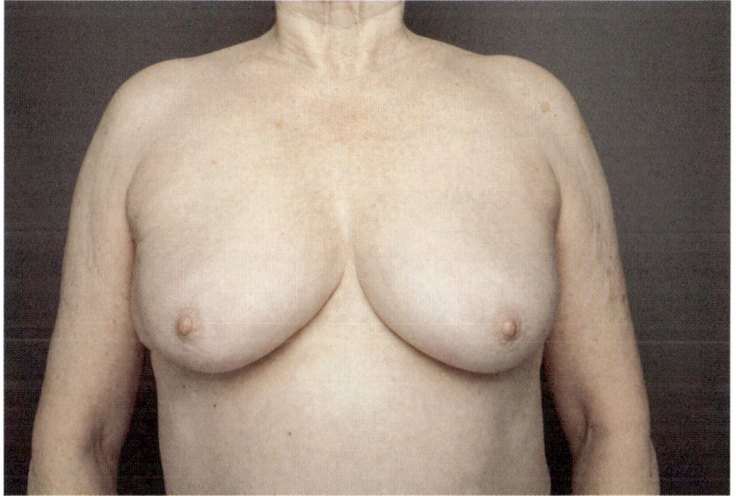

My breasts are quite small. I don't really think about them that much.
I could probably get away with not even wearing a bra. But I do! Because
they're small they're not down by my ankles or anything, there isn't enough
to sag.

My husband thinks my breasts are a bit of alright! He likes them.
They're not really an important part of our sex life. I know some women
like having their breasts fondled – they get some sort of feeling – but I don't
get any. I always wonder what men see in them. They're just there, aren't
they?

I left my bra off for today, and I probably won't bother putting it back on. I would if I went out. Around the house it's more comfortable. Bras are for a purpose, but I can get away without. It makes your clothes look nicer. If you get a bra that fits, it isn't that uncomfortable, but you are aware of it. Gossard Wonderbra, that was my lifesaver when I was younger.

I was at a dance in my teens, and they had those little pads you could sort of slide in. I was dancing on the dancefloor, and I looked down, and there was this pad. I knew it was my pad. I just kicked it away! 'Ooh, what's that!' As if I didn't know! I was annoyed really, because I wanted to put it back, but I didn't have the nerve to pick it up. So all the others I sewed in.

Surgical enhancements did cross my mind, but I was always frightened it might go wrong. If I was absolutely certain that it would have been a rip-roaring success, I would have done it. One of my girlfriends had it done. She got to 50 and she'd had two children, and they'd dropped. She had nice boobs anyway, she wanted them perked up. So they pulled them up. One went septic; it was terrible and she had to have it done again. She didn't have anything put in, but she had it all rearranged. They cut straight down from the nipple. Horrendous scarring.

I'm probably more body-conscious now than I've ever been. I was never body-conscious when I was younger. Some women are very aware of their bodies, and they take advantage of the way they look to better their life. I never did that, I was never aware that I had a nice figure, I just sort of got on with life. Then, when you start getting wrinkles you look back and think, 'I looked alright there!'

I wish I had been aware that I looked pretty alright. I think I might have … I wouldn't have done pole dancing, stuff like that, but I might have flirted more. I regret not using my womanly wiles.

When people talked about diets, I thought, 'Oh, for God's sake!' Because I never put an ounce on, I could eat anything. My girlfriends from when I was younger say, 'God we hated you, you looked so terrific.' No one told me I looked terrific at the time.

I don't know if I would have used my looks more. You could have all eyes on you because you look like a tart. Who would stick them out when they walk through a room? I wouldn't. I couldn't. I've never dressed to draw attention to my breasts. I've always had the best bra I can, to make the most of what I've got. But no, I would feel a bit cheap doing that. Which is probably why I didn't do it when I was younger. It wasn't something that ever entered my head. I don't think I've ever had anything that low-necked. I was just wondering where my life would have taken me, if I had!

I don't agree with airbrushing breasts. It makes people dissatisfied with what they've got. People put far too much stock on what people look like, rather than what they really are. I still buy expensive clothes, that is important to me. You have to make the best of what you've got. But it shouldn't be excessive. It's more important to be nice. I'm not interested in anybody else's body, just like I'm not interested in mine. I'm 65 now. I think children now are more aware than we were then.

———————

Age 65 | Three children

"My breasts are empowering, feminine, attractive and confident"

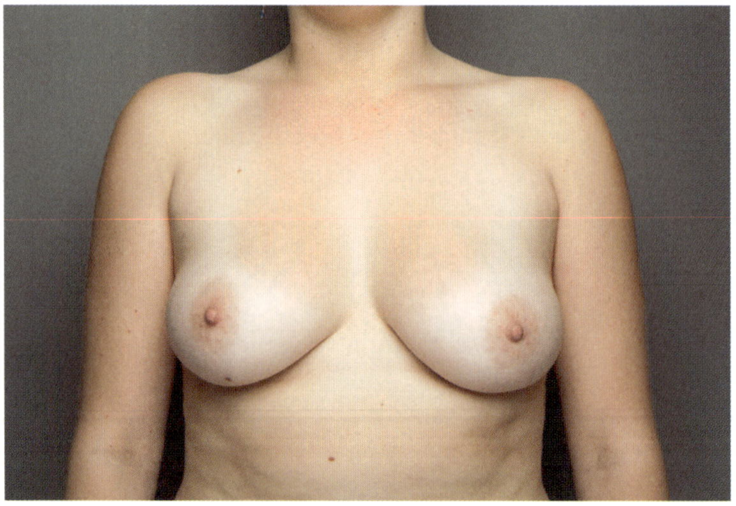

I love my boobs. What's the point in hating them? There's no point worrying about the niggles: 'Are my breasts big enough, are my nipples big enough?' They are a part of me and they make me feminine. They add curves, a bit of shape, and confidence when you're wearing a nice outfit.

I've grown up ith naturism. My mum was topless all the time when I was growing up. She's very open about it. When I'd just started secondary school, I invited my new friends over for the first time to a sleepover. Watch a movie, eat popcorn ... In the morning one of the girls said, 'Erm, your mum ...' I thought, 'God, what has she done now?'

She came bowling into the room, topless, flipping pancakes. No one knew where to look. But because she was so open with her body my friends found her easy to talk to. If they didn't speak to their own parents about things, they could speak to her. Everyone accepted her as she was: slightly kooky, and always naked.

Being topless has never been an issue for me. As kids you run around naked in the garden anyway. I came through the closed-off phase as a teenager quite quickly. My brother got a bit embarrassed for a while. I did feel like I needed to cover up a bit for him, so I'd be topless but wore pants.

I went to a naturist club with my mum once, and that was an experience. You don't know where to look. You are aware that you shouldn't stare, because it's rude, but everything is flying wildly and flapping about, and you can't help but do a double-take. After a little while it felt completely natural. I'm comfortable in my own body, but I don't feel the need to go to a naturist club and get it all out. I'm happy to be naked in my own home or on a nudist beach, but I don't need to play boules naked. That's the extreme of naturism – breakfast is naked, lunch is naked, everything is naked. Everyone takes their towels and sits on them, it's all very clean, British and proper!

I did a nude shoot once for a photography project and that was very empowering. I felt very strong afterwards. It's my body and I'll do what I want.

I've put on a 'uni stone' so I refuse to get my breasts measured. Bras are too expensive. I think I am a 36 or 38DD.

I play rugby, and everyone has a shower together afterwards. It's not sexual – everyone is just getting clean. I've become very accepting of bodies; you see a mass of people and compare yourself and realise you are normal.

You get some really nasty little cows who will deliberately pinch your breasts in a rugby scrum. Cruel. But the worst bits are the squidgy bits: the inner thigh and under the arm. I bruise easily in those areas. Sports bras are a must, you have to strap yourself down securely. Friends with very big breasts struggle a bit; they have to wear two bras. I tried playing a game in a normal bra once and it was painful as there was a lot of movement going on. I don't feel a particular need to protect my breasts. When I'm playing I don't think about anything else. Obviously you don't want an injury to your boobs, but it's not an area that gets much abuse, or much contact.

I get comments about being a female rugby player: some guys think it's hilarious. We have female coaches at our club, which has helped, because the guys are being coached by women as well. So the men respect the women's game and the women respect the men's game.

I also work behind a bar. I get, 'Give us a flash!' and 'You've got a pair of bazookas on you!' and the standard comments you'd expect, but you shouldn't have to expect it. If there's ever an issue, I say, 'I don't think that's appropriate', but I try and take it in good humour. I can respond about their male parts if I have to.

I'm bisexual, I'm not technically a lesbian. The rugby scene is very open and women in the sport have different sexualities. I'm in a relationship with a woman at the moment. I came out to my family a few months ago and they were brilliant. Mum fell on the floor laughing and told me about the time she was attracted to a woman. Dad gave me a hug and said it was fine whether it's a phase or not. I don't know if I'd be confident coming out to my grandparents though, that would be a shock to them.

We live in a more open environment now, particularly for women. All of my close friends have had at least one same-sex encounter, even if they wouldn't say they are bisexual, or have a relationship and come out to their family. It doesn't tear them up inside, it's just 'I'm a woman and I am attracted to women as well as men'.

My breasts are very important to me sexually, they feel a lot. What is different about being with a woman instead of a man is that women want to be with all of you, not just your vagina. Because women know their own bodies, they are more open to getting to know yours. It makes me happy when someone appreciates all of my body, when they want to pleasure my breasts, or the nook of my inner arm. I like that. Just holding someone's hand is a massive thing and gives you comfort.

My breasts are empowering, feminine, attractive and confident. They will change in time and I look forward to changing with them.

———————————

Age 22 | No children

"Men think they are the bee's knees"

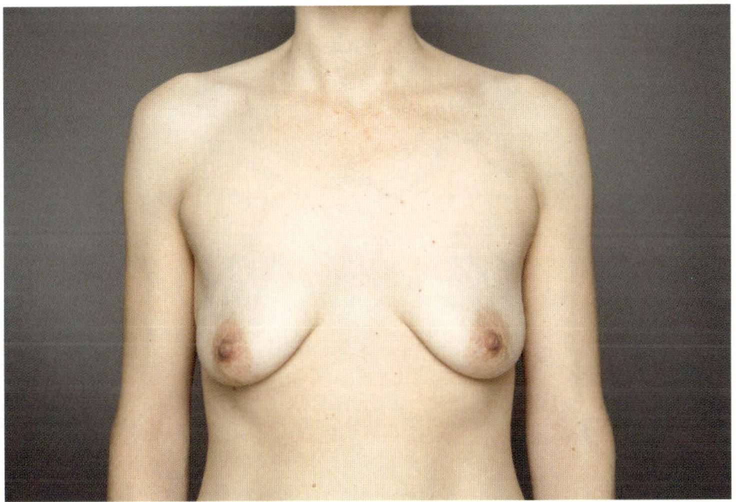

My breasts are OK. They are a little bit flat, but they'll do.

Gosh, I was a late developer. They started growing when I was about 14 and I was terribly shy. I hated the whole boob-growing process as a youngster. Home wasn't open, my parents weren't ones to talk about females developing and it wasn't discussed. Developing was an embarrassing taboo subject, and of course your breasts are the visual sign of puberty.

Because I was a late developer my friends were suddenly fascinated when it started. Comments were passed that I had 'bee stings'. I found it absolutely terrible that I was developing, and people were noticing, but they were just these tiny little bee stings. I didn't like it.

I remember my mother sighing, 'We're going to have to get you a bra now'. And you know what? She sent my father to get my first bra. She didn't come with me. Bless him, he's a geologist. He looks at me, and stares at my chest and stares at the bra sizes. Then he gets his hands and makes a cup and does this over my boobs and gets his hands and put them towards the bras, and that's how he measures. Then he picks up what he thinks is right.

If I didn't wear a bra I'd feel as if my boobs were touching my belly button. They have got a lot smaller with age; I've gone down two cup sizes. I'm a 36A. But it hasn't really bothered me, probably because I'm more mature in myself. They're part of who I am. But they have changed.

I thought my mother's breasts were big. I have a memory of her bending over, drying underneath these great big breasts, and slapping the baby powder everywhere, and fluffing up, and this plume of baby powder going everywhere, and then getting herself in a bra that looked so bloody awkward because she'd bend over and have to tuck all these rolls in.

Breastfeeding was lovely. In fact, my breastmilk has only recently dried up, and I stopped breastfeeding two years ago. But I found the whole breastfeeding thing was absolutely lovely, it was convenient, and it ticked all the boxes. They talk about the bond between mother and child, and you definitely have that. It's a lovely warm, natural thing that any woman who can do, should. It creates a lovely warm fuzzy feeling in your tummy. That is what I got from feeding my children. Also, you've got the sensation of the milk coming in. I enjoyed that, because I felt as if my body was doing something to feed this child, it felt as though the body was working, and doing what nature intended it to do. You can feel the milk being sucked out, when the child is in full suck, and you have that sensation of the milk letting down. I was a quick letter-downer!

My husband thinks my breasts are just fine. If I mumble about them he gets cross with me and tells me to stop it because he's quite happy with them. My breasts are important for him sexually, but they aren't for me. I don't get any sexual stimulation from them, or much stimulation at all, but obviously he does. I do wonder what turns him on, what he finds fascinating about them. I also wonder whether men are a completely different species, finding bizarre things like that fascinating. They're just bits of flesh hanging on you, that have breastfed, and they're not that attractive unless they are in a bra, really. But men think they are the bee's knees.

An ex-boyfriend once said to me he was very pleased not to be a woman, because if he was he would spend the entire time fondling his breasts. That's how he felt about them, he felt breasts were the best things since sliced bread, and all he wanted was to have his hands on them.

I think I would consider breast surgery, but I wouldn't actually do it. If it was nice and easy, nice and cheap, and had no nasty side effects, then yes, I would. But you could be scarred for life – why would you put yourself through that? When honestly my breasts are perfectly fine. My husband is the only one who really sees them and he's happy.

I think some breast surgery is perfectly ridiculous. When I was at the gym I was reading a nasty magazine and I saw a picture of Jordan and I thought, 'How blooming stupid'. It's just insane. I know a couple of people who've had enhancements. It's OK when they go up one or two sizes, but when they make them look completely artificial, it's just stupid. I can't say anymore about it. It just doesn't look nice.

Society would say the perfect pair of breasts is a generous C cup, with a cleavage that would pass the pencil test and probably evenly tanned. I don't think you get a perfect pair of breasts. I would like to have exactly what I've described, that would be lovely. I'd expose them! Well, I'd cover my nipples. I'd use them to my advantage! Because women are powerful people and we can use our sexuality. I'd exploit them. Sorry!

It's a good thing there is a taboo about our breasts, because otherwise men would be thinking with their penises all the time. If we were bare-chested, they'd be an absolute nuisance. They are fascinated with boobs, and for them they are sexual objects. If I walk around without a top on my husband is a bloody nuisance. I have to say go away please, so I can get dressed, otherwise he's just there fiddling and, you know …

If I had to lose a breast it would probably break my heart. I think it would break my husband's heart too.

———————

Age 40 | Three children

"Great liberation of the breasts needs to happen"

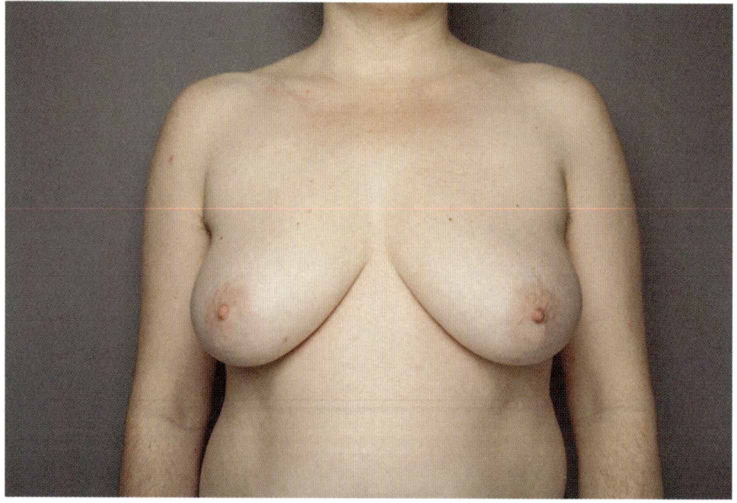

When I heard you were doing this project, I knew it would help liberate the breast.

I've ben a Buddhist nun in a monastery in Burma for eight years and I've just returned to English culture. One of the guys here buys *The Sun* regularly. There, on Page 3 was a picture of a woman and her boobs. Every single day they have this sleazy picture. I felt humiliated to see it. I thought, 'Wow, something is wrong in British society.' Breasts are beautiful and they symbolise the essence of women as nurturer and creator. To see them degraded in such a way was painful for me.

I am not prudish. When the weather is good I love to take my top off. I think when the weather is hot women should be able to take off their tops if they want. Don't tell the nuns in Burma that. *(laughs)* My friend and I go topless if it is hot and if there's only her partner or friends around, but we cover up if other blokes are around.

I've always been annoyed that I have to cover up on a hot day, that I can't take my top off. My male friends can walk down the street with their tops on. It's an illogical nonsense. I have to be uncomfortable, and the men don't. I could walk down the street topless but other people would probably react and lock me up! Which is a shame.

Because of the connections with motherhood, breasts shouldn't be hidden, they shouldn't be something to be shy about.

All of these things make me really frustrated with society. We have gone so far from the source, from nature. I think there would be less abuse and less assaults if the breasts were respected and cherished for what they are. I know breasts are a source of sexual arousal and enjoyment, for both men and women, but they should not only be seen in that light.

I was brought up as a Catholic in Ireland, with old-fashioned, conservative parents. My mother was very uncomfortable with her body and didn't give me healthy messages about my own body. If you repress something and make it taboo, it's a like a balloon which is squashed on one side and pops out on the other. In Ireland, healthy sexuality has been repressed, and there are so many instances of incest and sexual abuse.

I wasn't given a healthy template of myself as a sexual woman growing up, not only in the house I grew up in, but in the whole of Ireland. Sex wasn't talked about. Your vagina was seen as something a bit dirty. Thank you, St Patrick. It was so confusing for me when it came to first making love, because I had all these different desires. I had my own sensual sexuality but this conditioning telling me it was dirty.

I wasn't born a nun, I used to have a sexual life. I have been celibate for the last eight years. Celibacy is a lot more peaceful in many ways. Although when I decided to become celibate I was glad I'd had a satisfying sex life, I was pleased I didn't ordain as a virgin. There was a man I really loved, and I had a deep connection with him. I still love him. Our life paths were very different.

My breasts are erogenous. They were. They are. It's not like I'm dead and don't have any sexual feelings anymore, they're just not in use, they're on hold. *(laughs)*

I'm disrobing in two months. I will still be a buddhist but wish to do social work which I cannot do as a nun. I want to work more in society and with people in the world. As a nun you only meet people with a very deep calling, and I have a strong feeling in my heart that there are so many people who are going through hard times, and they will never get anywhere near a buddhist monastery. I need to go back into the world.

The monastic system is quite a male, patriarchal system and I don't like the timetable. It's like wearing a certain dress and the dress doesn't fit you anymore. The nun's life doesn't fit me anymore. You never have a rest day, there's no space for a day off when you are menstruating, if you need it. We need our timetables in sync with our cycles as human beings and women.

I feel the need to nurture myself when I am menstruating. I have heavy menstruation and very low energy and pain on the first two days. Before ordaining, when I was younger, I went through a phase where I would go into the forest with friends to menstruate. We would just bleed on to the ground.

It's uncomfortable being a nun. The monks are on a much higher social standing. I dealt with that as training for my humility. But they mix their cultural conditioning and their superstitious beliefs with the Dharma and the two are not the same. Burmese culture indoctrinates you that the woman's body is dirty.

You wear an outer robe, which is not practical or comfortable. The monks can go around topless when they are working if they are hot. But we had to wear these long sleeve shirts. I would often have my top button undone because I was hot. A nun would whisper to me as though they had a really important message, but it would just be a request to do my button up. I would be pulled aside for this very important message that I must do up my button.

You don't wear a bra or knickers as a buddhist nun, but you wear too many layers, you are always sweating. I was told my breasts were bouncing and showing. They'd have these discreet ways of telling me, I'd receive presents of new undershirts. I liked hanging out with the monks, and because I was western they didn't expect me to be the same as the Burmese nuns. They liked being about to talk to a woman who wasn't immersed in all these social ideas. It would have been lovely if I had learnt Buddhism aside from Burmese culture, but I had to accept their ways. Buddhist philosophy about the body is not negative at all. Nothing is bad: breasts, penis, vagina, they are just body parts. There is a teaching to transcend the body, not because the body is shameful, but because the body is a burden.

I hate wearing bras. I didn't wear a bra long before becoming a nun. You don't harm anyone by not wearing a bra. My becoming a nun is hilarious in itself, because I have always been very rebellious.

The two men who live near here are very nice guys. They are open-minded, but when they knew I was doing this photo shoot they were giggling a bit, there was a school-boyish thing going on. They joked they were going to come peeping in the windows. Actually they have both seen my breasts lots of time, because in the summer when it was very hot I took my top off. I laughed about it, but it struck me that they still have that mentality. I know breasts are sexually attractive and arousing, but at the same time I would like the men I am close to, to have a more wise approach and more informed understanding. Again, it brought home to me the unfortunate truth that breasts have been impressed upon us as purely sexual.

May breasts be free. I'm so inspired by Nelson Mandela at the moment, his life's mission was to free people. I feel like that about breasts, they need to be freed from degradation.

Great liberation of the breasts needs to happen. They need to be cherished and respected. They are a beautiful part of womanhood and motherhood, whether we give birth or not, whether we breastfeed or not, the potential is there.

Age 43 | No children

"It was wonderful that my son shaved my head for me"

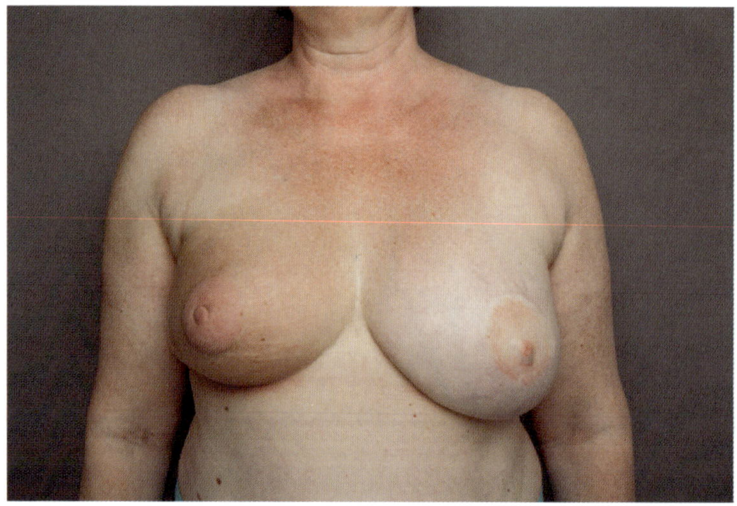

After my mother was diagnosed with breast cancer I decided I should be screened. It turned out I had very early breast cancer, all through my milk ducts. They said the only way to be absolutely sure to cure it was to have a mastectomy. It felt like my world fell apart.

I was told I cold have a reconstruction at the same time. It was a relief that I could concentrate on getting over cancer, I didn't have to worry about losing a breast and how it would affect me and my relationship with my husband. After 10 and a half hours of surgery I ended up with this magnificent breast. They took the nipple out, then the breast tissue, then put tummy fat in. Where my nipple was is now a piece of my tummy skin. I showed it off to everybody! I was so happy and so proud I had a breast. I think all my poor friends were like, 'Oh god, she's got it out again!' *(laughs)*

For about 18 months I didn't have a nipple. It didn't bother me, I sunbathed topless on holiday. I think my husband found it quite difficult, so I had the nipple tattooed for him. Because it didn't look normal it was a constant reminder I had cancer. We've been together a long time, and it's what you do when you love someone isn't it?

You can buy rubber nipples to stick on. Looking on the internet for these, we found some very interesting websites! My husband joked and said, 'I can just see the headline in the local paper, "Man Chokes on Rubber Nipple"!' But I didn't use it, it was completely ridiculous, it didn't look anything like my other nipple.

I had an amazing plastic surgeon, I had such confidence in him. You end up having a tummy tuck at the end of the day. It didn't feel like it at the time, but afterwards it was a double bonus! I didn't have cancer anymore and I had this lovely new body. I've never been particularly worried about my image, although I've tried to be reasonably slim and trim, but it was lovely being 44 and suddenly having a body of an 18 year old again. It didn't last very long! *(laughs)*

Life went on as normal, and then I was diagnosed with cancer again last year. After six years of yearly mammograms I was on my second year of no mammogram. I felt like I couldn't go another year. It's that safety thing.

They said there were irregularities. Everyone told me not to worry, and I couldn't feel anything, so I just went on my own to the appointment. They did more tests. I had cancer in my right breast this time. I was absolutely devastated. It was very deep in my breast which was why I hadn't felt it.

I was brought up as a catholic. I don't necessarily follow the catholic religion, but I do have beliefs and I truly think I have a guardian angel. There was no reason for me to want a mammogram, I couldn't feel a lump, I just felt I needed to.

I ended up having what they call a wide excision, where they take out a much larger area of your breast, and they took lymph nodes from under my arm. I had cancer in those as well so I had radiotherapy, chemotherapy and hormone therapy.

Chemotherapy was horrendous. The first week you feel absolutely wiped out, very sick, your sense of taste changes, you get mouth ulcers which make it difficult to eat. The anti-sickness drugs worked well so I didn't vomit a lot. But it feels like you are trying to think through gloop and walk through gloop. You get to the point where you start to feel reasonably OK again, and then you have to go for the next dose. You lose your fingernails, your toenails, and all your body hair, you get pins and needles in your feet and indescribable pain in your bones. The last three treatments made the rest feel like a breeze, they were absolutely wicked. At the end of the day you just have to hope its killed all the little buggers.

When I was 44, the thought of not having a breast was awful, but that didn't worry me when I was diagnosed at 52, I just wanted to get rid of the cancer. It's age, and being confident in your marriage and relationship, and confident in yourself as a person. I think it has taken me a long time to grow up as a person.

The main thing is to get rid of the cancer but the surgeons are amazing about saving as much of the breast as they can. They want women who have had breast cancer to feel as good about themselves as they can. I have a tiny scar you would never notice, although, yes, my breast is smaller than the other one. I can always go back at a later stage and they can even me up by giving me liposuction on the other one. From a practical point of view, finding bras to fit me now is really difficult. I must have 2 cup sizes difference. I will probably have a prosthesis to even me up, as I don't want any more surgery.

My treatment is all finished now. I went back to work recently, but I have pulled back from that as I have really struggled with fatigue and memory loss. I can't find the words sometimes. Maybe I will go back later this year. When I have to multitask my brain doesn't work very well.

All my friends keep saying to me, 'You're not Superwoman, stop worrying about work, they haven't worried about you very much. For gods sake, you have cancer, relax.' I have come to terms with that now, and it's helped me be kinder to myself. I was a PA to the same person for five years and been in the same job for 20 years. They didn't contact me for months, and that was only after my husband contacted them. In general, I think people don't know what to say. I want to get back to work and get on to the next stage of my life.

I have amazing friends and family and I've found strength in them. One day a friend came round with a hoover, made me a cup of tea and hoovered my house. A hanging basket had died, she took it away, re-planted it, and brought it back again.

The staff at The Royal Marsden Hospital were fantastic both times, angels. They have an open access clinic, so if at any time during the year you are worried you can see somebody to check you and reassure you.

Cancer brings you closer together as a family. On my phone I have the most wonderful photograph. You do this when your hair starts to fall out. *(runs her hand through her hair)* I got home one day and one of my sons said, 'Oh, mother, you can't go out looking like that, you've got a great big bald patch at the back of your head!' He went, 'Come on, today is the day we do the deed. You know it needs to happen.' So he went and got his clippers. My mum was staying with us too. They put me in front of the mirror and I had a large glass of wine. My mum had a large glass of wine too. My son shaved his head first, then mine. I could see my mum, and I said, 'Don't you dare, if you start crying you'll have to go. This is fine, it's got to be done.' And it really was fine actually. I thought I would be devastated, but in a way it was liberating. And it was wonderful that my son did it for me. I have this wonderful photograph of the two of us together. *(shows me the photograph)* He's a good lad.

My prognosis is really good, but it's almost impossible to say you are cancer free. Cancer never goes away, because it's in the back of your mind. You have to appreciate what you've got and not worry too much about the future. We need plans, but seize the day. 'The weather's lovely, let's just book a hotel and go away for the weekend.'

I don't think the changes to my breasts have affected my husband and our relationship. He's known me for 30 years, we're best friends. I think the hardest thing for him was the chemotherapy. He felt utterly helpless. When he heard the word chemotherapy, he thought I was going to die. Apart from being there, and feeding me soups and things there was nothing he could do. He still says I am beautiful, and it's never been an issue sexually. He was wary of touching me for a while because he didn't want to hurt me.

My breasts make me look nice when I am wearing clothes. At one time they were important, but they aren't now, they're just part of me. Body image is important to us when we're young, attracting our mates and all the rest of it, but it doesn't matter what you look like, it's about whats inside. Most partners don't love you because of your breasts, they love you because of who you are, and you just have to remember that.

―――――――――――

Age 53 | Two children

"My husband has bought me about 35 sets of matching underwear"

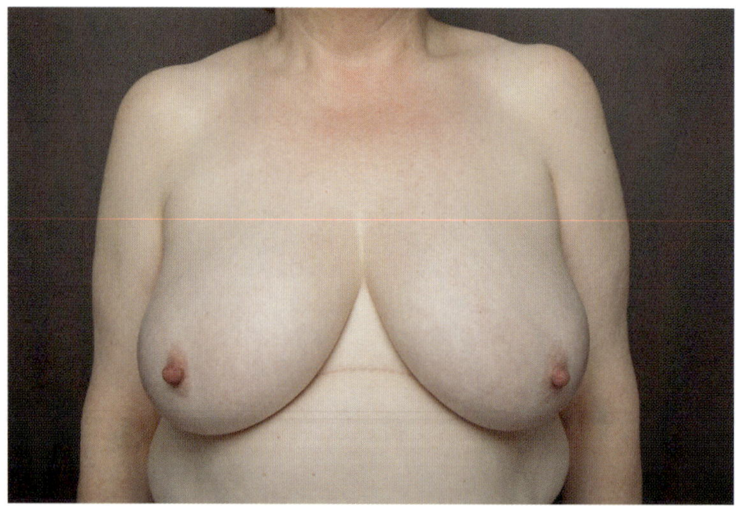

My breasts are my best commodity. My husband likes them. When I mentioned I was doing this he said, 'Go on, you've got very good breasts for your age.' I'm curious how he knows they're good ones for my age! *(laughs)* He'll be keen to see the pictures.

My husband has boght me about 35 sets of matching underwear, different brands. I counted them one day. I do prefer proper matching underwear. Mismatched underwear makes me feel scruffy, not properly dressed. I have no idea why he buys it!

He knows my size, but I don't. I couldn't tell you my size now. My daughter knows it because she measured me, she's a bra fitter. He buys me pretty but practical ones. I've trained him. Years ago he used to buy me those little skimpy ... dental floss things. I like big pants. I prefer underwire but my daughter has bought me non-wired bras. I was surprised how supportive they are. My first ever bra was 'Cross Your Heart'.

I work with youngsters in school and I work with teaching assistants. Their attitude to their weight and how they look is quite intense. If they put on seven pounds they're in a panic. How they look is a very big part of their life. So I think this project is important. I think they should just enjoy life, it's much easier. Even nine and 10-year-olds think about what they look like, and that does worry me. My friend's granddaughter was one of these bonny babies. My friend seemed to feel she had to mention she was bonny and apologise for it, even though she was a baby. Of course, she's grown up now and lost all that puppy fat.

Women are getting thinner as well as bigger-breasted in the media. I have no idea how! *(laughs)* I think it is achieved unnaturally. We've got more media now, especially the Internet. We get Freeview and it includes adult channels. I think that's awful. I remember years ago when 'Blue' films were on cine.

My breasts are an important part of sex, for both of us. I don't know what I'd do without them sexually. It doesn't feel like proper sex if they aren't touched, they are one of the most important erogenous zones.

I got married very young. I tried breastfeeding for the first baby and it was difficult, but with the second baby I didn't bother. Because my breasts were so important sexually I couldn't cope with breastfeeding. It was a mindset. One of my friends says she doesn't like anything about breastfeeding, she can't even talk about it. She is very anti. I find her fascinating, very black and white. But she is the most nurturing mother.

My daughter is very pro-breastfeeding and she gave me a lunchbox which has breastfeeding on it. I think breastfeeding is wonderful. I wish I'd had the input my daughter has. It's free, it's on tap, it's less hassle. Both my grandchildren are physically strong and contented and healthy. I think it's fantastic. I'm of the generation where it wasn't something you saw, but I'm used to it now. Breastfeeding wasn't on demand and it was done in a different room.

———————————————

Age 56 | Two children

"It's almost embarrassing when breasts are popping out at you"

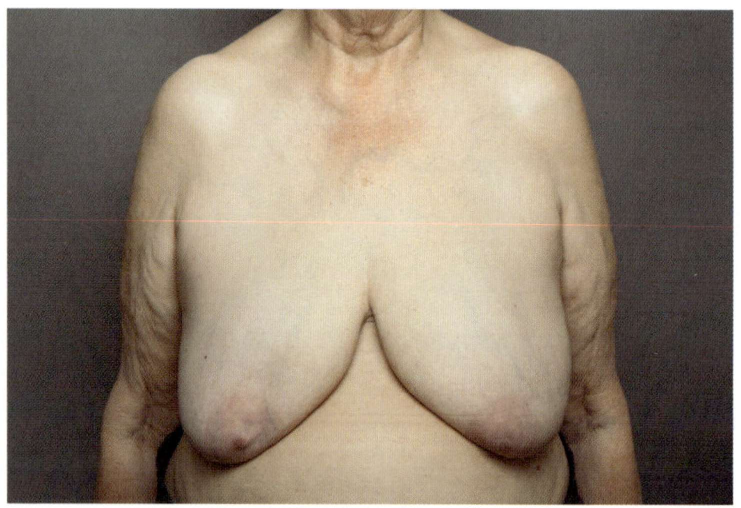

When I was younger I knew one lady with breast cancer, and that was it. What is causing all the breast cancer now? All types of cancer really?

When I was 35, I felt something wasn't quite right, although breasts can feel lumpy, can't they? I had a lumpectomy. No problem since. Two of my daughters have had breast cancer now. I have three daughters, so that's three out of four of us. They say there's no genetic connection. I don't understand it at all. I never thought I'd lose them, I thought positive. They had the chemotherapy, the radiotherapy, and the newspapers say the chances get better and better all the time. One of my daughters is still having treatment, she takes Tamoxifen.

You hear smoking and drinking aren't good for cancer. Well, none of my daughters smoke, or drink much. So, is it something in the food? When jars have a life of two years, what is added to them? My husband is in catering, and he has a thing about decaffeinated and 'no sugar' things, he says it's better not to drink them at all. I wonder if it's all the foods we eat these days.

Breasts weren't dramatically important to boys when I was growing up, not like these days. My Dad wouldn't have let me go out like girls dress now, in all honesty! I'm not a prude by any means, but when I see how some girls are dressed these days, you do worry they are flaunting themselves. It's almost embarrassing when breasts are popping out at you.

Wedding dresses are all off the shoulder, there's hardly any dress there. They think they look beautiful, and maybe they do, but to me a dress like Princess Kate wore is more attractive. I don't like tattoos on women either. I can't even look at my granddaughter's tattoos. I say to her, 'Your mum has gone through all that with her breasts and you are doing that to your skin, by choice?' I'm probably quite old-fashioned.

Breasts aren't extremely important in sex, they are just part of the general set-up. I have to say my husband is very good in that respect. If I wasn't interested he wouldn't push me because he wanted me to enjoy myself. Otherwise, it's like being a prostitute isn't it? It's so revolting to think a man would use your body just for his own pleasure.

I breastfed my children, no bottles or anything. I was paranoid about germs on bottles. Breastfeeding was easy and when the time came I put them on to little beakers. I was really glad I breastfed, and it was easy. Breastfeeding has gone out of fashion completely. These days many people put babies straight on the bottle. I think breastfeeding will come back into fashion, like growing vegetables has.

I used to have a set of scales in my bedroom, and one of my daughters stood on the scales. She wasn't very big but she wanted to lose weight. I said, 'Trouble is, all the weight is on your boobs.' I lifted her boobs up and the scales shot back. We burst out laughing. She's the one who had a mastectomy and when they took the breasts off it was quite a weight in grams.

————————————

Age 74 | Three children

"I felt more confident after the boob job"

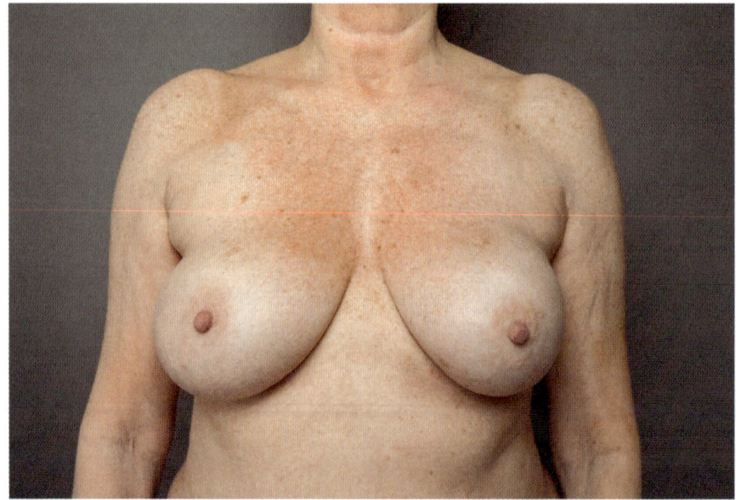

My breasts have aged, but everything does. Everything taken into account, I'm pleased with them.

Prior to the boob job I had such a big discrepancy in size between one side and the other, terribly noticeable. They were different shapes. One was conical and quite hard. The other one was more rounded and soft. When I was breastfeeding, that was the most productive one. My smaller one worked, but it was never as forthcoming as the other one.

When I was nine-years-old, in the last year of junior school, I was following someone through a swing door, and they let the door go back.

I had little sugar lumps growing, and it chopped the left sugar lump in half. Incredibly painful. I often wondered whether that caused it.

When I was growing up I was embarrassed about my breasts and the size discrepancy, I would never flaunt them. I would have a pre-formed cup if I had a swimming costume on. When I was older, I didn't flaunt them with sexual partners in that context, but no-one commented on them. I think they were being polite, they would have noticed the difference.

My mum wouldn't get me a bra. She kept saying I was too young. In the end, when I was 12 I went to stay with an aunt who said it was ridiculous I didn't have a bra. She went into the airing cupboard for some of my cousin's bras she'd outgrown. I was really pleased, I had three pairs of lovely bras.

Other than that, my mum didn't say much to me about my breasts and growing up, until I was about 16. It was the fashion to wear a string vest with your bra quite visible underneath, and I had a sky blue bra which was really nice. They had only just brought bras out in different colours. I was walking around the house wearing this string vest and bra underneath and she was furious and told me to cover up! And I said, 'It's only dad and my brother!' She said, 'It doesn't matter, they're still men!' I hadn't thought that my brother or father would look at it in the same way as other men because they were related. Looking back I understand, but at the time I didn't.

I was 40 when I had the boob job. I'm 34DD now. I could afford it, it was a convenient time, there was no man in my life, no-one to say yay or nay, and I found a very, very good surgeon. I didn't want to go over the top, I told the surgeon, 'I don't want a massively obvious boob job.' I just wanted to fit in. He didn't try to persuade me otherwise and it was done aesthetically to make sure it looked natural. The surgeon told me the silicon bag on the left was three times larger than the one he put in the right.

The operation was fine. No pain at all, seriously, no swelling or bruising, nothing. Instant result and no pain.

I look back on it as one of the best things I have done. Clothes hang so much better! Well, not so much now, because my backside and midriff have got bigger, but when I was 40 I had a nice figure, and that was the icing on the cake. I felt more confident. Before I was a shrinking violet, but afterwards I wasn't the least bit embarrassed about taking off my clothes. I felt more confident in every way. I felt people treated me differently although it could be related to having more confidence. I would say men took a more obvious interest in me. Men at work would be extra pleasant, extra considerate.

It's regrettable that people don't have the confidence to be as they are. But human nature being what it is, it's never going to be any different. So, if there's the opportunity to improve a situation, like I have, then it's fine.

I've never liked them touched. I dislike it intensely. I've never told anybody this before, but, I asked my first serious boyfriend not to touch them because I didn't like it. And he said, 'I know, you feel all lost and alone don't you, when I touch them.' And I said, 'Yes, how do you know?' and he didn't answer me. But it's a lost, lonely, horrible thing, I don't like it. No pleasurable sensations when they are touched.

I was breastfeeding one day and I had an orgasm. It only happened once, I was probably thinking about what's for dinner tonight, nothing sexual whatsoever. I know it was from breastfeeding. There was no preamble to it, no build up, it just happened, like a sneeze almost. No, even with a sneeze you can feel it coming on, and this just happened. I've heard about this happening, but it's not something I would have believed. It made me feel a bit disgusted with myself, that it was my baby, but it was the last thing on my mind, I wasn't thinking about such things.

I breastfed my first baby for eight-and-a-half months. I only stopped because of pressure from my ex-husband and mother-in-law. She said 'It's dreadful, you don't have to do this, you're not a cow, there are bottles, everything is safe and clean these days. Why do you do that?' My husband didn't like it. Maybe men are jealous of the baby. I don't know, I never questioned him on it. With my second I thought I'm not going to listen to anybody, I shall let the baby decide. And, well, she didn't decide, I did.

Three of us girls went on holiday together, and we all had babies. We were talking one night, and wondering what it's like to feed someone else's baby. We said the first baby to wake up, a different mother feed it. This woman's baby woke up, I picked him up, and he just latched straight on. She said, 'My son, my son!' and she took him back! My baby woke up later on and, as we both had to do it, she took my baby. My baby looked up at her, screamed and burst into tears, she had recognised a different face. Her baby was five months and mine was seven months. It could be because he was younger, or was hungry and didn't care. I burst out laughing! For years after that, whenever I saw her, I would say, 'My son, my son!' *(laughs)*

Because I have implants they always send me to the proper radiographer, not any old Tom, Dick or Harry. You know in the library car park they have a big lorry there sometimes? I couldn't go to one of those, because they have to be looked at carefully by a proper expert. My husband once said to me, 'Oh look, you could have a mammogram done in the car park. Why don't you go here, rather than the hospital?' I said, 'Oh that's because I once had a lump removed, and I'm treated as a special case now.' I did have a lump removed, but he doesn't know I've had implants you see. No one has ever known unless I told them.

The lump I had was a fibroadenoma, benign, and it never became malignant. They are sometimes called 'mouse tumours', because if you try to grab it, it slithers away. I had two others as well, but they were satisfied with mammograms that they were OK.

The implants are now 25 years old, I'm sure there are improvements going on all the time. This is a really old-fashioned pair I've got! You know how hard those plates squeeze when you have a mammogram? Really viciously hard, aren't they? I'm worried they are going to pop! They know at the mammogram department, and I say, 'Don't squeeze too hard, they're a pretty old pair, they could easily pop!'

I think that the ideal breasts are like mine were when they had just been done. I was really pleased with them, and I've been very happy with them for all these years since.

———————

Age 65 | Two children

"Porn takes the pressure away from finding relationships and sexual partners"

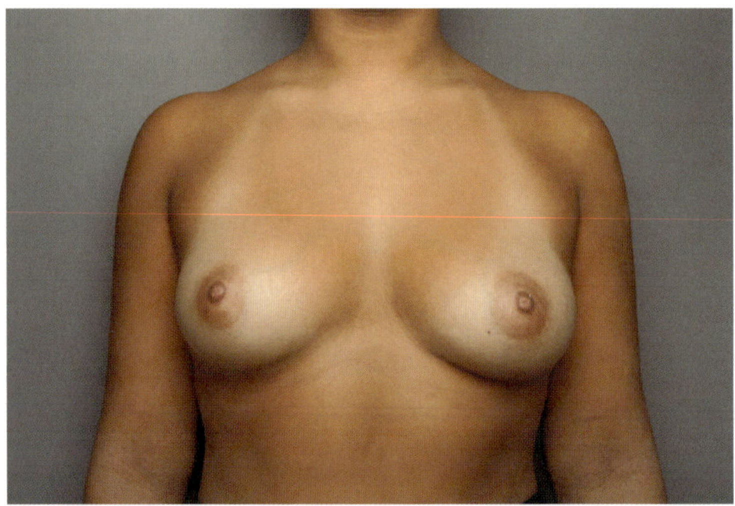

I'm happy with them. They could be bigger I suppose.

My sister looks older than me because she is busty, even though she is younger and has a younger face. We've been out for drinks in the evening and she gets quite harassed. At 17 she doesn't think she should get that attention, from men in their late 20s who are quite leery and lechy. She's my baby sister, so it's not nice to see. I went up to one guy and it came out all wrong, I said, 'Why are you gawping at her and not me?' *(laughs)* It sounded so tragic. He'd been staring at her tits. I told him she was 17. He said, 'Oh, I saw her tits and thought she was older than you.'

So, although I have thought my breasts could be a bit bigger, I came to the conclusion on my own that I am actually very happy with them. Phew, happy ending!

I'm not too big so I don't have to worry about clothes, they look very nice in a little jumper, it doesn't look like I am trying to make a statement. It is so ridiculous that women who are big look like they are making a statement in some clothes even when they aren't. It is so overwhelming that the size of your boobs can say so much about you. You should be defined by what is going on in your head and not your chest.

I've had people compliment them in bed. I had a strange comment from my ex-boyfriend. He said he really liked the colour of my nipples. I was like, 'What a bizarre thing to say!' I had never thought about the colour of my nipples.

One of my housemates is happy to be in her bra in front of the guys in the house. We've also got into the habit on a lazy day in the house of wearing T-shirts and no bra. The guys said, 'That's really strange, why don't you have bras on?' We were like, 'We've got our T-shirts on!' We thought it was interesting. If we're not going out why should we wear bras? They were strangely awkward about it. I wouldn't walk around topless with them, that would be inappropriate and strange.

There was one guy we fell out with in my last house-share. I don't want to stereotype but he was a massive jock. He said I was putting him off his breakfast, and asked if I was going to put a bra on. I don't normally lose my temper but I was so angry. I was in my pyjamas, but obviously I didn't have a bra on first thing. I've seen him topless! I found it insulting, and I don't know why he said it.

I have nothing against porn whatsoever. I watch about three hours of porn a week. One of my female housemates enjoys it too, but the other one hasn't seen it. She's nearly 22. She said she's always had a boyfriend so she doesn't need it, but that's no reason not to watch porn. I wouldn't believe someone else, but I believed her. So, bless her, we set her a little task last night. We said, 'Go to bed, go and search for some porn.' She came down this morning, it was just us girls, the guys had gone out. 'Tell us, what did you do?' And she was quite appalled, she said it was awful: 'The sex is so far from anything I've ever had.' She is quite a sexual being and had sex at quite a young age, but she said she couldn't relate to any of it, and therefore didn't find any of it arousing. She was dumbstruck and we felt really bad.

My housemate and I enjoy porn, and told her you can search for what you like. We like more arty porn showing real people having real sex. They are 'real' women, in the sense that they are natural. In porn you see and hear some terrible things, and the sounds that come out of their mouths are ridiculous. Pornhub is terrifying generally.

I don't know how many girls look at porn. I never did when I was at school. But it so happens I have friends now who are really open so it encourages you. I don't how but the topic always comes up at social events. I think some girls don't admit it.

I'm not very experienced. I have only slept with one person. I did have orgasms with the person I slept with, but I also faked them because it wasn't going to happen. When I orgasmed the first time I was silent. On porn the women cry out. I'm sure some women do cry out, but it seems so far off the truth. Because of the way they act I just thought it wouldn't happen to me.

Women on women porn is arousing because the women take time to pleasure each other. The first time I orgasmed wasn't from sex, it was from oral. I was terrified to tell him, I didn't say for months, but eventually I said, 'That's the only thing that seems to do it for me.' I was worried it would knock him.

My boyfriend and I had sex when I was 18. I could tell he was absolutely terrified. We were both virgins. He'd been my good friend for years. I was lying naked in bed, my first time, as vulnerable as you can be. He couldn't get an erection. I asked him what the matter was. He said, 'I'm not really sure what to do with you, because all I've got to go on is what I've seen on the web.' That was so sad. He wasn't looking at me, or thinking about what he wanted to do with me, he was trying to match what he'd seen to our situation and make it reality. I hadn't watched a lot of porn then, so it didn't ring true. Now I can imagine it was terrifying for an 18-year-old boy who's a virgin to match these male porn stars.

I haven't had sex at uni. The four girls I lived with last year were very sexually active – that's the nicest way to say it! I used to love hearing their stories. They said the demands from guys were unbelievable and they would put them in positions like a porn film. I didn't think it sounded OK. Porn is so hardcore. The home page of Pornhub is so scary, you have anal flashing in one box, double penetration in another, it's so daunting. I don't complain about porn because I watch it, but at the same time so much of the stuff is so vulgar.

Porn takes the pressure away from finding relationships and sexual partners. So many people hook up now with people they meet using apps like Tinder. I think people at university are looking to have sex, they aren't looking for relationships. Everybody is hyper-sexualised, everybody. It's nice if you get a match on Tinder, someone finds you attractive, that's great. But what you get is, 'I can come over in an hour.'

A date is retro now. I'm going on a date next week. My friends think it's cute. We're going for dinner. Surely that shouldn't be 'old school'?

———————

Age 20 | No children

"Women are much more likely to involve your breasts and to know what to do with them"

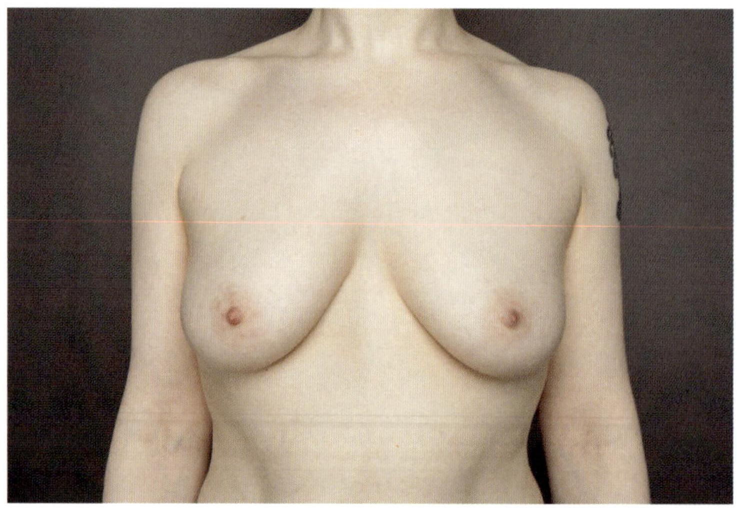

I'm quite pleased with my breasts at the moment. I'm doing all this exercise and they've become perter. I like that. My husband loves them.

My breasts are important to me as an erogenous zone. I like them to be kissed and have my nipples sucked. I'm not the sort of person who likes lots of delicate wispy touches, I like it rough! Definitive action.

Sexually, I've got what I like from both women and men. They're both capable, it's just some men need more instruction. I think popular culture's portrayal of sex gives men some very strange ideas about what's pleasurable and even anatomically possible. *(laughs)* I don't think men really appreciate subtlety. If I think about how sex is in films, TV and even fiction, people are immediately in the mood for it. Men, and the media, don't seem to appreciate there is a whole preamble; touching breasts, touching them before you've taken any clothes off even. But that doesn't come across.

Some women are tit women and some aren't. Women are much more likely to involve your breasts and to know what to do with them to create pleasure. Definitely. Also, they have some of their own! Women accept that a woman's whole body is an erogenous zone, which plenty of men have no clue about. They've got a map for where they might go which is much bigger and more detailed than men's maps are.

You assume men want breasts to be big, bouncy and round and all of that. But actually, half the time, men are so delighted to get near a pair, that they'll take whatever is on offer. Women don't have an ideal pair of breasts. They're more tolerant about different body shapes. It's about what's sold to the consumer. Men want big, juicy melons, because that's what's 'sold' to them in porn.

It's much more comfortable to be braless. I'm probably not wearing the right size bra. I tend to buy very cheap bras, and they fit badly. Whenever I've gone somewhere and had a fitting they always say you are some ridiculous size which you can't get off the rack. I think it's a con to make you spend more money. When I've tried on the bras that have been recommended, they don't feel comfortable, they feel tight and restrictive. I wonder if that's how they are meant to feel in order to be supporting you?

I went to Rigby and Peller. They ought to know about boobs, oughtn't they? They said I'm something daft like 30DD! I'm not a 30DD, come on, bugger off! Handily enough, it's a really difficult size to get, but they happened to have several premium brands. 'Oh really, do you really!'

I think clothes often look better if you have bras under them because of cultural conditioning. We expect them to be up here! *(indicates high up on chest)* I think to some extent, bras are not optional. Bralessness is non-conformist.

I don't inspect them as often as I should, I know this. I do try to do it, not least because a lot of medication I've taken increases your risk of breast cancer. I have had a heavy alcohol intake in the past, which increases your risk. I'm not going to have children, which increases my risk.

They're lumpier these days, maybe it's the ageing process. They're sort of fibrous, it feels like wet cotton wool. *(laughs)* I'm happy with ageing at the moment. I'm aware of the need to work harder. In my 20s I ate what I liked, I didn't bother exercising. Everything was fine, and my breasts were magnificent! Because they've lost size they feel a bit less impressive.

I don't want this magnificent rack on display like I did when I was in my 20s. It's just not very nice. I don't really want to wander about with my boobs out. Age is part of it and getting unwanted attention.

Men will engage with your breasts even if they're not interested in you. If you are under-dressed, or your breasts are visible, you might get men passing remarks to you, unimaginative, you know, 'Nice pair!' Women would definitely not do that. Even if you were in a lesbian club, where you might expect women to chat you up, they still wouldn't say something like that, it would be inappropriate, and not acceptable.

I would absolutely not consider breast enhancement surgery, I think it's completely unnecessary. I feel very strongly that general anaesthetics and surgery are not about vanity. This is serious stuff that's intended for saving and improving people's lives.

As a nurse, I think doctors who do this are exploiting peoples' weaknesses and it's a wicked thing to do. They charge so much money which could be spent on therapy to make you happier with yourself. It's a waste of medical education. Let us not forget, the state and the NHS pay for the medical education. Then they bugger off out of that.

It's a very unpleasant indictment of developed society that the cosmetic surgery industry thrives in the way it does. There is a lot of scandal over whether people are consenting properly and whether they understand the risks.

In the media, women's breasts are almost disassociated from the women they are attached to. They're such a commodity, used and exploited for selling just about everything. There's almost not a woman behind them. Recently GQ had 'People of the Year'. All the men were dressed, but Lana del Rey was naked. That summarises nicely for me how I feel about the media portrayal of boobs; it's about access. The media and the general public seem to have this entitlement to splash them about.

Towards the end of the relationship with my last female partner I became more feminine and I was thinking maybe I'd go back to men. Dressing more femininely meant making more of a feature of my breasts. Even jewellery can direct the view to your breasts.

During that time I had the same job, so my outward appearance changed at work. I noticed people I worked with behaved differently, depending on how I looked, and breasts were definitely part of that. They saw me as a sexual being in a way they hadn't when I was more androgynous. I noticed that people I was meeting for the first time were more likely to be cooperative, but less likely to take me seriously.

Another thing about breasts is they have a lot of comedy value. They are funny looking things! I probably notice the comedic value more with my male gay friends. I can think of situations with gay friends where there has been a lot of breast-related humour, and it's been a lot of fun. I think it's because they're gay, and it's safe. I often used to go clubbing in a bikini top, and they'd say, 'Nice Tits!' and I wouldn't be, 'How dare you, who do you think you are?' I think it's something to do with entitlement. Gay men don't feel they have an entitlement to access the breasts, but straight men do.

———————

Age 39 | No children

"I felt like I'd been eaten by a tiger"

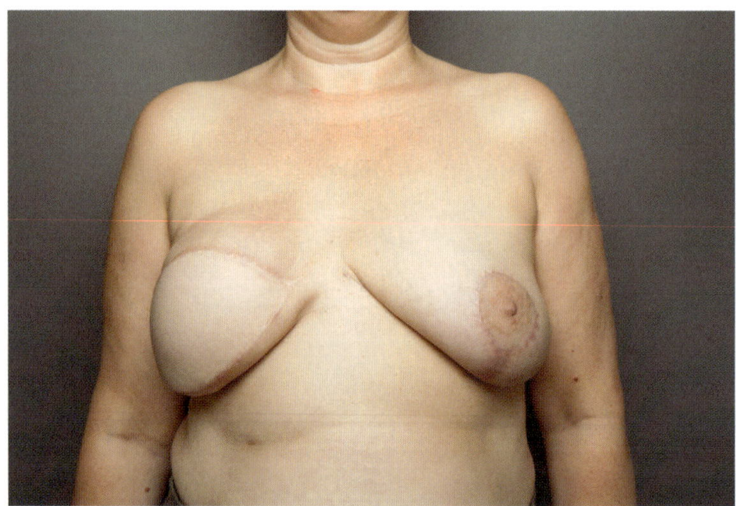

A couple of days before Christmas in 2009 I was sitting in the bath, looked down and noticed a lump sticking out of my chest. It had literally popped up overnight. It was tender when I pressed it. I thought it was a bruise. I decided to go to a walk-in clinic. The nurse said, 'Look, I'm not allowed to say, but I'm not worried about it.' I wasn't convinced.

I went to the doctor as soon as Christas was over. He said you never get lumps up there, but as my sister had just had breast cancer he said I needed a mammogram. By 7 January they had taken a lump out. I felt panicked about cancer. I told them to take the whole breast off, but they said they didn't need to. But by 30 January the breast was gone.

At that point I actually asked them to take both off. The surgeon wouldn't, he said it would give him a heart attack. They aren't supposed to remove a breast if it's healthy.

It was fine when I woke up with no breast. As soon as I came round I checked it was gone; to me it was the death area.

In 2011 I had a reconstruction. They took a flap out of my back and stitched that up. See the line? *(shows me her back)* It was the shape of an eye. They fed it under my arm so it was still attached, still alive. It was put on with a squidgy implant inside. I wanted the sort of reconstruction where they take fat from the stomach, because I've got loads of fat there, but they don't do it at the hospital I was at, because the graft can die off more easily.

I couldn't wear a bra because it was too uncomfortable, so I wore massive clothes. I didn't care, I felt like I had cheated death. Then I got a prosthesis. They try to match the weight so it was a big, heavy thing. I said to the breast care nurse that it seemed heavier than my real one, but she said it was actually lighter. I wore it once to my daughter's graduation, and that was all. I didn't wear it to my step-daughter's wedding, I wore a homemade foam thing that was better.

Because I was wearing huge tops I didn't think you could see my missing boob. My husband told me recently that you could see I had one huge boob and one flat side. I was oblivious, but he was worried people were looking. I wouldn't say he was embarrassed, but it bothered him. I think he might have been worried people would feel sorry for me. No one ever said anything to me.

I used to be a 36G. My right one was always a little bit bigger, so when I had a reduction on the other side a few months ago, I said to the surgeon, 'I know this is really picky, but is there any way you can make them match?' They were perfect. However, I've since found out I am pre-diabetic and I've lost lots of weight. My real one is tiny now and there is a massive difference.

I've had no breast and a huge one, a reconstruction and a huge one, and a reconstruction and a reduced one.

The reduction was a big operation. I had to give it a year for the skin to settle down after the radiotherapy. After that, I suddenly decided to do it. I didn't give myself too much time to think about it, or I might have backed out. It was really painful, I felt like I'd been eaten by a tiger. I don't remember any pain after the mastectomy. I managed to keep my nipple, which is good, because that's not guaranteed as they cut it off and put it back on.

It's all gone very quickly, even though it's been a few years. You can't stop to think. What helped me was that my sister had breast cancer two years before me. When she had it, I used to think, 'Oh my God, she's going to die'. We thought she was on borrowed time. When they said I had cancer I went to see her because I just wanted to see someone who had survived. I said to my husband, 'We have to change how we think'. We used to think anyone who had cancer died.

For a week after I got the results I seemed to stay in the same armchair. My husband never cooks, but he brought me my dinner every day in that armchair. In the end I said, 'What are you doing? I'm not ill.' Recently he told me he thought I was dying. *(laughs)*

I had chemotherapy because it had gone into my lymph nodes. They removed 13 lymph nodes. My daughter read about acupuncture so I tried that. Chemo brought on the menopause, so I've carried on with acupuncture because now it's helping me with my hot flushes.

You have to look on the bright side. I wasn't enamoured with 36Gs. They hurt, straps dug into my shoulders, I never ran. So I've had a breast reduction. And I used to have really heavy, bad periods, but the chemo stopped my periods.

I had massive bosoms and started wearing a bra when I was 11. My mum took me to the place where you got your school uniform and they sold these really old-fashioned cotton bras with no give in them. I remember being embarrassed because when we did maypole dancing my bra straps would fall down. I was the only one with a bra. I was known as 'Big 36' in my teens.

This man came into the place where I was working as the receptionist and I thought, 'God, you're lovely'. Apparently he thought, 'God, you've got lovely boobs'. Finally we started seeing each other, now we are married. My husband is definitely a boob man.

We passed this woman in the street, and she was probably about 50. I saw him look at her. He said, 'It doesn't matter how old they are, I still look.' That makes him sound really terrible but he's a lovely man. He jokes it's because he wasn't breastfed.

My breasts weren't important to me sexually till my I met my husband because I didn't actually like them. It took several years of him telling me how wonderful they were for me to think they were nice. I'd only settled into that for a few years before the lump.

My nipple has feeling, which is good. But the other breast doesn't feel anything. Both breasts have come back into play for my husband now. I said, 'What is the point of you squeezing it when we know about the thing they put in it?' I don't understand the point of a man feeling a woman's boobs when she's got implants.

My husband has found it much harder than me. He's pretended to me that it hasn't made any difference, but I don't know how he really felt about it when I had one. The night before the operation I made him say goodbye to the breast. He does find it amazing that I have two breasts back. I got him to admit he would have the bigger ones back if he could, but he's happy with these.

I prefer him to focus on the one with the nipple, and he knows that and does. That one gets the most attention, and the other one gets a little bit. I'm glad I had the reconstruction, I wouldn't want to just have a line.

I've got an extra nipple. Here it is. It looks like a little wart thing. Touch it! (*I do*) They are always in line with the nipples, like teats. When I had one of the operations the surgeon offered to cut it off, and of course when I came round it was still there. He forgot. He forgot the next time too, so I still have it.

I was keen to take part in this project. When I saw it, my instant thought was, 'It will be one-sided, there'll be all these perfect boobs. I need these mangled things to be in there.' I wanted there to be breasts with scars on.

———————————

Age 51 | Two children

"We're all trying to be the Special K woman"

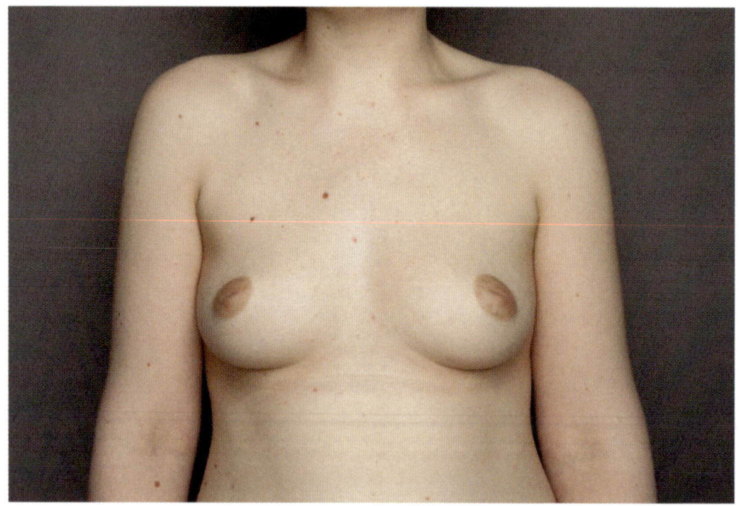

I love my breasts. I find it disappointing that my boyfriend doesn't want to look at them more. I want him to look at them, but he is quite happy for them to be in a bra. I just want to get them out! I think he is more interested in the experience of sex, but I want to be worshipped and adored and I like them as part of my body. I don't understand why he doesn't look at them and touch them more.

The modern woman looks lke she eats Special K, she's got the red dress on and no pointy nipples. She has a bump where her breasts are. She's very slim, goes in at the tummy. It's not fashionable to have a tummy. You don't see women in adverts who are average, they look perfect. Most people aren't quite like that. Some bras can give you a moulded shape so you look like a dummy in a shop.

I see things visually, I do like my art, I'm an artist.

I'm quite interested in my nipples. They are inverted a lot of the time. In a normal relaxed state they are flat, but when they are aroused they are inverted. I always think that looks like an arsehole.

I don't know anyone else with inverted nipples, I'll be interested to see if anyone else has them in your project. When I went into the changing rooms with my friend she used to say, 'Who'll have the biggest boobs when they are eighteen?' In the end she did, so she won one pound.

I think my boyfriend likes my boobs. I know he likes women, he says they're beautiful things. He doesn't praise me too much. I haven't asked my boyfriend what he thinks about me having inverted nipples. He says I am always going on about one thing or another, I don't think he wants to talk about breasts. I've got to be careful because he gets annoyed if I am disrespectful to him. I've got to try not to say the wrong things otherwise he will bark at me. He is nice to me.

I've lost quite a lot of weight, and I'm more attractive than I was, according to other people. According to myself I could still be much better, more slim. I need to lose more weight. This week I've lost five pounds. But I could be better, slimmer, sexier, get rid of fat on my legs. But I don't want my boobs to get smaller. We're all trying to be the Special K woman.

I do a lot of body combat dancing, my boobs bounce up and down a lot, so I find a sports bra useful. I go to the gym nearly every day now and I do five hours of classes a week. The company of other people is good for me. I've got to be careful of spending too much time alone because of my voices. They get stronger if you are unsociable. The voices are a hallucogenic symptom of schizophrenia. I have to be careful to be sociable.

I bought some nice lacy bras that were just £15 each. I was pleased because I think that is quite affordable. It's hard to choose your bra colours, you have to decide whether to be funky, or sexual and subtle. I love colour. My mum chose this bra for me. Sometimes it's hard when other people choose things for you, it's a different look. I like to go to to expensive shops and have luxury items. I feel good in slinky, lacy things, now I am old enough to be sexy.

If you go out in a T shirt and you don't have a bra on, it looks under-dressed and rude. When I went to a camp, a woman was wearing a halter neck and no bra and it looked crude.

If I had a baby I would want to breastfeed. But according to a lot of people I'm not allowed to have a baby because of my mental illness. They think I wouldn't make a good mother. That's how my family think. It's difficult for me because I quite fancy having a baby. I also wouldn't want it taken off me. I was living in a hostel and a woman had her baby taken from her. She was shouting, 'My baby! My baby has been taken away!' I don't want to have that. If I had a baby I would have to change all my medication. That would be a big problem for my mum. I love having nephews and nieces.

I like breasts, they are really nice. Men don't have them and I am really pleased they don't have them. It makes women special.

———————

Age 28 | No children

"I don't like the lumpy bits on my areolae"

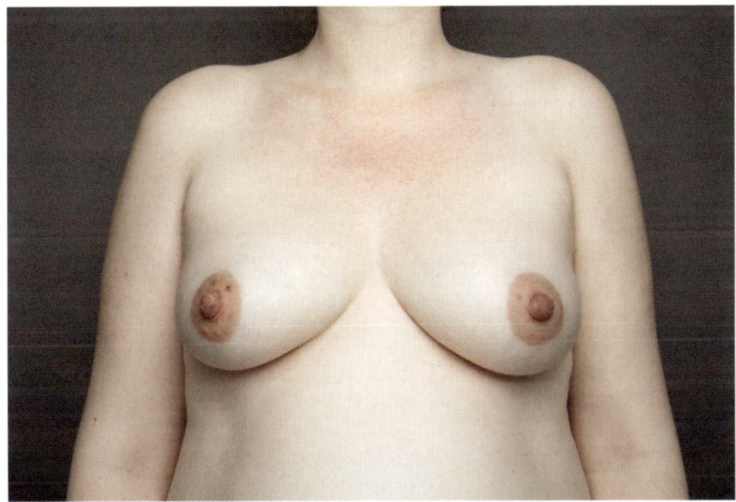

I think my boobs are alright. They are smallish and a bit saggy, but I've come to think they are OK.

When I was a teenager I didn't like my breasts. I lacked confidence, and that was focused on my breasts. I felt they were too small to be of any use. It took a long time to think they were OK. If I was going to worry about anything I realised it should be my bum and thighs and actually my breasts were fine! *(laughs)* It took a good 10 years to feel OK about my breasts.

There was an idea that boys only like big boobs. It was the prevailing idea from magazines, newspapers and boys at the time. Friends with bigger boobs had more attention, and that may have had more to do with personality or being prettier in general, but if they had bigger boobs that was my main focal point.

I don't like the lumpy bits on my areolae. I feel like they shouldn't be there, which is ridiculous because lots of people have bumpy bits. They look like spots, which sounds ludicrous – I ought not even admit to that. My breasts would be attractive without the bumps. If I see pictures of breasts in magazines or newspapers I always look to see if they have them too, but they always use fantastic looking boobs.

I don't think my partner is a boob man, but he does like them. They're not often a main focus for us. Maybe boobs are more of a niche thing, like feet? I think men appreciate them, but if the whole body is on offer, the boobs aren't necessarily a focus. The boobs are a taster for the rest of the body.

My boobs are variable. Sometimes I'm interested in involving them in sex, and sometimes I'm not bothered. I'm confident enough now to say one way or the other.

My partner and I talk about Page 3. In some ways I feel like I shouldn't like it, because it's demeaning, and why should boobs be in a newspaper? But then, there are a lots of things in a newspaper which are salacious and aren't news. Restrictions can be controlling and judgemental. If there are people who enjoy ogling, and women who want to pose, why shouldn't they? I wouldn't buy it, and I wouldn't let my children see it. My partner thinks it's a complete waste of time and money, and that it's for people of low intelligence.

I wouldn't want my daughter to be a glamour model. But then I wouldn't want her to be a politician or go into the army either. I suppose there are a lot of jobs I wouldn't want her to do! Maybe a teacher? I do think a lot about these things. I'd have more of an issue with her having a boob job because it would change her body permanently and it's risky. I suppose you could say being a glamour model or a stripper is risky psychologically too.

I never used to like breasts, but I do these days. I have an appreciation for a woman's body. Breasts make a shape. It's unfortunate for women who are flat, they would look better with breasts. Women are more attractive if they aren't overweight and if they have a shape, a bit of boob and bum.

———————

Age 32 | Two children, pregnant

"I can have an orgasm without my breasts, but it's a lot more satisfying if they are involved"

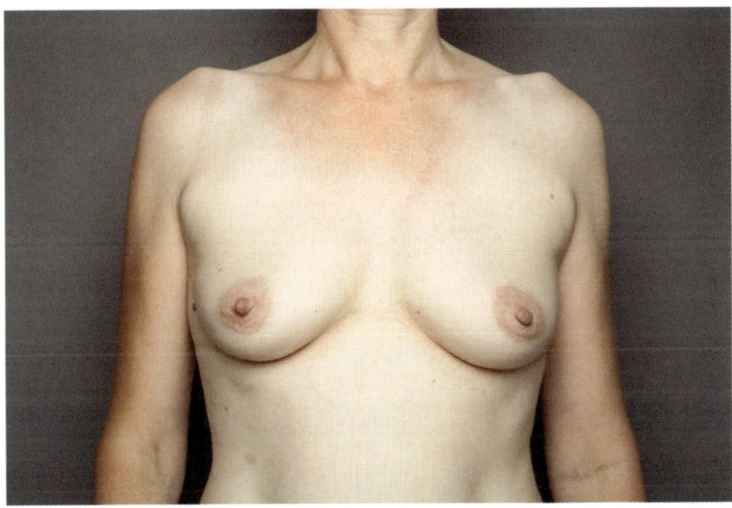

I've always quite liked my body as a whole, breasts included. I don't pay too much attention to them.

I do life modelling and obviously that means posing in the nude. I started about three years ago. I had friends that were doing it. I went to art college, and I've always had it at the back of my mind that I quite fancied doing it. I thought it seemed like a fun thing to do, and I wanted to know if I could do the nudity part. I wanted to know if it's comfortable to be naked in front of a crowd. It is, and if anything the ones who are embarrassed are the ones who are drawing you, especially the youngsters. Holding the poses is easy, especially if you are fit.

I like to leave a bit of hair down there, it feels too exposed otherwise. I just trim the sideburns, shape it a bit. I've had teenagers say, 'You're quite a natural woman,' and I think they mean my pubic hair.

When you take your clothes off it is so easy. I've sometimes thought the people doing the drawing should try it too. Being nude is as easy as wearing clothes. This whole thing about wearing clothes is so ridiculous in some ways. It feels nice to have a breeze and the sun on your skin.

I like to do different things and I like to push myself. I was brought up in a household where I never saw my parents naked. Affection was behind closed doors, we didn't see holding hands or kissing. Nudity, definitely not. I never saw my six brothers naked. Maybe I wanted to do life modelling and try being naked in front of a crowd because of my background.

It's always flattering when people paint you in a way which is attractive. I have some of them on my phone. You can think, 'Wow, do I look like that?' or, 'Do I really frown that much?' My back and legs are drawn quite consistently. My breasts are the least consistently drawn, maybe because I don't have big breasts which shout out to be noticed.

I breastfed each of my children for about a year and a half. That was an interesting experience because suddenly I had big breasts. *(laughs, indicating about 12 inches from her chest)*

I was quite embarrassed when my breasts first started growing. One breast started growing before the other one, so I felt lopsided. The other one quickly caught up. I wanted to hide them, it felt bizarre. I felt uncomfortable with my dad tickling me. I grew up in a household which was quite physical, but I started to feel embarrassed about it.

I remember very distinctly being out for a walk with my mum and I said, 'Oh, I'm going to be 12 soon!' And she said something about periods. My head started to swim and pound and I felt like I was on another planet. It was like an altered state of consciousness. I already knew a bit about periods – girls talk – but to hear my mum utter the words, I felt so mortally embarrassed. I think that's a real shame. I want to be able to talk to my daughter about these things.

When I asked my mum about things when I was small she gave me funny answers. Children are curious in a natural way, they just want to know. When I was five I asked my mum, 'I know a boy's is called a penis, what's a girl's called?' She wouldn't tell me. So, surprise, surprise, nothing was mentioned about breasts. Bras just appeared in my drawer. I felt weird about that. I am honest with my children.

I thought about asking my mum to come along today and take part in this project as well. I thought it could be healing, but then I thought, 'Do I really want to go there with her?' It's upsetting actually, but I wasn't aware of that till talking about it now.

Breasts are jolly lovely to be touched when you're having sex. For me, they are really important, a huge erogenous zone. It's nothing to do with size, thank God. I can have an orgasm without my breasts, but it's a lot quicker and a lot more satisfying if they are involved. They have to be part of the picture. It's like a triangle, a hotline. Lips too, I like being kissed a lot. I have experienced my breasts not being touched during sex and I found it strange and upsetting. It feels like that isn't accepting all of me. Breasts are such a part of being a woman, leaving them out of the picture is not accepting a huge part of her.

I can relate to women who can have an orgasm from their breasts. I've not met a man who is focused on doing that, it's not the main event for them. I've been so close to it on so many occasions; maybe I just haven't been able to quite let go enough, but I've nearly been there.

I've had an orgasm in a dream before. It shows how important the mind is. If you love your breasts and love them being stimulated, it's a huge turn-on. If you don't like them, then …

There was one man who had very erogenous breasts too, but I didn't particularly like that, I found it weird. I want the focus to be on my breasts! *(laughs)* I like hairy chests. I like the difference between men and women.

Breasts are also lovely to look at, even though I am attracted to men. I think it's because I love orbs and roundness, things that are mother-like and circular.

———————————

Age 46 | Two children

"I could look like a Page 3 girl, but I don't want to be a sexual commodity"

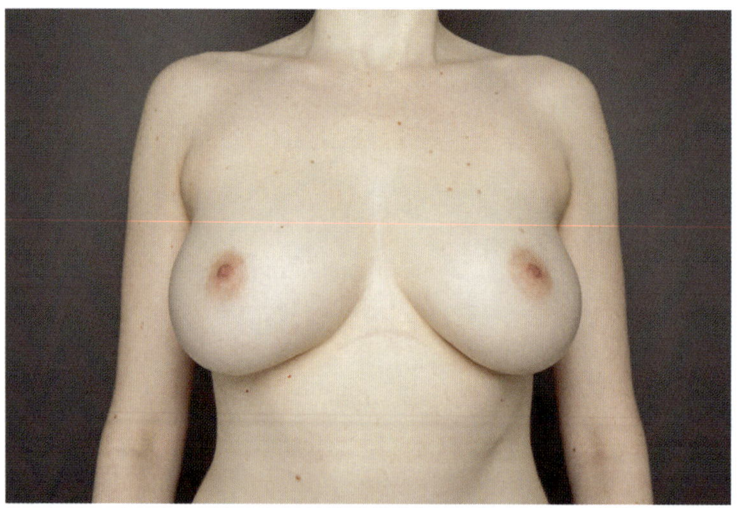

I started going to the gym about 16 months ago. It's funny how some women are quite body-conscious and wrap themselves up in towels and go into the little changing rooms in private. Other women have no inhibitions whatsoever. I think it's mainly the Eastern European women who are more open in the changing rooms, and also the ones who have spent a lot of time working out and are super-proud of their bodies. It's quite fascinating watching their behaviour, rather than watching them change. I can't face taking my bra off, I don't want to show off. I'm intrigued by my own behaviour because I didn't think I would be like that, but I am.

We have a very prudish attitude to breasts in the UK. When I was younger I went to swimming baths and everyone got completely naked in the showers. It was the first time I had seen my mum completely naked! I was stunned to stillness. I think we need to work on this in the UK.

I've got a funny relationship with my breasts. I was 13 or 14, when I started developing and I grew quickly. I was a DD when I was 16. Getting underwear was a mission, not an enjoyable experience. I would walk out in tears. Nothing fitted and it made me feel abnormal. I'm 32DD, which is fine nowadays, but in the mid 90s you couldn't get DD bras for love nor money. Anything above a D cup would have straps an inch thick, and that's not what you want when you're a teenage girl! You want underwear which makes you feel pretty and sexy. It's hard to imagine that now the high street is full of nice underwear. The lingerie industry has moved on and I think breast augmentation surgery has propelled that.

I never wear low-cut tops, I've always tried to disguise myself and keep myself hidden in baggy tops and shirts. Because of my body proportions, I'm a size six to eight, I feel like there is a lot up here. I feel like men will look at my chest and women will look at my chest, maybe enviously. I wanted people to talk to me, not my chest. Boys stared all the time, but I did a lot to try and prevent it.

I remember watching boy's behaviour over Page 3 at high school. I feel the way I do about my breasts because of the media. I could look like a Page 3 girl, but I don't want to be a sexual commodity, there's a lack of respect for that kind of woman. Big tits are like this seedy world, glamour, strippers, etc. That's not what I want to be associated with, but because of my body shape I felt like that's how I would be pigeon-holed.

Recently I have started wearing V-neck tops. I'm 32 now, it's taken me that long to become comfortable. Having big breasts doesn't make me body-confident. I've got the dimensions other women aspire to, but they don't boost my confidence. I've gone through a long period of hiding, hiding, hiding, but I'm coming into a more confident phase of life. I watch other women, and I think, 'I could be like that as well.' Not just celebrities, but women walking down the street.

Boyfriends have been quite surprised the first time they've seen them because I keep them quite well hidden. They're like, 'Wow!' Then smiles! That makes me feel good about myself, but it's a private setting, not a public setting. They like to feel them, squeeze them, suck nipples. I think some men have an inner-child thing. Lots of men are quite insecure inside, and it goes back to being breastfed. It almost turns you into a mother figure in a bizarre way, on certain occasions. Some men are very much more like that, they have a mother-type bond with my breasts, and other guys are much more sexual.

Someone wanted a tit wank once. I did do it. I didn't mind it, it was quite good fun, quite playful, and it was fitting at the time.

My breasts are sensitive so they play a big part for me sexually. How they feel depends on where I am in my cycle. If it's just before my period they are very sensitive, and I don't like them grabbed too hard. Other times, I like my nipples being squeezed. There's a pleasure-pain thing, and I might tell them to squeeze harder, or tell them it's too hard. I've always been quite confident to say what I like.

When I went back on the Pill my breasts were really painful, even walking up the stairs was sore. I actually had to hold them to run up the stairs, because wobbling made them sore. That's was when the nurse said I had to check myself, because contraception can change your breasts. Every time I go for an appointment about my pill she checks my breasts for me. The Pill definitely makes them bigger. There was searing pain through my breasts and nipples. But different pills have different effects, the one before literally made me mental. I would break down in tears for no reason, and fly off the handle. In terms of mental stability, this pill is fine, but for the first couple of months it made my boobs really sore.

Publicly I want to be treated as one of the lads, I don't want to use my female sexuality to advance myself, I want to be judged on merit. I've always worked in a very male-dominated space. Other girls do the power-dressing, chic but sexy, and use that to help themselves. Women in my industry are in a tiny minority. In some respects that gives you power because you can stand out in a crowd, but I have to walk a very fine line of femininity and professionalism, and it can be crossed oh so easily.

Nowadays at work I might wear a V-neck top, with a tiny little bit of chest showing, and more fitted shirts. I've sharpened up my image and I do attract different male attention than when I dressed in a baggy way. I'm now on that fine line of professional and sexy, and trying to keep it that way.

If I go to a conference and the guys have had a few drinks, they are all over me. The classic leaning in – men with wedding rings! They think they can get away with it, and with me! It can be quite uncomfortable. You can't make a scene, these are men who are quite powerful and influential so you don't want to piss them off. Some directors have an ego that goes along with the position they've attained, so they think, 'She's flashing it about, so she's game.' No, no, it's not like that!

Children would be the biggest change in store for my breasts. I'm worried in case they start sagging a lot, because they're not small pert breasts that can just stay up there! I don't think I'll be happy when they sag, but there's enough equipment to make them look like they're still up there. It wouldn't put me off breastfeeding though, it's good for baby. Breast is best, at least for the first six months.

I'm intrigued to know what a baby latching on and feeding from me will feel like, because I know how I like my nipples played with. I'm curious to know what the sensation and the bonding will be like! I may hate it, but I have no reservations about trying it.

I'll be 33 this year and I still don't have children, so I have 'virgin' breasts. My breasts didn't lose their 'virginity' when I first had sex, they'll lose their 'virginity' when I breastfeed, because breastfeeding is their primary function.

I'll say 'boobs' and 'breasts' but not 'tits' or 'knockers'. 'Knockers' isn't a nice, endearing word, whereas 'breasts' are nice, beautiful things. 'Knockers' sounds like the scrapper's yard. 'Tits' is a chavvy term. Sometimes I call my bra my 'boulder-holder'!

I have a very love-hate relationship with my breasts. When I look in the mirror, I think, 'Yes, pretty,' when I look down I think, 'Way too big!' When I'm walking and I can see them wobbling, I hate it. But then sometimes I catch sight, and I think, 'Wow!' A real love-hate relationship. My ideal breast size would be smaller, a B or C cup.

I wouldn't have a reduction. The only thing I'd have done is my nose! Your body is your body, you make the most of it. Some women, I can understand if they have specific hang ups and want to get things changed, but not personally.

I want to change my relationship with breasts, and get more comfortable with them. I want to shrug off what society thinks. Why does the MoonWalk *(breast cancer fundraising walk)* have to be moonlight, why can't it be daylight? Walking in the dark suggests there's something that has to be hidden. I'm a feminist, but femininity is a different thing.

I swim and jog, but about seven years ago a girlfriend and I took stripping classes. We were the first round of students who did it, it was a new craze. At the end we did a show, and I got my boyfriend and my mum, dad and sister to come and watch. You wore two bras, so you took one off, and you had another one underneath. You took the plain one off and you had a really elegant one underneath. It was quite good fun! The funny thing is, because I've had my own business I come up on Google, but there is also an article about the strip dance class!

I like burlesque, I think it's more of a turn on than strippers. Strippers get it all out and it doesn't leave anything to the imagination. Burlesque is much sexier!

———————————

Age 32 | No children

"When I bare my breasts I am trying to bare my soul"

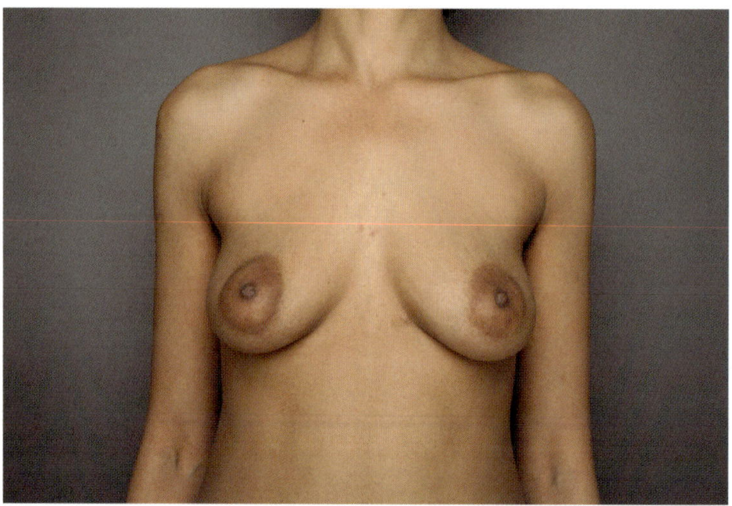

My breasts are small and pert, quite squidgy, with big areolae. I have a few hairs. I'm like, 'Should I tweeze them or leave them and be proud?' I've kept them. No one has commented on the hairs. I think if you are OK with what you have, other people are less likely to say something. Breast hairs are very fine, and they are a tiny detail. You might notice your own breast hairs but they are non-existent to other people.

I do like my breasts. They remind m of my femininity. It's nice and comforting to hold them. I'm quite proud of my breasts, I like them to be out there. I think more people should be proud of their breasts, whatever shape and size they are. I feel really good about mine and I just want everyone else to feel the same about theirs.

My friends who are bigger are less comfortable about being bare-breasted, either completely out, or on display with tit-tassels, or whatever. Because of the circles I am in, most people are completely OK with the 'breastage' being out, although not the nipples. Everyone is into the whole tit-tassel thing, but my friends rarely get them out completely. We go out to themed events and we might dress as, say, hula girls, with tit-tassels. You get hot so minimal clothes are good. I am known for being bare-breasted; my pseudonym is 'Captain Hello Titties'.

The 'Captain Hello Titties' outfit is a onesie, but with my boobs out, open Borat-style. It has a boob tube that is meant to go underneath but I removed that, because it kept slipping, and that's how 'Captain Hello Titties' was born. Lots of women said they were inspired by that outfit and were going to do the same thing.

At a party, I was going around dressed as 'Captain Hello Titties'. Some feminists came up to me and they said it was really wrong, that there must be something deep-rooted in me that made me want to go around like that, seeking attention. It was fascinating. I felt that they weren't comfortable in themselves and didn't know how to deal with my confidence and openness. They couldn't fathom it and thought there must be some darkness behind it. They even talked to my friends about it.

I wouldn't describe myself as a feminist, but I am pro-female, pro-people and pro-equality. I wouldn't use the word feminism because of encounters like that with people who label themselves as feminists.

I don't know if it's because there is something about me, but men are OK. I never feel disrespected or overly checked out. I feel like my body is being appreciated. It's never felt slimy.

I think the word 'titties' is funny. I can see how people would be offended, people who think seriously about these things, bodies and respect, but I think it's got comedy value. I think I need to do a bit more thinking about the 'Hello Titties' thing. People have asked me about the word 'titties' and the connotations around it. Do I need to look into it, or should I carry on? I'm intrigued by how words and playfulness can have a different effect on people.

When I bare my breasts and put on these crazy, wild performances I think I am trying to get to my soul, bare my soul. I'm trying to take everything off, and that's as far as I can get on a physical level. It's not in a sexual and provocative way, it's more about feeling liberated. It's never an easy thing to be completely comfortable with, I always feel a bit shaky when I do it, it's just something I push through. I like to challenge myself. I want to get to the core and uncover that; the clothes don't matter.

I try and encourage other people to do it too. Just a few weeks ago I got up on the stage when a band was jamming, and said, 'Right everyone, do it with me!' and I started stripping. I want everyone to be liberated. I feel really good when I've inspired someone else to do it, and they feel good that they've done it and surprised they worried so much beforehand. I think people should try it, don't worry about what other people think.

I love my clothes. I love fashion. But when I take my clothes off I am saying 'Yes' to transparency. I'll still be doing it when I'm old.

In sex, my breasts are fun. Different partners will focus on different things. When partners have focussed on boobage it has been nice, fun, even quite sensational sometimes! I like a little bit of biting, although I am not a pain person. I slept with a guy once who was very into his nipples being bitten and pinched hard. A few months ago I slept with a woman who particularly focused her attention on my breasts and expected the same in return. I'd never slept with anyone who liked that amount of attention. It was 70 per cent breast time, 30 per cent everything else.

I normally go braless; it feels better, more comfortable. I only wear bras if I am going to an important meeting and wearing a smarter outfit and need a push-up look. If I'm doing something a bit more corporate I'll wear a pencil skirt, shoes, a top and a jacket. I feel more full and raised with a bra and it looks better, maybe a more structured look.

Sometimes I wonder if I should shave my armpits, but luckily I haven't done it yet. I stopped shaving my armpits about a year and a half ago. I didn't like the process of shaving and the stinging and I was bored of it. I like the curliness, it's nice to play with, and my skin is more smooth.

Sometimes I do backstage fashion show management. I was telling some beautiful models what to do, and I noticed a general vibe. I was wearing one of my crazy onesies, not with my boobs out, but my armpit hair was showing. I could sense a gobsmacked reaction from these beauties. There was a loss of respect! I had to say, 'Look, I know I've got hair under my arms, but I'm OK with it.' I don't do it as a statement, it's laziness and comfort. It's funny when women aren't 'for' it. I don't shave 'down there' either.

———————

Age 27 | No children

"My husband's never really said how he feels"

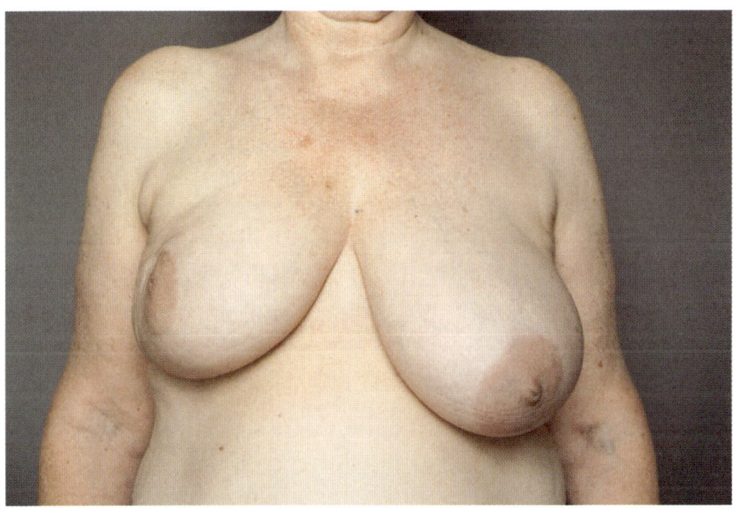

I got cancer. It was picked up at a screening. I had two lumpectomies and five years of treatment, which I am very pleased to have stopped. It was quite an aggressive cancer. After the biopsy came back, they decided I had to have a second operation to remove a larger area. It's about one-third smaller than the other now. I seem to be OK and that's it hopefully.

One breast is very cock-eyed, with the nipple going up sideways. I had the opportunity to have the other one reduced down to the same size, but I decided it was a lot of hassle and pain. I got fluid retention and had over a litre drawn off. It wasn't much fun actually, having the operations.

So I decided I'd just wear a jelly and look vaguely normal with that. I think you should accept yourself how you are. It's a bit cock-eyed, but it isn't on display to the world so, you know, I guess that's alright.

My husband's never really said how he feels. He's not one to discuss his feelings, unfortunately. He doesn't do that sort of discussion.

I breastfed my children, all of them. I did get mastitis a few times. I had flat nipples, so it was very painful to begin with, particularly with one child who sucked hard. It actually sent excruciating shivers down me. I breastfed her for a year and I gradually got used to it. I did feel it was best, so I persevered. They all breastfed differently. The others breastfed for between eight and 18 months.

I'm glad I breastfed. It's a lovely feeling. Except one child, she didn't put on weight like the others, and was whingy and difficult. It was probably because I had two other small children as well, and I had caesareans, and they were quite difficult to get over. I had cracked and bleeding nipples and that possibly made it difficult.

I carried on because I believed there are so many beneficial things in breastmilk that you don't get any other way. It was a pleasant and bonding feeling. I believe my grandmother got quite ecstatic with her breastfeeding. I didn't get ecstatic, but it was pleasant enough. 'Oh, Granny was over the moon about it, I never was,' said my mother.

Once I was feeling ill and I was fed up with this child who wanted to be feeding all the time and I gave it to another friend to breastfeed. It didn't bother me, although she felt uncomfortable about it. But she did it and the child was perfectly happy, it didn't care where it got its milk actually. I would have been quite happy to feed someone else's child, it wouldn't bother me.

There was a case in Africa where a woman was feeding a pig on one side and a baby on the other, but the pig got fed first because it was very valuable. Another old lady had fed so many kids, her breasts were so long she could tie them in knots.

Did I see my mother's breasts? Occasionally. She was private. Nobody went around the house naked. I saw her getting dressed from time to time. She did have a corset that I had to lace up. I had to do up the hooks at the back, because you couldn't have a stomach. When I came home from England she said, 'We must go and get your stomach pulled in, you can't have a stomach'. These things were so tight and expensive. I only wore it about twice, I couldn't bear it. It wasn't a corset, but one of those tight pull-you-ins.

I remember the boys at school killing themselves laughing because we were doing long jump and, of course, when you are developing you start to bounce up and down. They were cackling among themselves. I went to my mother and I said, 'You've got to get me a bra, I can't be coping with this any longer.' She thought it was hysterically funny, but next time we went to town, which was a matter of catching a bus quite a long way, we could get a bra. I was 13. I was quite pleased to be developing, but I didn't like being laughed at. I had a friend who used to wear sticking plaster over her nipples. She was quite small and didn't bother with bras, but she didn't want to look too obvious.

My breasts are OK. They certainly improve the look of a dress! It's to do with overall shape and our concept of what looks good. I wouldn't mind if I'd had smaller breasts. I'd rather have had smaller hips, and they go together. A lot of fashion fits people with smaller boobs better, quite frankly.

When you're growing up you like to try different necklines, and it's exciting to think you are sexy. But the breasts aren't in isolation. I see them as part of the overall thing.

I don't do what's 'perfect'. I just think people should be happy with themselves as they are and not be so obsessed with their looks or their breasts. They should be more concerned with their personality, and being caring and loving people.

One of my daughters was considering breast surgery. I said she could do what she liked, but that it's a wicked waste of money. She should be happy with who she is, and if she's not she should do what she can to improve, like lose a bit of weight and dress well.

I don't feel my boobs, I can't be bothered with all that. I just imagine there are lumps all over the place. And in fact, when I did get breast cancer, it was small and I wouldn't have felt it anyway. I just think people get a bit obsessed with themselves, quite honestly. Maybe checking breasts is good for some, but it's not something I can be bothered with.

———————————

Age 65 | Four children

"He literally stood there for five minutes massaging my breasts in one direction"

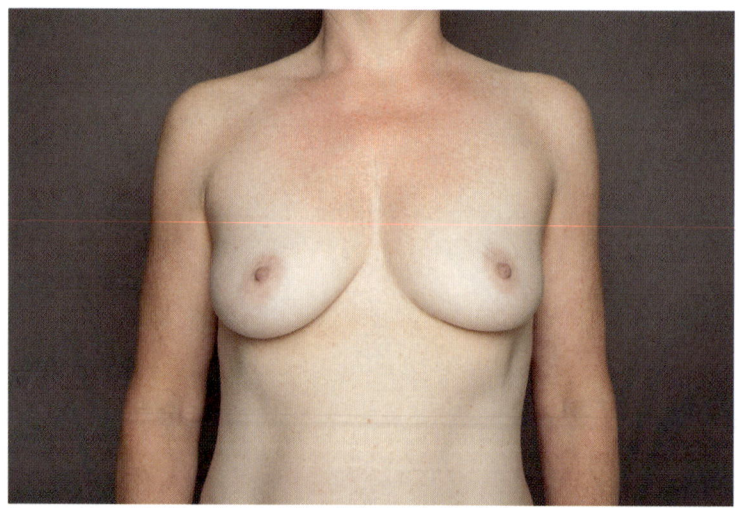

I like my breasts very much. I've always thought it would be nice to have slightly larger breasts at night and smaller breasts during the day. At night time you can wear plunge tops and get them out a bit more. Generally having smaller breasts is advantageous for clothing.

My partner says he adores my breasts. Whther or not he truly does I don't know, but he would be an idiot to say if he didn't. As I get older I realise other people's perceptions of your breasts are unimportant; it's how you feel about them that matters.

I have to buy quite a lot of underwear for my job as a professional escort. I have a large selection, and spend a lot of time trawling online. Pages and pages of tall leggy blondes with huge boobs and implants leave me cold. I try to go for classy rather than slutty underwear. Stockings, little lace teddies, not necessarily underwired or cupped, show my breasts to their best, and anything from teeny G-strings to beautiful satin pants.

As long as you look fairly smart, and I always wear high heels, it doesn't matter. I'm careful to note what I wear so I don't repeat it next time I see them. Men don't really notice though, each time it's a novelty! Even my partner would have no idea what's in my underwear drawer, he wouldn't be able to describe anything.

I can't afford to buy very expensive underwear as I change it a lot. I spend about £700 a year on my work underwear. I spend a bit more per item on my own underwear. I keep it all separate – I'm conscious of that for my partner – although I never let him see me get ready to go out.

Men are visual creatures, so what boobs look like is important, but what's behind them is more important, for sure. I have mentioned to men in my professional capacity that I would like my breasts to be a bit larger and they have said, 'For God's sake, whatever you do, do not have implants in your breasts.' They find them ugly. That gave me confidence to say, 'They are what they are'. That's a recent discovery for me. You become more confident as you get older.

Men lust after women like Gwyneth Paltrow, Emma Watson, Keira Knightley – they haven't got big breasts, but they look smiley and friendly. I think we over-estimate the importance men place on breasts. Although if a big-breasted woman walked into a bar, men would say 'Phwoar!' with that male rugby mentality.

Clients have said they've seen women with poor boob jobs, with nipples facing the wrong way, scars and ridges down the side. Breast jobs also aren't forever, they can go hard. They may look good, but when you feel them they aren't nice, not feminine.

Men have been from one end of the scale to another with my breasts. Some haven't even asked me to take my bra off and have totally ignored them. I've been paid hundreds of pounds to just sit in a room for an hour and never even taken my clothes off. They may have just asked to have a wank while I show them my pants. That's one end of the scale. Fantasy land. And at the other end of the scale some men pay a lot of attention to my breasts. My breasts are nothing spectacular, they're not out of this world, but men are willing to pay £100 an hour or £1,000 a night to spend time with me. It's proof that you do not have to be a size eight, leggy blonde for a man to want to spend time with you. Almost anybody could do it, not that everybody wants to.

Some repeat customers come from all over; one comes from Switzerland. I don't see myself as amazingly beautiful – so what does he see? Obviously there has to be some sort of sexual attraction and some sexual skill, but it's also about having someone to chat to. He doesn't have to make any effort or ask me one single question about myself all night long. It's all about him. I have to smile and go, 'Oh, you're so interesting!' And often they are.

But that's only one reason; there are lots of reasons why men see escorts. It might be that there are sexual acts their wife won't do. One man said, 'You must think I am a complete heel for seeing you, but I just needed to do this so when I am older and sitting in my rocking chair I have something to look back on.' They want to have time for themselves. Or they haven't got time for a relationship because of their lifestyle.

Some men do actually want to give you pleasure. I met a very inexperienced young man in his 20s. I had to take the lead a little. I stood up and took my top and skirt off and put his hands on my breasts. He literally stood there for five minutes massaging my breasts in one direction. Then he massaged them back the other way. He was clueless about what a woman would enjoy. The five minutes left and right did my head in. In the end, I transferred his hands to my bum. It was dreadful. I don't know how I didn't laugh.

I don't give tit wanks because my boobs aren't very big and I find it quite awkward. You have to get into a very awkward position to do that. It's uncomfortable and I don't really like it. If a man was choosing someone for that they would probably go for a larger rack than mine. Men quite like it if you keep your bra or your top on. There's something naughty about it. 'Ooh, that looks naughty, a glimpse of nipple.'

Some men are very gentle, some are a bit rougher. My natural sexual orientation is to be slightly submissive. But with rough sex it should be incremental. You start gentle and then build up. If I felt threatened in any way I would terminate the appointment. I've never had to do that. Normally I would say, 'That feels nice, but please don't leave marks because I really don't want to have to explain those to my children when I get out of the shower tomorrow.' That will stop it straight away, because then they see you as a mother and not just as a sexual object. With my own partner we enjoy bouts of quite rough sex, and I quite like him to manhandle me a bit, but again it's incremental and I trust him to stop.

It's surprising how many men like their breasts sucked and licked, and treated more like women's boobs. I will explore their nipples and then I will say, 'Do you like your nipples sucked or licked?' You can hear in their voice how far you can go.

My partner hates me being an escort, but I was doing it before him. It's caused us trouble, but it's part of my plan. I am not prepared to work 36 hours a week for the same money as I do now. I don't want to do it long term. I'm very lucky that I am in a financial position where I can pick and choose, I am not hand-to-mouth. I can think about my safety and self-respect, I have that choice.

It's hard to know whether my breasts have affected who I am. Would my life have been different if I had massive knockers? How would I have been treated? I used to work in the city, and when I came across women in the workplace who displayed a lot of cleavage, a lot of tit, I always found that unprofessional. Why do that in the workplace? Unless you are barmaid.

My partner said to me, 'You look at men's crotches all the time'. I do not! He thinks all women do, but he is really wrong, women don't look. I was horrified he thought that of me. I'd probably done it a few times in my life inadvertently but, since he said it, I've done it more! It feels really lecherous. If his jeans are tight he feels self-conscious.

I'm very proud of breastfeeding. I fed my first baby for six months and my second child for a year. It hurt at the beginning, I had mastitis. I was trying to stay off antibiotics so I tried cabbage leaves. Fresh, cold cabbage leaves stuck down my bra. There might have been some success with it, but I took paracetamol as well.

I got sick of the sight of my tits when I was breastfeeding and they became totally non-sexual. Then one day I felt like I had my boobs back, maybe about six months after I finished breastfeeding.

Some men love the idea of a woman producing milk, almost as if it's still for them. I read somewhere that men like breasts because they remind them of a backside. I think it's because they are an intrinsic part of being a woman. A lot of men are turned on by lactating. It's dirty and mummy-like all at the same time.

Age 46 | Two children

"Breasts can come into sex in BDSM in the form of nipple play or nipple torture"

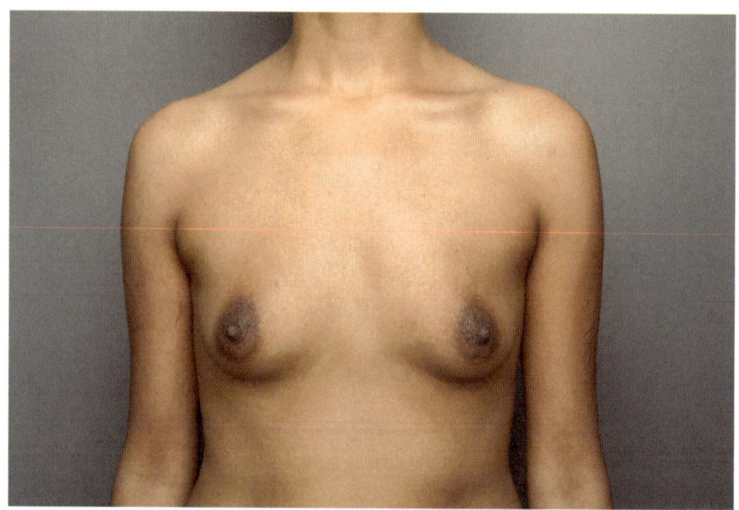

I think my breasts are too small, I would like them to be larger and perkier. I've noticed that they have little nodules – lumps – and I'd rather not have those. *(She means Montgomery glands.)*

In my culture (I am of south-east Asian origin), it is more attractive to be paler. I have Indian, Pakistani and a bit of African in there. I didn't like my dark colour when I was younger, but as I've grown older I've grown to love it. I really like my dark nipples.

My family are Muslim, but I am not. I have rejected the whole concept due to life experiences. The concept of there being a God is not to my liking. My family don't like me rejecting religion, but they haven't argued against it. I have so many mental health problems it has allowed me to 'get away' with certain opinions. I don't live with family, I'm not married, I don't have kids; this is not traditional in my culture. But because I have these issues and I have said I want to study, and I can get treatment in this area, it has allowed me to get away from them.

My family prefer me not to express my choices in front of other family members. It's not the done thing that someone rejects their religion in our culture, it is seen as dishonourable and embarrassing. I just keep quiet. When other people are praying I pretend I am on my period and go into another room. When you have your period you can't really pray. This is what I heard when I was a kid.

I feel my breasts could look better if they were bigger, so I go for certain bras which have a plunge and a gel. I haven't tried the chicken fillets yet; I think the bras do an OK job so far. Society thinks women look more in proportion if they are bigger. I don't think my breasts are in proportion to my frame at the moment.

I have several mental health issues, which are interlinked. I have body dysmorphic disorder, anorexia and bulimia. I also self-harm as a way of coping with emotional pain. My eating disorder is about control and coping with emotional pain, and it's linked into body dysmorphic disorder. For me to take part in this project is massive.

I've had my struggles, but compared to stories from other south-east Asian lesbians, I consider myself very lucky. My mum knows I am a lesbian, but she is in denial. My dad and one of my brothers don't know. It's a big family secret. My mum is so ashamed of it.

I've pretty much always been a lesbian, even though for a long time I didn't realise it. I'm a switch but at the moment I am in service to a professional dominatrix.

A BDSM mistress looked at a picture of my body on Skype and asked if I would consider having breast implants if she paid. It made me think. It was the first time someone had suggested that, and the first time I had thought of them as that small. And yeah, maybe I would. She finds me attractive, but would find me more attractive with larger breasts. There could be a dynamic where she wanted more control over me, but it didn't enter my head at the time.

There were complications with her and I had to block her on this website. But she created a new profile and contacted me again, saying she had missed me and I am so unique and stuff. She wanted to re-establish a connection, but because of the things she had said to me in the past, and out of respect to the mistress I am serving at the moment, I had to decline that. I don't know what she finds attractive. Obviously my breasts didn't put her off that much.

Men and women both prefer the hourglass figure, which I don't have. People have mentioned to me that I need to put on weight. I am borderline anorexic. The first thing you notice if I lose weight is my collarbone, which is very prominent, and my breasts, which shrink. I want bigger breasts but I have an eating disorder. The two don't go together unless I get implants.

I've heard a lot of horror stories about implants, that they can rupture or leak, and after a certain number of years they aren't safe. That and the money put me off.

Breasts can come into sex in BDSM in the form of nipple play or nipple torture. I don't like torture on my nipples, even though I like being hurt generally. My nipples just seem very sensitive. The experience I have had is clothes pegs on my nipples for a substantial amount of time. It really hurts when you take them off. Some people love it.

The first time I was properly dominated, it was online, by my ex. I'd never done it before, so I thought 'Why not?' I was being obedient and submissive. She made me wear them for longer than I would like, but I liked her harsh, dominating nature. What she did to me was harder than what other people do to me in reality. Maybe that fulfils my self-destructive side. But it made me realise that nipple torture is not my thing. I've told my mistress that's one thing I don't like, so she has said she won't do that to me.

In the past I haven't enjoyed people sucking my nipples, but I've found that whether it turns me on or not is to do with the person. If they are properly caressing me and then touch my nipples at the same time, it can either heighten my sensuality or turn me off. It depends on the person and my mood.

Breasts are great! The look and the feel of them are sexually appealing. I've never mentioned this before… I get very paranoid when I am playing with someone else's breasts with my mouth or my tongue, and giving them a pleasurable sensation, because in my experience, girls don't vocalise their pleasure in moaning, whereas I do. The majority of girls I have been with don't make a noise. I feel more confident when I go to the vagina, but I don't feel I get much of a reaction from playing with breasts.

Getting into BDSM involves showing my body naked, sometimes in front of several people. The very first time I did it I was mortified. I've done it several times since. I'm just hoping it will give me more confidence about my body. I would expect people to be repelled by me, and be disgusted by what they see. I didn't hear those comments, so hopefully it will sink in that I am not so bad. Maybe I am grasping for anything to find confidence and self-esteem. Doing things the vanilla way hasn't brought me much confidence, so I am trying something that will shape me and give me confidence.

There are a couple of people who are interested in me at the moment, but for some reason they are men. I don't seem to have much luck with women: after a few meetings they seem to disappear. I've been single for about four years now. It's sad. I hope it will change. One thing that really gets to you is loneliness, but it doesn't stop me trying to interact with people. I've been to the south-east Asian gay clubs, Desi clubs, nothing to do with BDSM or fetish, but I haven't had any luck there. I've tried different avenues.

———————

Age 35 | No children

"All boobs go south"

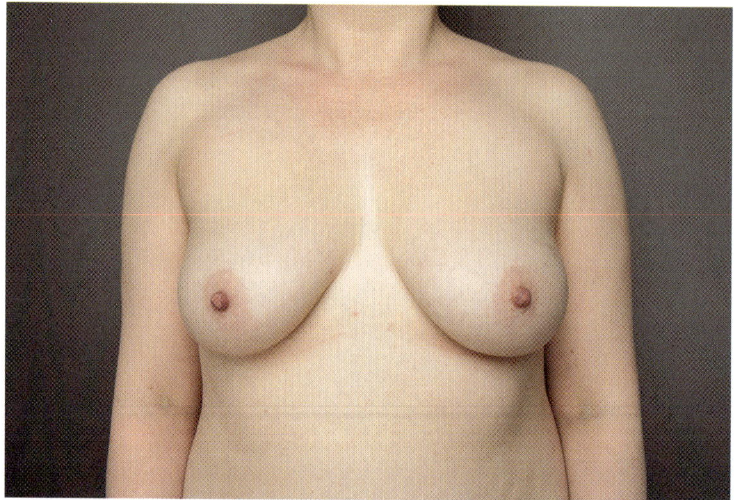

My breasts are not too large and not too small; they're OK for my size.
They are quite pert, they don't droop. There's enough of them to get a
decent cleavage in a decent bra I suppose. Overall I think I do like them.

When my partner and I first met he aid, 'I always thought I was a leg
man'. I said, 'Oh, well, I'm only 5ft 2in so that's a bit of a shame!' *(laughs)*
He said, 'No, I think I'm a boob man now!' So he likes them, although he
hasn't exactly commented on them a lot. I may have converted him!

When I'm out I always wear a bra, or I'd feel very uncomfortable. I'll
tell you why. I've got incredibly sensitive nipples. If I am not wearing a

bra you can completely tell and it just looks ridiculous. I have these bullets sticking out of my T-shirt. My nipples are very sensitive and are rarely smooth.

I think the shape and the look is nicer when breasts are smooth. I'd like mine to look buxom, not like they're cold with two shrivelled, obvious points, otherwise you just get people looking at them. I would look.

I don't know why men like breasts sexually, but I'll be honest, I do as well. Not sexually necessarily, but I'll look and go, 'I'd like a cleavage like that!'

You can appreciate the female form. They're a nice thing to have. You can think, 'Nice curves, nice dress.' I don't have an issue with men thinking that too! There are certain ways you can appeal to men and be quite provocative. I think it's just instinct really.

The whole thing I have an issue with is airbrushing. Boobs, wrinkles, taking off four stone, whatever. I like the Dove adverts that portray women as we see ourselves. We all know we've got one boob bigger than the other, so I just try and ignore that kind of airbrushing. I think it creates a feeling of inadequacy for people.

When I was younger I used to work in an old people's residential home. So I've seen a lot of naked women's bodies. I don't want the big droopy boob thing down to my waist, but it's going to happen! *(laughs)* There were ladies with really small chests and ladies with really big boobs and it doesn't matter, all boobs go south. We all end up like that.

I think there's a stereotypical view of what I might be like. I've got the bum, the boobs, blond hair, lighter-coloured eyes. I'm kind of the epitome of a bimbo. The boobs have played a part in that. But then people talk to me and realise I'm not. But I do use them and they are part of me, dressing in a way that makes me feel the most confident.

I think I'm quite lucky with my boobs.

____

Age 35 | No children

"I grew up with scars on my breasts"

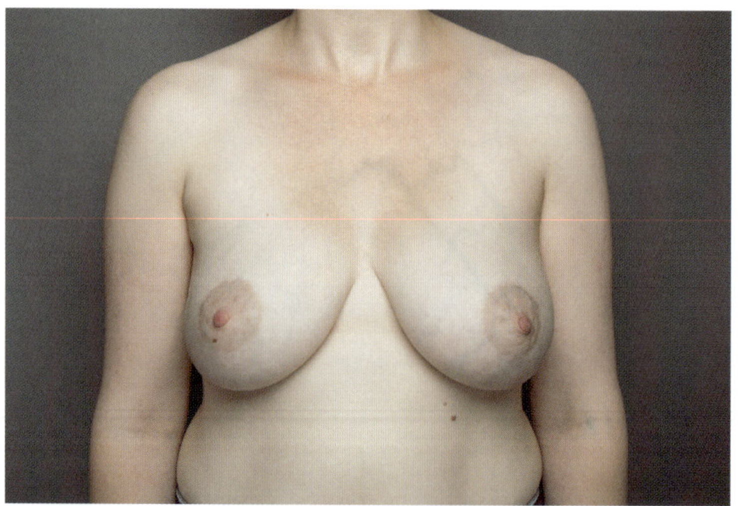

I lost my mother to breast cancer. She died about six months after I was born. I was born very prematurely because of her cancer. I think I was induced, but my dad never spoke about it, and he is dead too now. I can't really find out what happened because they don't have records that go back that far. Breasts can be dangerous because of cancer, but they can be positive because you feed your children.

I have scarring on my breasts because my lungs collapsed when I was born. Do you see that discolouration? *(shows me a scar)* It looks smaller now because my breasts are bigger, but when I was a child it was more noticeable.

I see it as a positive reminder that I am lucky to be here. I survived at 27 weeks, 33 years ago. I'm healthy, I've had children and been able to breastfeed. I didn't know if my breasts would work properly because of the damage.

It's hard not knowing the full story about my mum and my birth. It bothered me when I had my daughter. You can't miss what you haven't had, but that was the first time I had real grief because I realised I had been this small and my mum hadn't been there.

When I was pregnant with my first daughter I was paranoid that there could be some dormant gene. We don't know if breast cancer is in the family because there isn't anyone to ask. My older sisters get screened, but I don't.

When I was a teenager I was self-conscious about my scars with boyfriends. I felt like I looked different. Women in films and on TV didn't have scars. Mind you, I felt generally embarrassed all over! The scars aren't too noticeable and they don't affect the shape of my breasts. They don't bother me at all any more.

My husband reads *The Sun*. I've always thought if women want to be on Page 3 that's their choice. But since breastfeeding and having two girls I feel a bit more put out by it. I don't think it promotes a very positive image of breasts. It's as though breasts are just there to be looked at, and they're not. I think the only point of it is so men can go 'phwoar'. I talked to my husband about it. He says it's a British institution and you can't get rid of it. I'd hate my daughters to see the pictures, think that's what breasts are for, and feel like they aren't good enough.

Before, my breasts were to look good for men. I wore clothes and push-up bras to make them look better. Mine aren't going to look that good again, they've lost their stuffing. I joke to my husband that if there's a strong breeze I'll fly off, because they flap in the wind.

In some ways, certain men (and women?) can be very easily manipulated by breasts, almost as if they have some sort of magical power! I know I've used my breasts, by dressing in a certain way, to get my own way with men. However right or wrong that may be! I worked in the building industry for a number of years, and felt it was easy to manipulate situations, like moving deadlines, or getting items cheaper, by using appearance. I'm not sure how magical I feel mine are now, but I certainly used to feel quite proud of how they looked. After having two babies I would now describe my breasts as amazing.

Doing this project has made me feel outrageous, because of how my friends have reacted. None of them would have taken part.

Age 33 | Two children, breastfeeding six-month-old

"I'm a burlesque dancer who doesn't fit the beauty archetype"

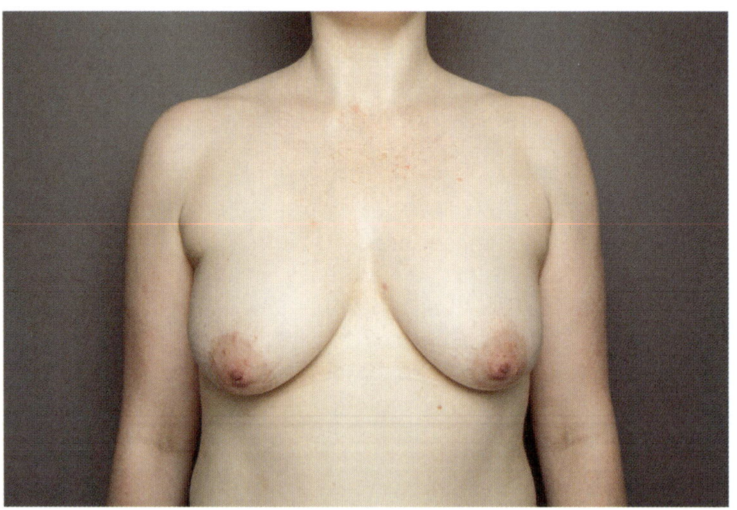

It's interesting to talk about breasts separately from the rest of my body because I have never conceived of them that way. When I look in the mirror I see an hourglass shape composed of my breasts and my hips. It is that line that I connect with. It's not a shape you would see on billboards as a perfect physique, although I like it. When I thought about this interview I realised I had never conceived of my breasts separately. When I perform and dress as a burlesquer, my breasts are just part of a reveal of many parts of my body.

Burlesque is a real litmus test for a lot of people in how they feel about women controlling and enjoying their bodies, or using them as a tool in an intellectual performance. Men are normally quite embarrassed to be there and they are not sure how they are supposed to react to a burlesque performance in front of other women. Women have a whole spectrum of responses.

After the performance you socialise at the bar and meet the audience. This group of young girls came up to me, and funnily enough one of them happened to be my bikini waxer. She has seen a lot more of me than I have of her! She is a beautiful young woman, she meets a lot of the standards of a beauty idol. She was saying, 'That was amazing. I would like to do some lessons, but I don't think I can perform. My breasts are too small.' I thought they looked perfectly in proportion, but she is slim. She leant in and said, 'You can see, all my friends have really big breasts, and I would love big breasts.' I had never experienced someone not doing something they want to do because of a perception about their breasts. The burlesque show she had just watched featured a woman who's had a mastectomy, with one breast, a woman in a wheelchair, and me, size 14, plus a woman in her 50s and a couple of men. So I thought, 'Where did you put yourself on the spectrum when you decided you couldn't fit in?' It was sad.

It's interesting how women react when they see a burlesque dancer who doesn't fit the beauty archetype. Very early on in my career, a young girl came up to me and said, 'It's so nice to see someone overweight do burlesque.' I'm not an orthodox beauty. She enjoyed the performance but was still policing it. Bless her, she was very inebriated. The comment was a double-edged sword. But it was her hang-up, not mine.

My mother's reaction when I took up burlesque was, 'What! Are you going to be taking your top off on stage?' I never thought I couldn't do it. I go down to nipple covers and knickers for some of my acts. I have friends who do full nudity, and some don't take off any clothes at all. Some burlesque acts are sensual, some are comedic. Sometimes if they use big fans they don't take off any clothes, it's tease and reveal, but no clothes come off. It's a different play on expectations.

In most of the venues I perform in, they don't allow nipples to be uncovered as they don't have that sort of licence. The reveal of flesh on show is a determining factor, so nipple covers get round that. In truth, burlesque and gentlemen's stripping clubs are worlds apart. I think the real difference between them is that men have a low opinion of women at strip clubs. They pay women to submit to their desire to strip for them. In a burlesque club you are performing for an audience, it's not one-to-one and it's not for arousal. It's a theatrical performance that has elements of sensuality.

Nipple covers can be part of the costume. For instance, in a Christmas act the nipple covers might be giant snowflakes, or in an act about eating cake the nipple covers might be cupcakes. Sometimes the nipple covers fall off by mistake, it's just one of those things. Normally the audience laughs if that happens. I have large areola. I couldn't trade nipple covers with other girls back stage, as theirs wouldn't cover my areolae.

Burlesque is part of the cabaret genre. It's subversive, a bohemian form of entertainment. It can be glamorous and feminine, political commentary, satire, any number of tableaux. You can see surprise at the end of the show, the women in the audience haven't felt threatened at any point. The body isn't reduced to a clinical object.

The boom of burlesque, following the success of Dita von Tees and Pussycat Dolls, has led to a new wave of performers who are part of pop culture, rather than the subculture that existed before. They are bringing in body image and self-esteem issues, and we are not used to that in burlesque.

Burlesque is not empowering in itself. You should be empowered and then you do burlesque. It is a literally and metaphorically exposing thing to do and if you are insecure off stage you will also be insecure on it. Newer performers are more aware of the male gaze. I have noticed that the demographic in some audiences is changing, and groups of men are coming on their own. So burlesque is facing some challenges at the moment.

It's hard to make money from burlesque. A lot of the new performers won't last the distance, it's hard to earn a living and their insecurities will push them out. The audience can sense insecurity in a performer. They won't respond positively if they sense you don't connect emotionally to your body. They won't 'boo', but you might get a gentle smattering of applause. Right now burlesque is in fashion, but it will go back to being a subculture again. It thrives on not being mainstream. In the longer term, sexualisation of society might be more of a problem for burlesque.

There are an awful lot of single burlesque performers. Does being a sexually confident woman intimidate men? I don't tell people what I do until I know I am definitely with someone I want to spend time with, because of the expectations it creates. They wouldn't get past it. The burlesque becomes their object of attention, not me.

Female burlesquers are the most confident I know. They don't waste time, and they don't need male attention, they don't crave it. But whenever we have social media profiles we are deluged with aggressive, sad individuals. Very sad, very lonely men, who spend their lives emailing women to tell them how pretty they are and trying to meet up with them. They think it's safe to approach you because you are a burlesquer. Social media gives them an impression of access and they assume you are open-minded. Men send you unsolicited pictures of their penises and vulgar language. They think if you take your clothes off on stage you must be a goer in bed.

Boyfriends have been wowed by the idea of burlesque while I am off stage and they love the confidence. But there aren't many boyfriends who will go and watch a performance. The ones who do are the ones who last. Men almost seem slightly cowed by it, as though the women are too confident for them. They can't cope with the confidence.

My breasts are important to me sexually, but not more or less than any other part of my body. It's interesting that men can be very clumsy about sensual eroticism. Breasts are always a great focus for men, and I have to show them that the back of my neck, the touch of my skin, are as sensual as my nipples. It's as if I have to train men to see my body as an erotic whole, not cut and pasted into body sections.

———————

Age 36 | No children

"I'm the one with the huge breasts, that's my thing"

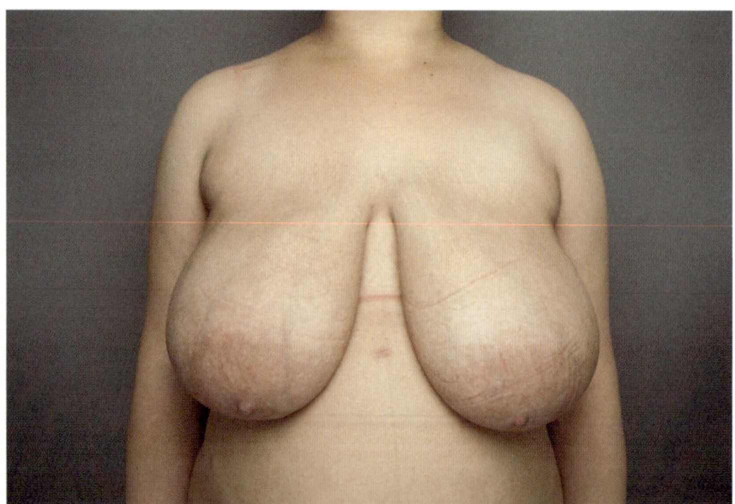

I'm the one with the huge breasts, that's my thing, and they are part of my identity. I'd like my boobs to be higher up. Realistically they couldn't be, it would be ridiculous. For my size and my age they are fine and I am quite pleased with them. I'm not prepared to go through the effort and cost of changing them, so I have to accept them.

I wouldn't have a redction. I don't think they'd go down to a level that would be much more manageable. They'd still be big, and it would be a serious operation. I don't have back problems.

People don't mention them immediately, but if I mention them later on, people tell me they noticed my boobs. I don't get rude comments, but they come up in conversation. I don't think it's a bad thing; maybe it's an odd thing to be proud of, but it's not something to be ashamed of. My breasts are noticed, but people get past them. That's the crucial thing, they aren't the reason people continue to speak to me.

I'm a 32HH. I've been reading the Everyday Sexism project on Twitter and it made me think that I don't get those comments. Or I worry that I am getting comments about my breasts and I don't notice! Perhaps I have a self-defence mechanism and I block out the sexist comments. I have a naturally angry-looking face and I think people wouldn't want to shout things at me. I think I have an intense look, and I walk tall, so I may look more confident than I am.

I think my race protects me from sexism in a way. I don't notice women of colour being retweeted through Everyday Sexism; maybe they would define their problems as racist, not sexist. This is part of my problem with feminism. It is often very white, very middle-class. So I might have had sexist comments about my breasts and just not taken it on board.

I am only 5ft 1in and quite busty. I think my build is meant to be smaller, but because of the breast issue I seem wider than I am. I know I'm not as wide as I think I am. There can only be so much on your frame, so my breasts go outwards, and it changes what I think my shape should be. My ideal cup size would be E or F – substantial, pert, but not as big as I am.

I wear clothes with stretch in. I've accepted that if I buy a top it will be a lot more cleavagey than it is on a mannequin, because the material won't cover as much of me. Luckily, because I am in an academic job I can wear something low-cut and it seems less 'dodgy'. I've never felt self-conscious wearing anything low-cut to work. My breasts are always going to be there, so people will see them – unless I strap them down or something ridiculous.

At a job interview I'd worry more if there was a woman on the panel that it would seem like I was showing off, a dolly bird coming in with my large breasts. It should be about my skills, but first impressions count. I think people have been taken aback by how I look physically, but I don't know if that's a racial thing, because they weren't expecting me to be mixed race, or because they're thinking, 'She's got much bigger breasts than me'.

When I meet any new woman I check that her breasts aren't bigger than mine. It's the one thing I have to have, the biggest breasts in the room. It's a positive part of my identity. But if they have got breasts as big as mine it's good because we can talk about how hard it is to get bras. It's not that I'll shut off a woman who has large breasts, but I do find myself eyeing up new people. It's become competitive, even though it's not something to be competitive about.

On dates I wear quite low-cut tops, but I don't know why because I don't want that to be noticeable. I've been doing some online dating recently, and I met up with someone. He said, 'Why didn't you mention on your online profile that you have large breasts?' I said, 'Because I'd get weirdos!' *(laughs)* It was bizarre, he seemed like an intelligent man otherwise. Did he think I should have warned him? I think he liked my breasts but he was thrown that I had them. When you put your profile up you put basic things like your height and your race, your interests. All my pictures are head and shoulders. I just think it would attract the wrong types, and it shouldn't be a crucial part of how I sell myself. You wouldn't ask a man to post pictures of his penis.

I don't think men have been great with my breasts sexually. They always concentrate on the nipples, because that's what they think the important zone is, but I don't have much feeling in my nipples. People think that because my breasts are big they will be erogenous, but they're not really. Maybe their sexual potential hasn't been unlocked! They don't know what to do with them, like it's a level of intimidation. Maybe I've just been with men who are like rabbits in headlights. Or maybe I just can't get that aroused by them.

I don't agree with the 'No More Page 3' campaign. Partly because the feminist in me asks why shouldn't they use their body to make money? Are we going to ban modelling or pornography? If that's how a woman can make money, why not, if they are happy doing it? It's not like prostitution or pornography where women can be forced into it. They don't get paid very well for it, so that is a bigger issue. I don't feel other people should belittle it. If a Page 3 model says it's a horrible scenario then let's re-evaluate it. It seems to be a better environment for the models than fashion modelling.

The Sun doesn't have the topless picture on Page 3 on a Saturday as it's a family edition, children may see it. That's an issue: why shouldn't children see breasts? They might have been breastfed, they may see their mother or sister naked. You can't protect people from seeing breasts, and why should they be protected? Maybe it needs to be looked at in a way, but not a blanket ban.

Page 3 doesn't reflect the ethnicity of the country at all. Are women of colour auditioning for Page 3? Or do readers not want to see black and Asian women on Page 3? Is it a cultural thing? I can't imagine an Asian Page 3 any time soon because of cultural norms, it would bring shame. My background is Jamaican and Jamaicans can be very conservative and religious. Maybe there aren't many women from a Caribbean background who would feel comfortable doing Page 3.

Maybe *The Sun* don't have many black readers, or think they don't. It's aimed at white middle-class men, in their 50s upwards.

Even high fashion agencies don't have many women of colour on their books. You don't see many black faces on the runway or in magazines. The mainstream isn't ready for people who don't look like them. But that's ridiculous, that is what we look like.

I didn't tell friends I was doing this. I told people I was busy but kept it mysterious. I didn't want anyone to put me off because I was excited about it. I didn't want anyone to think it was strange and put doubts in my head. The project was mentioned to me by a friend. It sounded really interesting and original. I want to say 'yes' to more things in life. I felt I could help people by taking part.

Age 25 | No children

"They're not bad, are they?"

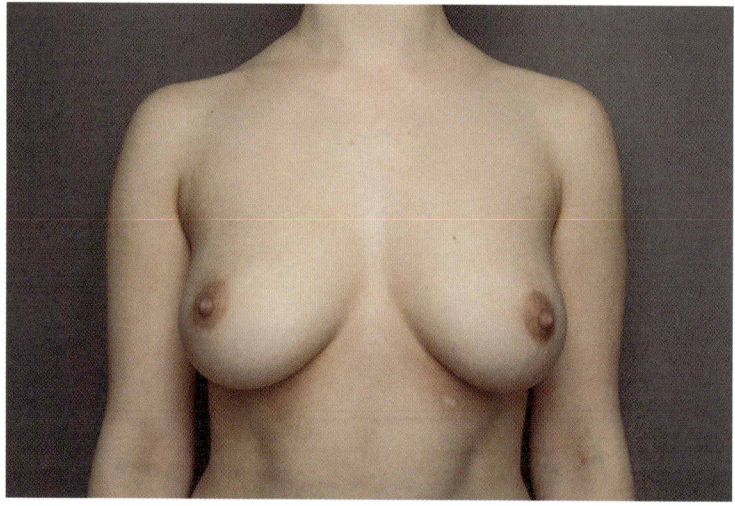

I like my breasts. They are a good size. They arrived early and I was afraid they would be too big, but they stopped. I've been told a few times they are the perfect size.

I don't get hit on much. I exude, 'Don't talk to me.' I just don't like it. I wore glasses till recently, when I had laser eye surgery. More than anything that has changed how people look at me. I think I would have had more sleazy attention if it wasn't for the glasses. But I'm not a girly girl. I wear trainers, and sports clothes, and I don't flaunt my boobs.

The girls were more powerful in the sixth form; they know they have power over the boys. There were quite a few girls who would flaunt themselves.

I'd say my breasts are important sexually. I prefer my breasts to play a part in sex, but the problem is guys get a lot of stuff wrong. I've only realised in the last couple of years that I want breasts to be a part of it, because before that it was clumsy. I don't always know how I want them touched. Men don't think about how it feels for women. They just grope for their pleasure.

Once I experienced really, really horrible hard sucking. It was, like, violent, it almost hurt. I think he thought it was nice. I never admitted that to anyone else! It was awful. I thought, 'What are you doing?' You know when you don't feel present, and you are looking at a situation? I think I was just looking, I became an observer. I only saw him for a little while when I was about 18.

When I was about 14 I had a cyst in my breast. I watched a programme about breast lumps and that night I had a feel and I found a lump. I ran to show my mum. The first doctor I saw was very young, quite nervous, she prodded me and said I was fine, but she just used her fingertips, she didn't examine me properly. She sent me on my way. We went to see another doctor and she referred me straight away. I had a biopsy, which hurt, using a really, really long needle. It was benign, but because it was big it had to be removed.

There was no crying – I was very excited about getting a week off school! I told one of my closest friends at the time I had a lump. I was worried he would laugh. He responded by telling me his mum had a lump on her big toe once. Exactly the same! *(laughs)*

I felt guilty because I was in a ward with three other kids who had cancer, having chemo, no hair. I was sitting there, all my hair, no cancer. I felt like I shouldn't be there.

I had a very ugly boob after the operation. It was bruised, yellow, brown and blue, with stitches. My friends were horrified, disgusted! *(laughs)* The scar has never bothered me since. The only time I cried was when they took the drain out. It felt like they were taking out something that went right through the middle of me. Maybe that's when all the emotion came out, because I had a crying session.

I had another biopsy recently; it's still benign. I still have the same lump, it hurts when I get my period. It's weird. It doesn't seem to be straightforward.

I'm comfortable taking my clothes off in front of my friends. I lived in Germany for a while and they are much more comfortable with nudity.

People swam naked in the river there. When I went on holiday to Croatia with my boyfriend, we went out for the day with Croatian friends, island-hopping on their speedboat. They said, 'We're going to be naked all day, do you care?' And we were all naked all day. It was so nice, so relaxed. Just jumping into the sea, finding little coves.

As a psychology graduate, I believe that breasts need to be more understood by men. They are a part of us which isn't necessarily always sexual. It would be nice to sunbathe topless without being perved on. It would be nice for girls who develop breasts early not to get beeped at by white vans. It happened to me, it happens to most schoolgirls. Forty-year-old men perv on schoolgirls. Why do men like breasts? Probably because they don't have them. Maybe it's just because they are told they are sexy. We sexualise breasts by covering them up with clothes, and wearing clothes that emphasise them.

____

Age 25 | No children

"I still hate my body, but I've always loved my boobs"

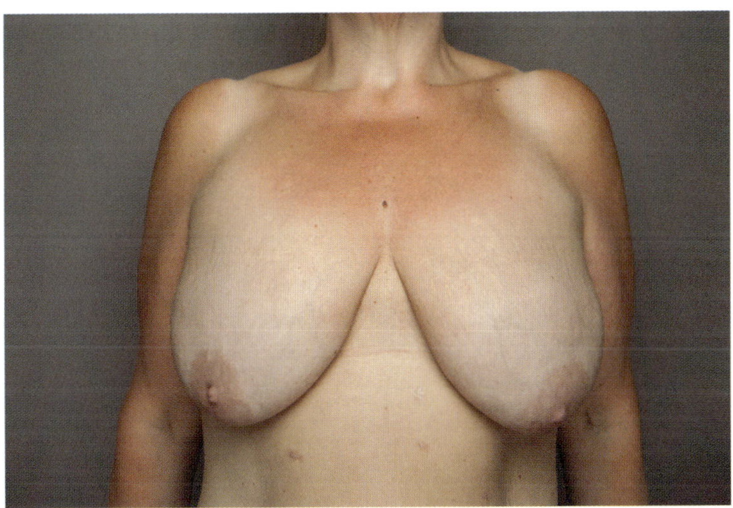

My breasts are old and saggy; they've seen better days. When I was younger they were gorgeous, perfect.

I love being well-endowed. My husband loves my boobs. I'm really bad about checking my breasts, but my husband is forever touching them. He is just boob-obsessed. He's dreadful. If I'm just about to put my bra on in the bedroom he runs up to me, and I'm like, 'Get off!'

I breastfed all three children. I would have liked more children, but my husband didn't want any more. Breastfeeding completely changes breasts, but I wouldn't have had it any other way. They are my children.

I'm also a lazy person, so it was easier than bottle-feeding.

Certain things are easier for the young today, and certain things are harder. There is much more pressure on them to look good. Celebrity culture is a bad thing. We want our children to have everything and we buy them too much.

Men of my age thought themselves lucky if they caught a peek of their dad's porn under the bed. With the internet you can click on porn easily by mistake, even without looking for it. When my eldest daughter was 17, she had sex for the first time. She's a model and she's beautiful. Afterwards he turned around and said to her, 'You haven't got a good figure, you're not like the porn stars.' Boys have huge expectations now. I'm lucky I have such a good relationship with my girls that we talked about it and I was able to say, 'What an absolute wanker. Don't be stupid, you've got a lovely figure. Forget him, he's a dickhead.' It was tragic. They are cruel and nasty, far worse than when I was young.

Things are different for girls now. Both of my girls are beautiful, but they are also quite respectful about themselves, they don't sleep around. I'm so lucky they are sensible. It's scary when you realise what the young get up to.

My other daughter knows she has good boobs and is absolutely striking, but she doesn't have a very good body image. Her friends tell her she has perfect boobs. Mind you, if you combined her body now with the confidence of women our age, it would be dangerous!

I had a gastric bypass about 18 months ago and I've lost 10 stone. I always said if I lost my boobs I would have plastic surgery, but they haven't shrunk at all. I thought they'd shrivel to nothing. I'd just want a lift, I wouldn't want anything put in. They literally cut and pull up, but it leaves you with a scar. It's a long way down the line, two or three years. We'll see.

I've been big all my life. I have three very thin sisters and a very nasty mother. From the age of seven she put it into my head that I was this huge person. I wasn't, I just had a bigger build. She gave me psychological problems, and I've achieved what she said and become a big person. Two of my sisters have bulimia. I definitely think this was because of my mother. At Easter she said to one of my daughters, in front of the whole family, 'You've put on a lot of weight.' She hadn't even said hello.

I still hate my body, but I've always loved my boobs.

———————

Age 49 | Three children

"My breasts are still intact. I am grateful for them"

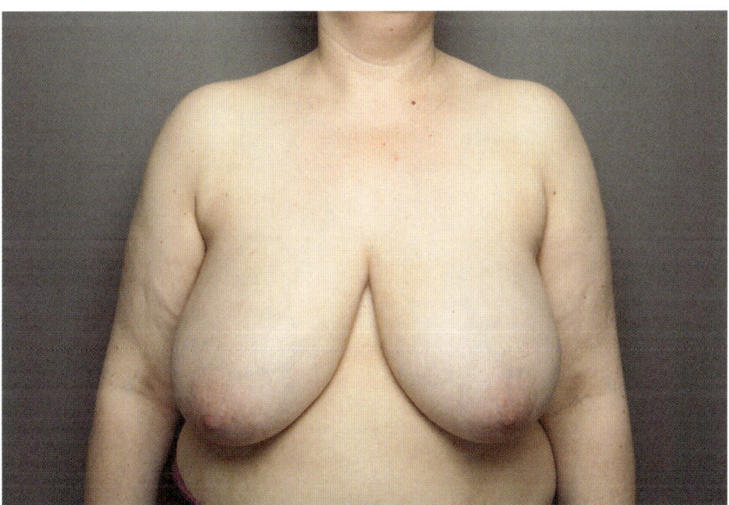

I feel differently about my breasts since my sisters, mother-in-law and sister-in-law have had breast cancer. My husband's mum and my sister-in-law sadly died.

I had to detach a bit from my sister-in-law's experience and death because one of my sisters was diagnosed at the same time, and it was too depressing.

A few years ago I would have liked them to be smaller and perkier; they just hang now. Since seeing what my sisters have been through, I think I am lucky I haven't gone through that. I don't feel that vain about them anymore. My breasts are still intact. I am grateful for them, grateful they are here. My sister used to call hers pendulous before her operation. We have to get it in proportion in our heads. They are here, I am here.

Cancer moved from my sister-in-law's breasts to her skin and ate away at her. I changed her dressings. It's so trivial to say my breasts are droopy. It doesn't matter.

I did worry about myself. I have annual checks. I have a mammogram and then angst till the results come. I don't worry quite as much now, I think it can make you ill just worrying. I check in between but the annual check gives me peace of mind.

I don't put a huge importance on my breasts sexually. I'm quite neutral about them. I quite often get my husband to check my breasts. My fear of checking them actually stops me from doing it. For us as a couple my breasts are more of a concern than sexy. That's how it's evolved.

For a while one sister had only one breast and it was hard. I'm lucky that I have two breasts to add shape. If someone said I was at risk of breast cancer and my breasts should be removed, I would be upset but I would accept it.

I don't know how it came about but my sister and I were trying clothes on. One of our daughters said, 'Your breasts are the same.' For some reason we decided to take a picture of just the breasts and see if our husbands could tell the difference. We thought it was hilarious, but I don't think they found it funny at all. They found it odd they were looking at our breasts. They guessed right. *(laughs)*

What's happened in the family has grounded my daughter. She got really upset about cosmetics advertising after her aunt died. 'How can they spend all this money on advertising when it could go to cancer research?' She wants to look nice, but she knows there are more important things than face cream. She found the grief difficult to handle, seeing her aunt ill and die, and then see her other two aunties with breast cancer. She still struggles with the grief. I am sure in the years to come she will turn it into something positive. I can see her campaigning in the future.

Age 41 | Two children

"At night, I use the left breast for the babies, and the right one is for sex"

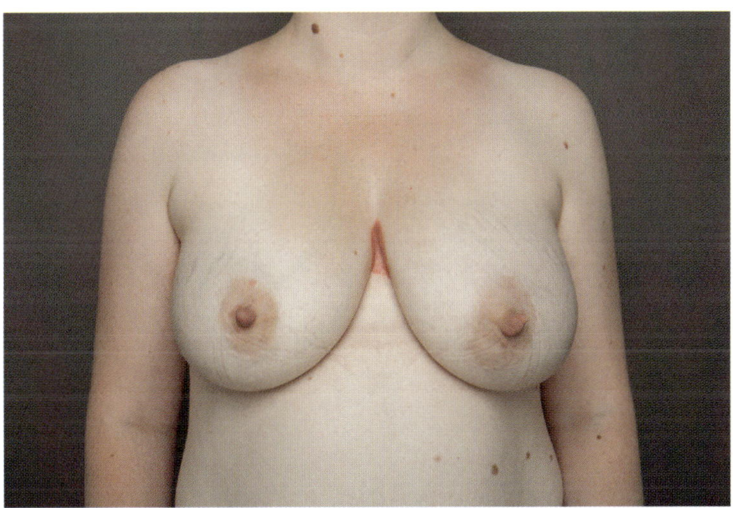

Before I had kids my breasts were one of my favourite features. They haven't been mine for a little while, so it's hard to know what I think about them now. They have a different use now.

They have changed a lot. They have stretch marks. My nipples are a lot bigger. Women see the changes in their breasts more than other people do though. I've had psoriasis for about six years, but it started on my breasts after my second daughter was born two years ago. I wasn't particularly stressed when it started on my breasts, in fact I was more relaxed this time round. It's between my breasts and underneath, in the crease. Every so often it's a bit itchy and uncomfortable, but I don't generally notice it. No one can ever see it when I'm wearing clothes. I don't wear low tops. I forget it during the day, it's just a bit itchy at night.

My son has just turned five and he was breastfed till just before he was four. I tandem breastfed my son and my daughter for seven months. She's two and she is still breastfeeding now. It was a great transition from one to two children. I have two boobs: my son was only using one boob, and the baby was on the other. He was really generous that way. *(laughs)* He didn't have to feel left out. In fact he took full advantage of the fact that I was sitting down feeding his sister, so he would come over and feed too. He was more of a daddy's boy at the time, but his interest in breastfeeding increased after my daughter was born. I could breastfeed him at night too and he didn't have to feel left out.

At times I felt a little 'touched out' – I didn't want to be touched for a while. But the tandem feeding really quietened down.

I have a photo of us in hospital when my son met the baby for the first time, and there is a teeny head breastfeeding, and a big toddler head. It did look kind of weird.

I started bra-fitting as part of a programme that was incentivising breastfeeding when I was in the US. I now have my own company selling nursing bras online and I do in-home fittings.

The majority of women are comfortable with me seeing their breasts. Some women leave the room to try the bra on and I might not see it on. It's harder to assess the fit if I can't see, but some people are self-conscious. I have pictures of me on my website in a bra. I don't like them, but who else was I going to persuade to pose for me?

I always really liked my breasts. They are a really sensitive part of my body, and sexually that's my area. My husband is a tits man. They still play a part sexually, but there is a bit of a weird crossover going on. I don't necessarily want my husband's bacteria from his mouth on my nipples. At night, I use the left breast for the babies, and the right one is for sex.

———————

Age 33 | Two children, breastfeeding two-year-old

"I've streaked at half time at proper big matches"

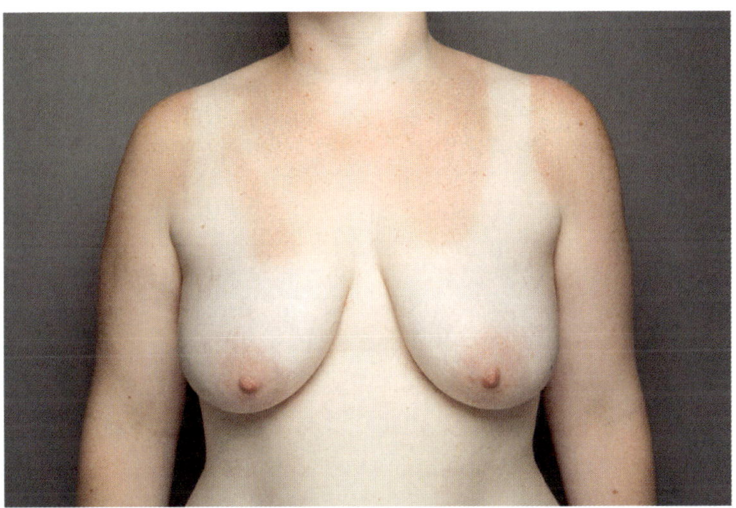

I don't mind my breasts. I don't mind getting them out. I streak at rugby tournaments and at my rugby club. I have a few beers, then anyone can dare me and I'll do it. I don't mind. You have to pick your moments so that everyone remembers it, normally after a few beers when everyone is outside having a cigarette. I've streaked at half-time at proper big matches, when you aren't interrupting the game. Then everyone gets a half-time show!

It's fun getting your body out. When I was younger I wasn't that confident in myself, and it's helped me get over fear of my body.

The first time I did it I didn't really have much of a choice. It was Valentine's Day and my birthday, and one of my teammates said, 'If it's your birthday you have to streak.' I was like, 'Really? You are taking the piss?' They said I had to take all my clothes off, but I was allowed to leave my shoes on because the floor was wet in the bar. I disturbed quite a few romantic couples with my naked body running through the club house.

One of the guys came up to me, and he said he wanted to do just one streak in his lifetime. 'Yep, I can see why you were sent to me!' I said. I told him to take one swig of his beer, take all his clothes off, and with no holding, no cupping, run across the field. Then I said we should walk back. I did it with him to give him confidence. It's about being accepting of the human body. I could tone up a bit more, but at the end of the day I can't be bothered.

I wasn't comfortable with the showers when I was 17. I knew who I was but I hadn't come out. They all knew though! I went through that for a year, waiting to come out. That's when the streaking occurred. I think I streaked because I had come out. Your teammates are your family, so whatever you do doesn't matter. They give you so much confidence.

Some of the younger ones shower in their pants. I don't think they are worried about lesbians. I think women feel that men will look at them more than lesbians. They are just nervous about their body being out in front of anybody. As a gay person you are conscious of not offending anyone and don't look at anyone, but straight people don't care and they look. *(laughs)*

There was a straight girl who commented on my pubes. I was like, 'What, you looked?' She knew what everyone's pubes were like. I said, 'Are you sure you're not bi-curious?' *(laughs)* She has that reputation now for looking. That came from a straight girl, but I wouldn't look, because I wouldn't want people to think I was coming on to them. I would feel naked without pubic hair. As long as you are clean and tidy it's good. I prefer to have a little bit.

I'm a 38DD. I have breasts! Obviously you need a really good sports bra. If you have a bad one it's all you can think about when you're running. They can be reinforced and pad you in, with a mesh to hold you in and protect you. When you tackle somebody you get them round the waist, not the breasts. It's only when you land you can hurt your breasts, but the bras can help with the impact.

It's our choice at the end of the day. If we want to box, play rugby, play netball, be a supermodel, it's up to us.

I used to play for Scotland. At my rugby club now, there are a few old farts who don't think women should play rugby. One of my coaches says,

'You know how I feel about women playing the sport, but I do threaten the boys with bringing you along to tackle practice. If you were a man you'd be in the First team.' I've seen such a change in 13 years. The guys are very supportive, and we watch each other. The guys play on Saturday and we play on Sunday. I don't like playing on Sunday. It's just ridiculous for us that team bonding is on a Sunday night and we have work the next day. It's a big commitment for us, more than the blokes. I think they should stagger the kick-off times. We have enough changing-rooms: we could play on the first team pitch at 12pm and they could play on it at 3pm.

I definitely enjoy my breasts being fondled during the act of sex. They are part of my body, so I love them. But my arse is my favourite part of my body. I'm into face, bums and legs. Whatever size women are is fine. I appreciate a nice athletic figure. I don't want to sound superficial, personality has to be behind it.

Guys say they like a good handful, but I like breasts to just fit in my hand. I do have chats with the guys. Some guys like them overspilling both their hands and get tucked in. *(indicates putting face into a cleavage)* Some men like them quite small and gently play with them. One guy said he liked a good handful to fondle when he's doing it doggy style. They like tit wanks. There you have it! They all seem to like boobs, but the obsession with breasts isn't as bad as women think it is. They love talking about women. In the rugby club they do talk about them like objects, but when the girls are there it's different. But it's the same with the girls. They talk about the guys just as badly. Maybe it's rugby club culture.

I hope everyone can accept their breasts. They're great, and there's a purpose for them, but they are sensual too. And if you don't like your breasts you can do something about it. But at the end of the day, someone will fall in love with you – because everyone is looking for love.

———————

Age 30 | No children

"People say they want to motorboat them"

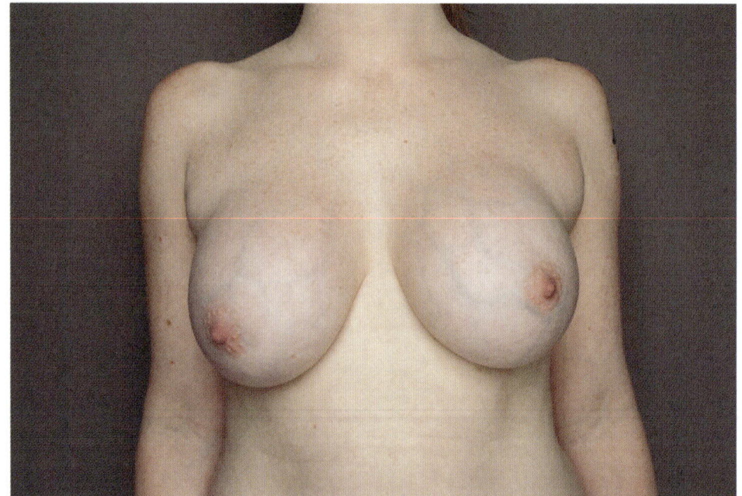

My breasts are pendulous. There are days when they get in the way, banging against doors. Because they sag, when my daughter gets into bed she'll lean on them and it can be quite painful.

After I had my daughter I had an episiotomy down below and it got infected. It wasn't very nice. I suffered postnatal depression as well. I put on just over a stone, and most of that went on my boobs. The stretch marks were ridiculous because my breasts were so big. The skin looked horrid, like chicken skin. My boobs were the only thing I could change. The surgeon wanted me to go to an F because there was so much skin, but I thought that would be too big, so we went up to DD. I didn't want the 'stuck on' ones that look like jelly tots. They're like a fake cake: nice to look at, but you wouldn't want to take a bite.

I only breastfed for a few weeks. I was a single parent at the time. My mum said she was on the breast all the time and other people wanted to hold her. She was a hungry baby. I'm pregnant again but I'm not sure if I'll be able to breastfeed this time with the implants. If I can, then I will definitely. I do think it's important that women try, there's no real excuse not to. It wasn't something that bothered me at the time I had the surgery. I'd just had a sprog, and I wasn't thinking about the next one.

I remember the very first time I looked down at them, and it was like, 'Oh my God, I have breasts again, what happened?' It felt like I had two little men on my chest. They were sore, but I didn't care because they looked good. It changed how I was feeling and my confidence.

My pre-baby boobs looked fake and I liked them best. If I lay down I still had a whiff of cleavage. They were pretty cool. I like the implants next best. I didn't like my saggy post-baby boobs.

I'll consider more breast surgery. What I would probably like to do is have them nipped and tucked, have them a bit smaller. There would be a lot of scarring, but they would be better. They take the nipple off, make the breast smaller, stitch it back. But if I have more implants, then there's only one way to go, and that's up. I don't want to be lugging two pendulous GGs around when I'm 60. I've seen pictures of older women with implants and it looks disgusting, really saggy skin and the implants hanging there.

When I look in the mirror I see wonky eyes, wonky boobs, massive teeth. I look like a rabbit. But I do quite like my breasts.

My breasts aren't mega-important to me sexually. I think they're good for tit wanks. I don't mind, they're quite enjoyable. The best way to do it is to get a bra that's got a little gap, then you can fit it between and do it that way. To be fair, it doesn't last long when I do it.

I'm a lap dancer. I don't think I'm planning on doing it anymore when I have the next little one. I'm 32 now and when I started this, I didn't think, 'Woohoo, I want a career as a lapdancer!' It was just a way to get some cash and meet some friends. Once everything starts going south, my face, my boobs … I don't want to be the oldest stripper in town. I think some customers notice. It's an industry based on looks.

I can't believe the attitudes of the young girls. They moan if they don't earn enough money, they think they are governing the bloody country or something. 'No, you just flash your gash for cash.' They're two a penny.

I was 22 when I started dancing. I had a breakdown and my mum took me on holiday. I couldn't face going back. I said, 'I can't deal with this shit now.' I didn't want people looking down on me or being over-sympathetic. I followed this Spanish guy to Tenerife, but he turned out to be a violent bully. I moved out, and I thought I could either go back to England with my tail between my legs or I could make something of my life, whatever that might be. I started PR-ing. A guy I liked was all over this lap dancer, so I decided to try it. I was a size six to eight, I had natural white blonde hair. I'd never even gone topless on the beach. I haven't looked back since. I've taken sabbaticals, but the minute a bill comes through the door and you don't have the money …

I was shitting it before my first lap dance, so nervous. I've always been a sensual dancer, but I was mortified when I did my first one, because the guy turned round to someone and said I was dancing too fast. And someone else said I didn't dance close enough. But I earned my first €50 note, so I didn't give a shit to be honest. I earn a bloody good living out of it.

The backlash you get from it is ridiculous. You'd think you were going out sucking off reverends! You're not beating children for a living, you're taking your clothes off in an environment that's safe. It's the younger women who wear too much make-up, and put pictures of themselves up on Facebook, who get nasty. People have called me a 'whore' and a 'sex worker'. I call myself an 'erotic gymnast'. It's not sex work, we're the 'warm up act' or one for the 'wank bank'.

Brasses and lap dancers should not work together. I've got friends who are prostitutes. If someone is going to pay you £20 for a dance, or nosh you off 50, there's no comparison for me. But it doesn't work in unison, there need to be boundaries. With dancing there is no touching, otherwise it's prostitution.

I'm quite a bitch. The moment someone comes into the private room with me I push them down and say, 'Spread your legs, bitch' with eye contact, and I take control. 'You sit there and shut the fuck up.' You have to believe it, otherwise they will try things, put their fingers up you or touch you. You are standing there stark naked. If someone touches you, you led them on. It's your fault, because you weren't in charge from the beginning. I warn people that if they touch me I will spear their bollocks to the chair. I've done it before. I used my heel to pin his trouser to the chair, I missed his skin by this much. *(indicates a few mm)* You have to have a mouth in this job.

Men love my breasts, they get good comments. People say they want to motorboat them and bury themselves in them. I take it as a compliment,

I never take offence. Some girls are bitchy and say they look fake. If men aren't sure I do this. *(moves breasts around with hands, making them wobble)* When I lick my own nipple, they're freaked out! I can hang my G-string on my nipples too. Occasionally I do it during a dance. I wear a push-up bra and take it off to dance. I take it off slowly, hold my boobs up and then slowly lower them down, so they don't suddenly drop down. I'm very suggestive. I'll put my fingers in my mouth, then look at their crotch, then put my fingers on my boobs. That makes them gasp. It's quite amusing. I get turned on slightly by the power. I am gobsmacked by the effect breasts have on men. 'You used to suck your mum's and now you love mine.' I put it down to comfort.

Having my boobs done made no difference to my money at all. I was quite surprised about that, but it doesn't work that way. Your looks attract them, but your personality keeps them, similar to a relationship. You can have stunning girls, but if they are up their own arses then they're not going to earn.

I think a lot of the guys are lonely. Some come in for respite. It's a treat, a bit of titillation, like a dirty mag, or getting a scratch card. Boobs and fanny. It wouldn't phase me if my partner had a lap dance; it wouldn't bother me at all. I organised the stripper for his stag night. But he says, 'Why go out for beefburgers when I've got steak at home?'

I think Page 3 is fab, I absolutely love it. It's a fucking industry, an institution: Sam Fox, Linda Lusardi, Jo Guest. All this women's lib, what's the point in burning our bras if we don't get our tits out? It's liberating for women. It cheers builders up, sitting there eating their breakfast.

The Sun does what it says on the tin. It's a paper for men. It's not a family paper. I don't find it offensive. What else are they going to put on Page 3?

Once a guy bit my boob. I swear to God, I have never punched anyone so hard in my life. It was a bit of a shitty club. I said, 'You kick him out or I'm going to fucking walk. Get him out now.' Eventually they threw him out. I think he must have detested women and thought it was OK to hurt me. There aren't as many of those as you'd think. And you normally find they are fat, ugly and old. It's a power trip for them.

Good-looking customers tend to be more arrogant. They think they would pull you in a club and they ask to meet you later so they don't have to pay for a dance. 'No darling.'

———————

Age 32 | One child, pregnant

"Sometimes I think they are too flat and nothingy"

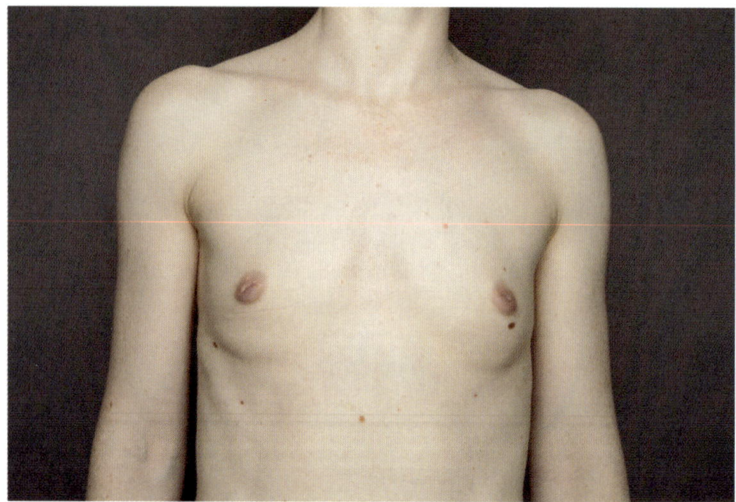

My breasts are very little. They're quite plain and they're white. Sometimes I think they are too flat and nothingy. I'm a 36AAA. Overall I am happy with them.

I pluck hairs off my breasts. I get short black hairs around the pink bits of my nipples. I have to do it about once a week. I think if I left them they'd go curly. They grow fast. I try to make sure they aren't seen.

I wear a bra because I want to be normal. Wearing a bra is part of being normal. I want them to look like a normal size, although really I am too small to look like normal. I also think they would sag more if I didn't wear one.

When I was pregnant I went to get a nursing bra at a fitter's house. But she said, 'They aren't really for people like you. They aren't for your size.' She didn't have any bras for me, although she claimed she could fit anyone. I was too small for a breastfeeding bra. That wasn't very nice.

My breasts were big when I was breastfeeding! They were hard and stuck out. Someone described them as 'melon-like'. Yay! If I could have kept them that size I would have. I think that my breasts are even flatter since breastfeeding, if that's possible. There's more skin than flesh.

I've got inverted nipples. One side was better for feeding than the other. It was a bit difficult. My nipples were quite painful for about a year. I got splits in them and bleeding. I was pleased I managed to breastfeed and it made me feel better about my boobs. Tick. Thank God for that.

It was hard to get my son to latch on at the beginning, I think because of the inverted nipples. I wish the hospital had given me more help. They just gave me a syringe to put drops of milk into his mouth. They could have been a bit nicer, but never mind.

My nipples are sensitive, but my breasts aren't. When I am aroused or cold, they come out for a short time, just as if they are feeling frisky! I find them helpful sexually. I've tried to find out if my partner likes them. I think he is just trying to be nice; he doesn't want to say they are too little.

Having little boobs keeps you shrinking away. You don't dress the same or act the same as other girls. It was awkward in the changing rooms at school. I would avoid the whole subject. I'd exclude myself from any conversations about boobs, bras and boys. I couldn't join in because I wasn't the same. I don't think anyone else was as small as me. In sport training you have to do press-ups so your boobs touch the ground. Which is really fair, isn't it? *(laughs)*

My breasts have definitely affected me. It starts with how I behave around people. I'm not as confident with other people. I don't feel equal. Small boobs really affect how people see you. I'd have been a different person if I was bigger: more outgoing, more comfortable. I think if you have bigger breasts you are more in charge, more matronly, more shoulders back, 'This is me', a ruler.

Age 34 | One child

"My first true love made me feel good about myself"

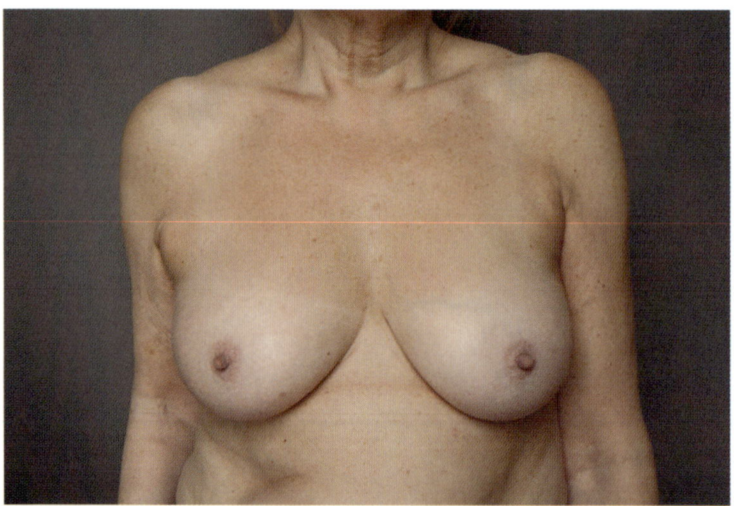

I love my breasts. No complaints.

My first true love made me feel good about myself and my body. He appreciated my breasts. I was always very shy and he brought me out of myself and made me feel good about my body. I wasn't fat, but I was teased by my brothers who called me 'fatty' constantly. He said I wasn't fat, and not to listen to my brothers. From then onwards I was much happier, and would even sunbathe topless. Before him I wouldn't wear a bikini. He made me realise you should enjoy your body no matter what shape and size you are.

My daughters' father would never touch my breasts and I would think, 'What's wrong with them?' I did ask him once and he wouldn't give me an answer. I thought it was strange that he never fondled my breasts, nothing at all. He wouldn't touch me when I was pregnant, wouldn't come near me. He never made me feel good about myself. He put me down.

I had a caesarean with my first daughter. I was out of it the first day, and the hospital bottle-fed her. And I knew I was going back to work quite quickly. She seemed happy on the bottle, so I didn't see any point in trying to breastfeed. Breastfeeding wasn't promoted like it is now. My sisters didn't breastfeed either, or my sisters-in-law, and none of my friends. It's encouraged now, they say it's better for the baby: maybe it is, but none of our children have had any problems being bottle-fed, so I can't say either way. Everyone to their own, that's what I say. Even my mother said it was my decision.

I would go braless years ago, but I have a thing about it now. My sister died of breast cancer. For about three years leading up to her death she would come in from work and take off her bra, saying her boobs were hurting. And I wonder now if it was a sign she had breast cancer. At weekends she would never wear a bra, she said it was uncomfortable. So now I think if I started not wearing a bra it might mean there was something wrong with my boobs. Even though I check myself and have mammograms.

I examine my breasts more now. Before I did it occasionally, but now I do it every week. But my sister was the first one in the family. I encourage my daughters to check too.

———————

Age 62 | Two children

"The only thing I see in the mirror which looks like I think it should, are my breasts"

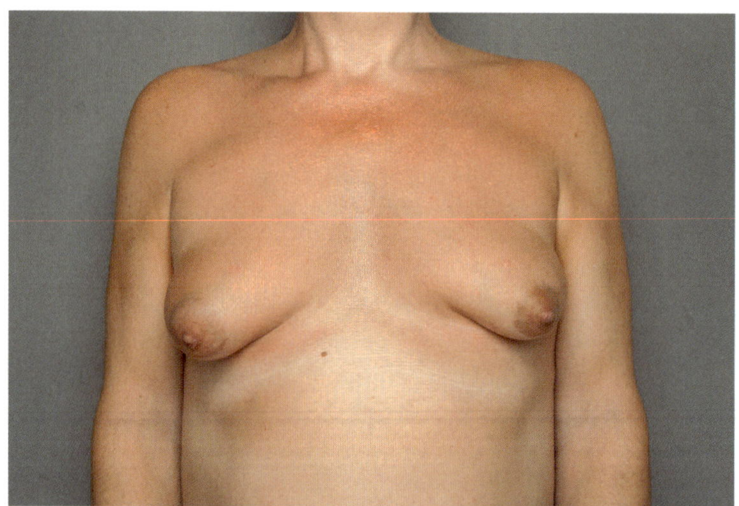

I'm partially transitioned. At the moment I describe myself as being in an androgynous state. Mentally I'm the same as I've always been, female. I hate those gender tick boxes with a passion.

I resisted being female very strongly. My father wouldn't have tolerated any expression of it. Life was very black and white in the 70s. I think my dad would have beaten me up and then thrown me out. That sounds harsh but it's what would have happened. So you bury it, to be safe. And it was scary because I didn't understand it.

You had to play rugby at my school, you didn't have the choice. I've always been quite sporty. I thought if I had to do it I'm going to do it as well as I can. It was quite blokey, but I did as much that wasn't blokey as I could. I was in the choir and poetry clubs. I think a lot of people thought I was gay.

I left school. In an attempt to get away from home and bury my femininity, I joined the Navy. Which meant I went from one worst-case scenario to another. At sea it was a nightmare, 24 hours a day in an all-male environment. In those days women didn't go to sea. Nobody ever used the expression 'gay', as it was illegal in the armed forces then. I think they just saw me as being different but they couldn't quite put their finger on why. Looking back I could see I was in very strong denial and hiding it from myself.

I went to the Falklands and marched across with a group of Marines because that's who I was attached to at the time. For months I was just scared. It was so far removed from reality that the gender thing didn't come into it.

I'm someone who never learns from their mistakes! *(laughs)* When I left the Navy, I joined the Fire Brigade. Another macho culture. Apparently this is a classic thing for gender dysphoric people. It's classic self-deception. I'm still in the fire service. It's one reason I am holding back on the full transition. Some people know. There haven't been any malicious comments, but that's partly because of the rank I am.

I went through a phase when I thought I was a transvestite rather than a transsexual, and I would cross-dress. It was hugely unsatisfying, it didn't solve the problem. Most transvestite men are happy being men. I realised it was about what was inside me.

To start with I removed body hair, but lived a 'proper' man's life. I met the person I am married to during that period. When we became serious I explained to her about my situation. She cut me off, and said, 'It's alright, I already sussed that out for myself.' I wouldn't have called it gender dysphoria then, but I knew I had issues. It made things easier.

You don't have to conform to a black and white image of gender. You don't have to be one or the other, you can be on a spectrum. But when I go to the Gender Identity Clinic I feel I need to make an effort to be feminine. The worry is if you don't look like you are trying hard to be a woman, you won't be taken seriously. It's total sexism. You're not a real woman unless you're going all out.

My wife fell in love with a person, not a gender. The most important thing about our relationship is being friends and soul-mates. But however open-minded you are, the idea of the person you are with transitioning is not the dream you have when you walk up the aisle.

We do have an active sex life. We had a bit of a heart-to-heart about my breasts, and she touches them now in that context. My nipples are erogenous and sensitive since having hormones. It's nice. It works on two levels, it's sharing with someone you love, and it's also an acknowledgement of my femininity.

I 'tick' bisexual. I don't think I can honestly describe myself as a lesbian, because of my androgynous state. Inside I see myself as a woman who is attracted to women. I went through a phase that my wife found difficult where we didn't have penetrative sex at all. She likes it, so she found it difficult, but I hated my body reacting as a male. I didn't like that 'obvious maleness' that occurs. I've been in a bath and seriously thought about taking a razor and cutting it off. I have to see a penis as a big clitoris. We do have penetrative sex now, but it's not what sex is all about, it's just what happens sometimes.

The only thing I see in the mirror which looks like I think it should, are my breasts. When my breasts started budding and were painful I was almost whooping. They will never be perfect and I've got some way to go. I've got a big male rib cage so they are further apart than they would be on a born woman. I'd like a more pleasing feminine shape.

About three years ago I went through a bad period of PTSD (post-traumatic stress disorder) and depression, it was very bad. I was in the Baltic Exchange. I still have nightmares and flashbacks. We went into the building and we hadn't been told it wasn't safe to search. It collapsed around us. We were in there for several hours, it was horrible. When we were coming out we came across the body of a young girl who had been killed. I had no reaction to it for about a year. The PTSD surfaced later.

I was also at the Soho Admiral Duncan bomb. The body of a woman that was killed there was also left in the road, uncovered. After incidents like that, the bodies are left in situ for forensics. It felt like a real violation. Both times I wanted to go to them and protect them. The two women at the two incidents had remarkably similar injuries. For a moment when I saw the body at the Admiral Duncan I thought it was a flashback to the Baltic Exchange.

I've been through two suicidal phases; taken overdoses and had to be resuscitated. My wife said she knew it was only a matter of time before I attempted it, but she didn't know how to stop it.

People double-take me in the street now. To start with only women noticed; now men do as well. When people first started looking it was a really positive affirmation. Sometimes it is a longer glance and that is more uncomfortable. Occasionally men look a bit aggressive. Women look more puzzled if I am out with my natural hair and no make-up. My face looks more feminine now. I used to have a very heavy beard shadow, and I've had that lasered. But it's by no means a feminine face. I look at it in the mirror and go, 'Fuck off!' But people have worse afflictions in life. At least I have nice legs!

Nobody knows all the details about this... My wife doesn't know about this. I was on a residential course. On the last night everyone decided to go out for a drink. There were these two blokes I had been aware of during the week. Quite early on they made a comment about my eyebrows being shaped. They made comments about me fluffing my hair too. I can't remember what I said, but along the lines of 'Wankers', and how exhausting it must be for them to be so in-your-face masculine all the time. They clearly didn't like it.

We all staggered back to the accommodation. I got ready for bed and went to the loo, which was up the corridor. If I hadn't gone my life would be so much better. When I came back I noticed them standing in the corridor. I remember feeling slightly anxious and uneasy. You tend not to linger in corridors, don't you? As I walked past them they grabbed me. At first I thought they were going to rough me up a bit and prove how masculine they were, retribution for me insulting them in the pub. But they dragged me into a bedroom. They were insulting me, called me 'poof'. I wasn't transitioning then, but they were making comments about me being effeminate. One was holding me and one was punching me from behind. It was shocking. It froze me.

Then they started saying I needed to learn what it's like to be a proper man. One of them pulled off my shorts. At that point I realised what they had in mind. I froze, I didn't fight, or shout or scream. *(cries)*

I was pressed face down into the floor and one of them was on top of me, pinning me down. The other bloke did what he did, which was basically, you know ... He raped me. Physically it was painful and horrible, but he was also saying stuff the whole time, insulting stuff. 'You poof, you need to learn how to be a proper man. You fucking sad tart, playing with your hair.' That sort of stuff. How did that teach me not to be effeminate? I would have liked to shout, 'I don't want to be proper man,' but I didn't talk at all.

I didn't want to report it or tell anyone. You think it's your fault, you didn't put up enough of a fight. I felt dirty, violated.

Age 52 | One child

"We are goddesses, we create life"

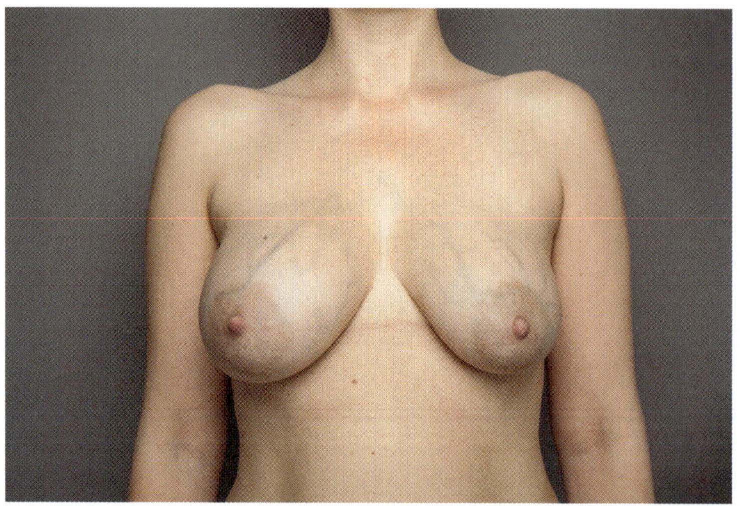

I love my breasts. I am very grateful for them. I think they have their own intelligence. Now I am a mother and breastfeeding, I have watched my baby grow from eight pounds to double that, purely from what my body has made for him. It's totally incredible to see him come from my body and watch him grow.

I think the body in general has its own intelligence. I probably didn't realise how much until I had a baby. It's not just an object, there is consciousness to the body.

It's difficult to remember how I felt about my breasts before I had my baby. But I wrote a poem about breasts nearly 10 years ago and that shows I thought there was an intelligence to them then.

I had some lumps when I was 19. I went to the doctor and she asked if I was doing enough of the things I liked doing and I realised I probably wasn't. So I went off and did more yoga and writing, and that definitely helped. She was unusual, an Indian lady, and she was spot on. So I have that kind of 'conversation' with my breasts. I had irregular periods and my breasts would tell me when I was coming on, and tell me when I was ovulating. My breasts give me signs, it's like a conversation.

My mum has a breast lump now. My aunt died from breast cancer, and there is also ovarian cancer in the family. So that's a bit worrying.

I was an A cup before I was pregnant and now I'm an E. It's how I knew I was pregnant. I knew about four days after I conceived because my breasts grew and I felt sick. I'd been pregnant and had a miscarriage before so I recognised the signs.

My sister who is 10 years younger than me has been considering breast enhancement. I wouldn't want her to anyway, but seeing how much I've grown I've told her not to. She can't know how her body will evolve after she has a baby, and also it could affect breastfeeding. My mum says to me, 'I can't believe you've got boobs now!' Whatever happens when I stop breastfeeding, I can't believe they will go back to an A.

I haven't had sex since I had him, which is four months now – not because we don't want to, we just haven't had a chance. Before, my breasts were very much part of sex for me. I would find it hard to orgasm without my breasts being stimulated in any way. I don't know if being bigger will make me feel more sexual or not.

My husband said he doesn't remember them being smaller. I don't know what's going on in his head. Before I was pregnant he said I had the nicest breasts in the world, and he wouldn't lie about something like that, he must have thought it. It was really nice and confidence boosting. He has said they are definitely saggy now, and that I'm like a cow now. I said, 'Why am I like a cow because I am making milk, why can't I be like a human making milk?' But that's just the normal association, people tend to drink cows' milk.

He hasn't said it out of nastiness, it's humour. He has a lot of respect for what I went through initially with breastfeeding. He knows the benefits as well. He's only being silly. But I do find it interesting that humans associate milk with a totally different species.

I've been a vegetarian since I was eight, but since having my son I switched to totally non-dairy. I really know now how hard it would be to have your young taken away from day one, and have constant mastitis. The first six weeks of breastfeeding were way more painful than birth. And artificial insemination is kind of like rape really. I think having a baby has raised my vibrations. I've always been conscious of things, but more so now. I always liked cheese a lot, but now I don't miss it. Apparently we consume a lot of carcinogens through dairy as well.

Because I am still breastfeeding I feel like we are one entity, I don't feel we have totally separated as two people yet. There is something that goes on between his body and needs and my boobs, and I don't know how to describe it fully. In its rawest form it is supply and demand, but I think it's more than that.

I tried going to yoga recently. After about 45 minutes I felt my baby was crying and said I had to go. I walked home as fast as I could, holding my boobs because it would hurt to run with them. I got back home and just as I was walking through the door I got a text from my husband asking me to come home. I asked if he had been crying for seven to eight minutes and he had. I am sure I had picked up on his crying somehow, I knew he needed me. I wonder if I could have been like that if I wasn't breastfeeding. I think breastfeeding maintains a physical link.

'Biological nurturing' is an amazing position for achieving a deep latch. One of the main reasons women give up breastfeeding is because they can't achieve a deep latch and their nipples are sore. When my son came off me and my nipples were misshapen and sore I knew it was a latch problem, but the midwives told me it was fine. I phoned a lactation consultant in tears one night because I needed help. She was really kind and spent time with me on the phone explaining biological nurturing, which is when he sits up, goes astride my leg, I lean back a bit, and gravity makes him open the bottom lip and open wide. When they are tiny they bob around a bit like a kitten or a puppy. Because they are doing it themselves they get it right, rather than when we try and force them on. I don't know why the NHS midwives and health visitors don't promote it. The position also avoids reflux. You can do it from birth, babies can crawl up you and find the nipple. I wouldn't do it because because it is quite full-on, I'd feel it was a bit cruel, but they can do it, it's amazing. I was so keen to tell you about it because it's a shame it's not more widely known.

I don't have stretch marks on my tummy but I do on my breasts. I think it's wonderful, it shows how my body changed to grow another person. Any changes are part of the story of my body.

What used to turn me on most was that ultimately the drive from the man I was making love with was to procreate, even if that wasn't on their mind. I think we are goddesses, we create life. My breasts are part of the ability to be a goddess.

———————

Age 31 | One child, breastfeeding four-month-old, breastfed on one side before the photograph

"One is quite shy. One is like a roaring teenager and up for anything!"

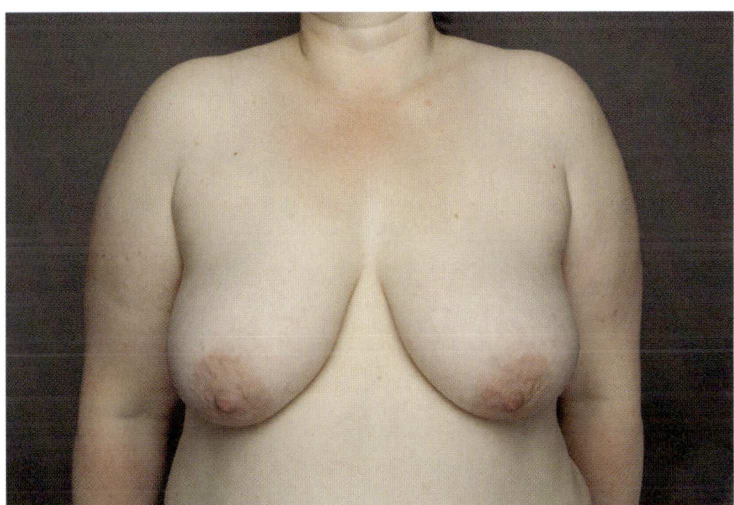

I'm not sure how connected I am to my breasts now. When I had children I felt very connected to them because they served such an amazing purpose. Now they are just part of my shape.

They're great for sex! *(laughs)* That's probably their main function now. They are erotic, and sensitive and sensual. One breast is much more sensitive than the other. One is quite shy. One is like a roaring teenager and up for anything! The other one is more considered and she likes to have a cup of tea and take it nice and slowly, and then she eventually turns into a raging teenager later. I can't believe I just told you that! It's just general sensitivity, they are wired differently. I think it's connected to brain functioning.

The sensitivity from my breasts is very important to making love, and they are important to my husband too in a very tender way.

When I was breastfeeding I had copious amounts of milk, it was obscene, I could probably have breastfed twins. When I went back to work I froze expressed milk but I was dubious about it - it can't taste as good! *(laughs)* My next child didn't really want to be breastfed at all. Even now she doesn't like milk much. We had a fight for about 12 weeks, I wanted to do it for that long so she would have immunity, but then I just didn't want to fight her. She constantly turned away, fought me, she was colicky, and preferred a bottle. Then she became a hungry baby.

I didn't feel rejected, she just knew in her own body what she wanted. I was a bit sad, I did want to breastfeed her, but we came to a mutual agreement. She was distant from me, it was like she didn't want to bond with me, she was a daddy's girl. As she gets older, she really needs and wants me, so she knows I am there for her. When she was younger if she fell over and hurt her knee, she would always want her dad, but now she says she tells me everything. My son was a complete mummy's boy, but now he has unlatched himself. They balanced each other out!

As a nurse, I've noticed that a lot of women have smelly breasts. It's the first thing that comes to mind. On the surgical ward, women would get thrush under their breasts where they were hot and sweaty, that was quite a theme. I had to wash women and treat under their breasts. Being on antibiotics makes you more susceptible to thrush.

My body image has been affected by seeing lots of naked men and women while nursing. Bodies are just bodies, you don't judge them because you see so many. I've seen how different everyone is. In an ideal world I might want my body to be a bit different, but it's my body and there's nothing wrong with it. I think nurses know how amazing the human body is, and they might have better body image potentially.

All old women's breasts go the same way. It's not bad, it's natural. They do go downwards, like material, like a sheet, with the breast tissue just hanging. Mine felt a bit like that after breastfeeding, when you deflate.

They sell wired bras for girls as young as 10 and 11. They don't need a wired bra, I think it's disgusting. Some of my daughter's friends wore shaped and padded bras when they were budding. 'But you're 10, you're a little girl, you don't need that shape!' People buy them because that's what in the shops so they think that's what you do. I think when you are growing is too early for matching knickers, wired and shaped bras. It will make her look more sexually developed than she is and make her vulnerable to a situation she isn't ready for.

It's hard to find bras which aren't padded – apparently nipples have to be hidden! We have such confused, mixed-up messages. You can find pictures of women everywhere, but we mustn't show our nipples.

Girls' magazines show girls in these little crop tops. They are kind of alright, they feature normal people, but they are all slim, not hugely curvy, and then there are the models. I had to explain to my daughter, and my son as well, how much photoshop it takes to make them look like that. It's sunk in now. I think looking at perfect images all the time is hard work.

———————

Age 40 | Two children

"I had plenty of unwanted attention in the typing pool"

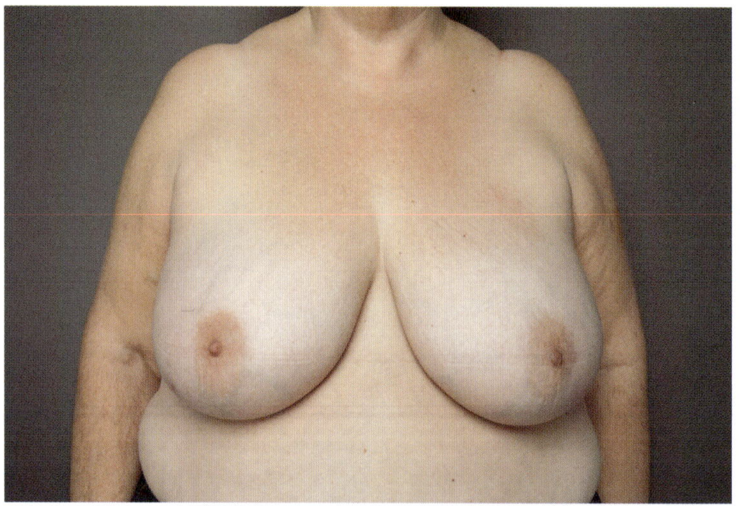

I've always liked my boobs. In fact, they're the best part of my body. They've always been a good shape. Obviously when I was younger they were an even better shape. My husband says they've always been a good size.

There wasn't the range of bras in the 60s. You went to a haberdasher's shop, you couldn't try them on, you just bought a bra you thought was your size. They weren't comfortable, and they had tight straps, not elastic ones. They used to cut into you quite a lot. Unless you went to Rigby and Peller – that posh shop in London – you never got a fitting.

The bra's purpose was to give you a good shape, which was pointed, very pointed. Almost Madonna-like. I remember my English teacher at school had the most pointy pair of breasts I have ever seen, even I couldn't help looking at them, they were so pointed. We've gone for a more natural shape now, bras are more comfortable now.

My mum wouldn't have taken me for my first bra. It was very different then. My mum said to me on my wedding day, 'Is there anything you need to know about?' You didn't discuss breast size, periods or anything. What she probably did, knowing mum, was to buy one, leave it on the bed and say, 'You're wearing that now.' I had two bras, one in the wash and one wearing. And you wore them till they wore out and got replaced.

I didn't have a serious boyfriend till I'd left school and was at work. I didn't think I was very pretty, I didn't have the confidence. They'd go in for a feel on my breasts. It wasn't the done thing, because it was that era, and I was a nice girl. But I quite liked it. A nice tingly feel, a pleasant feeling. But I was frightened it would lead to other things and contraception wasn't around. The 60s didn't come to this town! The buses stopped at half past nine and there was nowhere to go anyway.

My husband and I have had a good sexual relationship. That's why I've kept him around! *(laughs)* I think my breasts have been important for him. I liked a cuddle, even if there wasn't full sex. A hand coming over in the night was nice.

In my younger days I had comments at parties, like 'Ooh, they're a nice pair', from men, usually when they were drunk. I was quite chuffed. Everyone likes a compliment don't they?

I had plenty of unwanted attention in the typing pool in the office, especially in the early days. You used to get blokes leaning over you. The manager of the typing pool did it and touched my breast. Was it an accident? Now I'm older I know it wasn't, it was inappropriate touching. You know it's wrong, you have to deal with it straight away. Because I'm tall I have a physical presence. If I felt that someone was being a bit of a lech I'd stand up and move towards them and they'd back off. He'd get the message. Because it was the typing pool there were lots of women around me and that empowered me.

———————

Age 64 | Two children

"The piercings make my boobs look pretty"

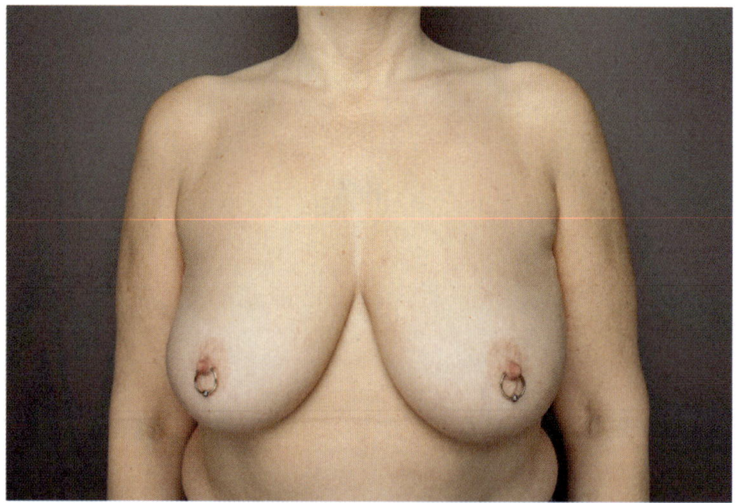

I'm OK with my breasts, I like them. I feel comfortable with them. The only thing I am unhappy about is that they're lopsided. When I look in the mirror one appears slightly higher. If I put on weight they're fuller, but if I lose weight it's more noticeable.

I got my nipples pierced about 15 years ago, in Camden. I had them pierced for me, not for anyone else. I think they make my boobs look more pretty. It was a bit of a dare with my husband. He was going on a lad's holiday and said, 'Don't get them pierced when I'm not there.' So I put two fingers up really, and got them done. The first one wasn't too bad because

I didn't know what to expect, but the second one was excruciating. They clamp the breast and then it's pierced with a needle.

When I told my husband, he didn't believe me. He didn't think I'd have the courage. When I first had them pierced I had to sleep with a bra on. No one could come near me, the pain was horrendous. I must admit, it was me being stubborn that kept them in. It was me saying, 'I told you I could do it.'

They hurt for nine months when I had them pierced, and it was more painful around the time of ovulation. They would leak a white fluid, almost like milk. I don't know whether it was to do with the menstrual cycle. I had a full hysterectomy at 40; that could have a lot to do with why I don't get the leaking anymore.

I'm pleased I had it done, but the piercings I've got are the originals. I'm too scared to change them, because of the pain, and also in case I can't get them back in. I'm getting to the age where I'm thinking, 'Why have I got them, am I too old now?' I had them done in my early 30s and I'm 46 now. I feel I should take them out, but my husband's like, 'Oh no, keep them!' He thinks they're pretty.

I'm quite proud of them. It's funny, when I have been topless on holiday people have stared. You see women with one nipple pierced, but you don't often see women with two.

I got tattoos and nipple piercings at the same time. It was self-expression, a bit of 'me' coming out. My first marriage was when I was very young and I wasn't allowed to do anything. I married my second husband when I was 30, and I was allowed to be me. I used to colour my hair crazy colours too.

My breasts can be an important part of my sex life, depending what mood we're in. We don't just ignore them. They are more sensitive and sensual with the piercings. I have to be careful not to catch them because it can be painful if they are pulled.

My daughters were quite shocked when I had them done. My elder daughter had one, but she took it out during her pregnancy because her boobs became so swollen that the nipple piercing almost disappeared. It didn't affect the breastfeeding, but you can't breastfeed with them in. She won't have it done again.

My piercings show through clothes sometimes, depending on the bra I'm wearing. It does show through more in the summer, when you're wearing T-shirts. It doesn't bother me, but it bothers some of the girls I work with, they say it looks like I've got four nipples. They have more of a hang-up than I do.

My breasts can get me more attention from men, they're quite a thrill in some ways. I'm not ashamed of them, and when I tell people they don't believe me! Same with my tattoos, they are quite a shock factor. Men look like they've got a smile on their face. I think they like it because not many women have got it done.

I gave up breastfeeding after a week. I didn't produce enough milk, maybe because I was very slim or because I was stressed. I really wanted to breastfeed, but for some reason I couldn't. It was very painful for me as well. I went on to the bottle. I just gave up, I didn't see the point.

Personally, I don't like very large boobs. I find they overtake the image of a woman: all you see is boobs. On the other hand, I feel for people who don't have any boobs. I don't know how they feel, but I think when you look at a woman with hardly any boobs it can look quite manly.

I like Page 3! I don't skip it, I enjoy it. I like looking at the face as well as the breasts. I find it interesting, no jealousy or envy, just thinking 'She has a nice body, nice boobs, nice face.' I'm open-minded enough to look at things like that, it doesn't embarrass me.

I don't know why we're interested in looking at other women's breasts, whether we're thinking, 'Are ours like that?' All the Page 3 girls are young. It would be interesting if you had an older generation Page 3! *(laughs)* I probably wouldn't look actually. I've never had pert boobs like some of them.

Breast implants scare me in some ways. I'm not unhappy enough with my breasts to have surgery and I just don't think they look natural. But, if it makes that person happier … You hear about them leaking, health problems. I know a few people who have had implants and they were unhappy with the shape, it didn't go right. One friend had terrible trouble with infections, she had to have it done again to correct the problems. That scares the life out of me. I wouldn't put my body through that just for my boobs. I'll let nature take its course. If God had intended us to have false breasts, he would have given them to us! I'm not against other women having them done, but I don't think there should be a need for them.

My elder daughter would consider it. In the family she's got the smallest. We've not made fun, but we have said she's not got our side of the family's boobs, and we probably have made her conscious of it. I wouldn't like her to have it done, because of the risk factors. I'm not sure it's safe.

I never think of my breasts as being big. But if I wear a tight top, men have said, 'You've got a good pair, a big pair.' I take it as a compliment, I like it. I had comments from strangers like, 'Nice tits!' when I was younger. I don't like that, I find that offensive. I think, 'Are you just seeing my boobs, are you not seeing me, my eyes, my hair, who I am?' I'm not theirs to comment on. It could be one reason why I cover up. My personal opinion is that when you see older women, they shouldn't have them flopping out. It doesn't look nice.

I've always joked I don't need to have a boob job done. I could put string through my piercings and lift them up and that would give them an uplift! *(laughs)* They're not small, and I wouldn't want them bigger, but they have lost that pertness and it's that, if anything, I would want back.

———————

Age 46 | Two children

"I was reborn as a 'Drag Goddess'"

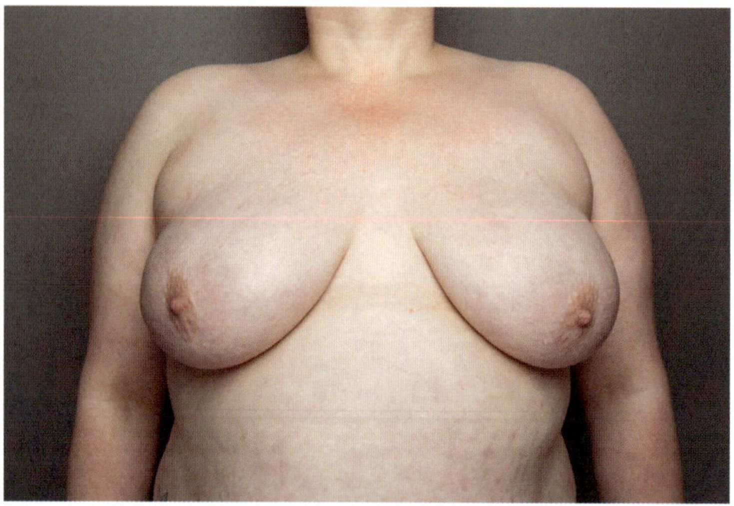

I won't have children so I'll never use my breasts. They aren't part of my identity. They aren't erogenous. There have been times they have hurt because they are quite big. I'd rather not have to wear a bloody bra.

I define myself as queer. There havebeen times in my life when I would rather have been male. I would have found it easier to be a trans male person and have my breasts removed, because they are such a huge signifier of so-called femininity. Over the years I have accepted who I am, and I don't feel the need to transition. I am happy being a biological female. I don't choose to identify 100 per cent as female. I have the breasts and genitals of a woman, but internally lots of parts of me are more male. If I could have waved a magic wand I would have removed them in the past, but now I have accepted they are part of who I am, and I like who I am.

I really thought about transitioning. I get mistaken for a man in my day-to-day life a lot. I get called 'Sir'. I have a lot of facial hair, I have to shave every day. Maybe it's my size, my hair, the fact I don't wear any make-up during the day, or the way I hold myself, I don't know. People have looked at me funny in the toilets. It offended me sometimes when I was younger, but now I don't care about other people's hang-ups about gender. It's their issue not mine.

I left school at 16 with nothing. I discovered drugs, sex and rave. My parents put me under the typical heteronormative pressure, 'You will grow up and have children, that's your life'. School said, 'Go and do a menial job, that's all you're good for'. So I spent a lot of time ignoring all that and getting high. Then one day I woke up and needed security. I joined the army for two years.

When I was in the army my breasts were very small. I was fit and lean. At the time I thought I was straight. I knew there was something different in me, but I pushed it down. There were dykes everywhere in the army. I was always very aggressive towards lesbians, because I was fighting my demons. Then I came out of the army and finally thought, 'What the hell am I doing?' I came out of the army and came out of myself.

I did a photography degree and I got into art and critical thinking. I became a professional dominatrix for a while. I worked as a receptionist in a brothel for a while. I was an assistant on heterosexual porn. My artwork was very sex-influenced. At the same time I was coming out properly, so it was a creative and sexual evolution.

The porn photography was quite strange. Women would do a 'single pinkie', where they pull their outer labia away, or a 'double pinkie', which would be pulling the inner and outer labia back and showing the vagina. Apparently this is what men want to see in porn. I decided to subvert this for my degree and take photographs of men showing their arseholes. The college hated it, obviously.

I was a dominatrix for 10 years. It's like theatre, you constantly have to be creative. Mainly men, but occasionally women. There was no sex on my part, but they could do what they wanted to do at the end. It was about exploring the mental, rather than the physical.

I would use my breasts as a teasing tool. Ten years as a dominatrix taught me that men are very easily turned on. You could tie them up and literally brush past them, lean in to them a bit. 'Ooh, breasts!' Straight away a penis-brain reaction. Bless their hearts, much as I adore men they are very visual and very easy. Women are much more cerebral and more effort. None of my clients ever saw my breasts. I wasn't a huge one for traditional outfits. Everyone else would wear leather and latex but I had a smart, business-like, stern headmistress look.

A lot of women know if they want something from a man their breasts are a tool to use. As a dominatrix I had what I wanted: they were subjugated and under my spell. I don't feel any regret for using my breasts to do that.

Men are very childlike in their approach to breasts. They don't know what to do with them, and they play with them like dough. They do that adolescent thing of snogging you and going for the tit straight away, like a textbook progression. Men are more needy with breasts than women; they want them as a nurturing, mothering thing.

I don't have any erogenous feeling in my breasts. I love breasts, but my own are just lumps of flesh, they have no sensitivity. I had them pierced years ago, and I was told that can increase sensitivity. It didn't do a damn thing. I haven't written them off, I have tried to enjoy them.

I moved to Vienna to be an artist. I thought it would be decadent and fabulous. It was there I started gender-bending and performing. The timeline of my work went from sex to S&M and gender. I was reborn as a 'Drag Goddess'.

I am a female drag queen, or a 'Tranny with a Fanny', or a 'Drag Goddess'. I saw some really bad drag queens, and thought I could do that. People said I couldn't because I am a woman, but I thought, 'Why not, gender isn't black and white'. I also think some drag queens are really misogynist. It's sad that someone who is emulating a woman, a fabulous, over the top, larger than life woman, can be rude about women. 'Ooh, it's really fishy in here, there must be some lesbians!' That was one of the main things that inspired me to do what I do. I thought, 'Hang on, you're wearing a frock. Why are you being so insulting to women?' I fucking loathe the definition of 'fishy'. I hate it. Defining a woman by saying her vagina smells of fish is vile, hugely derogatory.

I've had gigs cancelled when people find out I am a woman, because they want a man in a dress. I come across it a lot. But I'm like, 'Were you entertained?' I think promoters under-estimate their audiences, they think they only want a straight switch over.

There's also fear. If you listen to young, cackling, gay men talking about women, they have a fear of the female. They think we have teeth down there. They have been conditioned to be far away from the female, so their sexuality is trussed up in their own genitals. Men have to be masculine and they fight their own femininity almost. There is a huge amount of misogyny among gay men.

There's an idea that drag performers have to have big tits, and I am lucky that I work in a community of queer performers who don't wear bras, or don't tuck; they just wear a wig and a dress. They don't necessarily feel they have to have breasts, and that makes me more comfortable that I don't need to display my breasts.

When I dress in drag I wear more supportive bras than in the daytime. During the day I wear sports bras or T-shirt bras, but when I am working I wear supportive bras and hold them up a little more, to improve the silhouette. That's not for anyone else though.

In the US a lot of girls, biological women, use their breasts as part of their act. I choose to hide them completely. In the US they are called Faux Queens, but I am not fake anything.

In my work I like to leave something to the imagination. If I get my tits out they instantly know, this is what I am. But the whole purpose of what I do is to make people question what they think they know about gender. I used to sit in a window on a high street to do my make-up for two hours. People walking past would be watching me in various states of drag. The reactions of the public were fascinating. 'Is that a man? Is that a woman?' For me it was interesting to see how they perceive gender. Why should it be have to be binary?

My tits are quite inhibited and shy, they don't come out very often. Ten years ago I wouldn't have done this, but now I am more relaxed about my breasts, more ambivalent. They're just tits. Today is the first time I have got my tits out for anybody! *(laughs)*

———————————

Age 37 | No children

"I used to dream a lot about being naked in public"

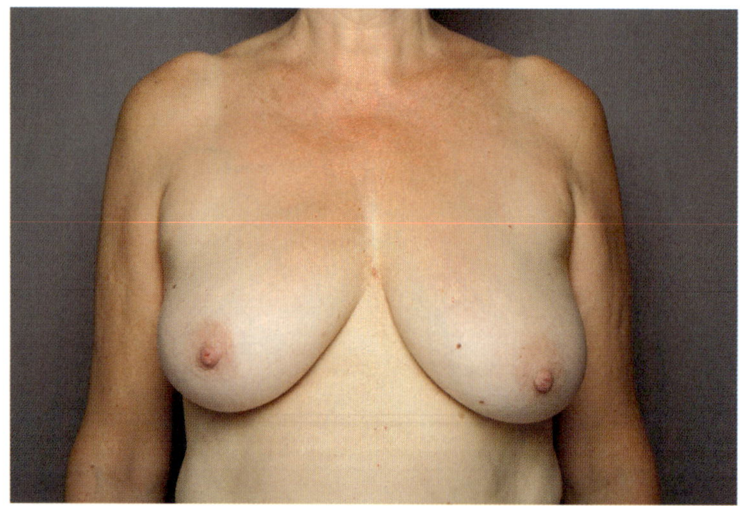

My breasts are healthy and I'm happy with them. They haven't changed much.

My partner who I was with for 20 years used to call them 'little dachshunds'. It was said affectionately, I knew they were relatively pendulous. We laughed a lot about a film where a man has an affair with an older woman. When she first takes her bra off he sees her rather pendulous breasts and he says, 'And they dropped like two hanged men'. My partner didn't say it to me every time I took my bra off, but that line in the film was referred to a significant number of times. I can see with hindsight it wasn't very nice of him. There was more going on under the surface of our relationship.

There was a time when I was struggling with my shop. It wasn't making any money and I needed to earn some income. I had a friend who told me about life modelling. Before my mind censored me, I asked her what she was paid. She said it was £25 for a couple of hours. Having gaily said I wouldn't mind having a go at it, my friend asked me to stand in for her when she couldn't make a class. I was nervous, but they were all absolutely delightful.

It's pretty good money but its not regular and it's for short periods of time. The work comes and goes. The environments are always pleasant to work in. It's normally warm, quiet, people are concentrating. It's not nice if it's chilly.

Life modelling was the first time I had been naked in front of a group of people. In privately run art groups there are quite a lot of blokes. But it makes no difference to me modelling for men or women.

I'm intrigued by the drawings of me. If I know they are doing it for the first time I don't immediately go and hover because I am aware they may be self-conscious. You get a range of abilities in a class. I've heard that some life models don't look at the work, which I find surprising because I'm always curious. And apparently some life models get offended, which I find extraordinary. People are just trying their best. I've had a go and I know how incredibly difficult it is. If somebody is less experienced and able they may not be looking at what's actually in front of them; they just draw what they think a breast looks like.

After being a life model for a couple of years, I am quite used to getting my clothes off quickly. I'm so used to turning up to places, putting my bag down and whoosh, it's all off. I do different jobs, cleaning jobs, various bits and pieces, and sometimes I wonder, 'Am I doing this in the right place? Am I getting naked when I should have brought my bucket?'

I used to dream a lot about being naked in public. In the dream everyone would be totally OK about me being naked, and I was never cold. Several years after starting life modelling I realised I hadn't had that dream for a long time. It felt it was like a 'preview'.

––––––––––––––

Age 60 | No children

"It's worrying when you get padded and push up bras for growing breasts"

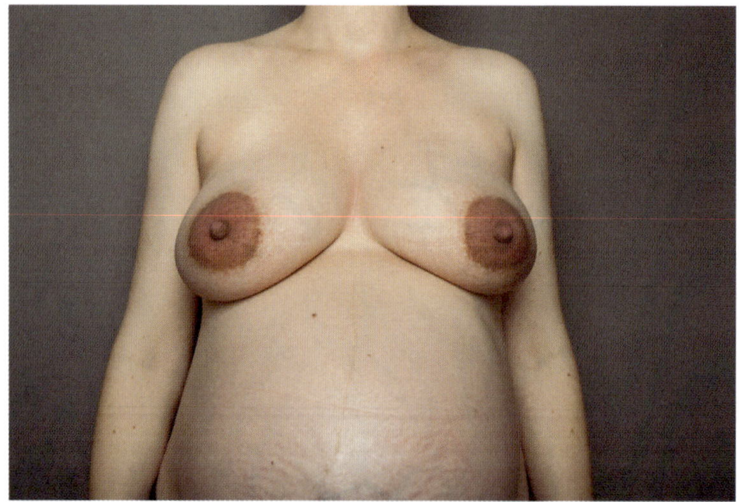

Mine are OK. I'm not unusually proud of them, I'm not upset by them, they're just there.

They're more rounded at the moment, obviously. Before I was pregnant this time they were a lot flatter and droopier. But that doesn't upset me. In a way I quite like it because it's a badge of honour of having had my children and fed my children.

They feel rounder, heavier and more dense when I'm pregnant. They're definitely fuller at this stage – that's the blood flow and the milk ducts getting ready.

In our society breasts are generally viewed as an extension of sexuality, rather than as a function. My breasts are less sexual for me than they used to be, and I think having children has changed that. They were erogenous before children, but they feel less so now. Since having children I think of them as functional. I'd say my husband feels the same too, or maybe it's just our relationship is different. Before you've had children – I'm guessing we're typical of most people – sex is much more important, it's much higher up the agenda. Whereas when you've got young children, it slips right down, more like, 'Actually do you know what, I'm tired and I'd rather you took the bins out than we had sex!' *(laughs)* I think my husband is pretty happy with them. It's not something that we talk about a lot, it's not dinner conversation!

I would never consider breast surgery for a non-medical reason. I think it's sad if people have such major issues that can only be conquered by having breast surgery. I think that's a very sad place for them to be, that their breasts make them that unhappy. They have surgery and then miraculously they are happy? I think it's a worrying trend in society to have unrealistically large boobs.

If my daughters wanted it done in the future I would be very sad that their physical appearance was making them so unhappy. It's certainly not something I would want them to go into lightly and I would perhaps suggest that they have some counselling first to see if there were any underlying issues they could sort out with themselves. If you're not happy with yourself underneath then there will be something else that you're not happy about after your breasts.

It's worrying when you get padded and push-up bras for growing breasts. It's part of the sexualisation of childhood, being aware of breast size at a scarily young age. It's telling girls that what they've got isn't enough, right from the start. I think it's horrible.

Generally there is quite a negative portrayal of breasts in the media. Page 3 is a horrible phenomenon and I don't understand why it still has a place in a national newspaper. I would actively move it away from my daughters if it was there and I thought they were going to open it. If we were getting on a train and there was someone sitting there reading *The Sun* with Page 3 open we would choose to sit somewhere else. I don't want them to think that that's normal.

Age 36 | Two children, pregnant

"Large breasts are seen as amazing when actually they are an extreme pain"

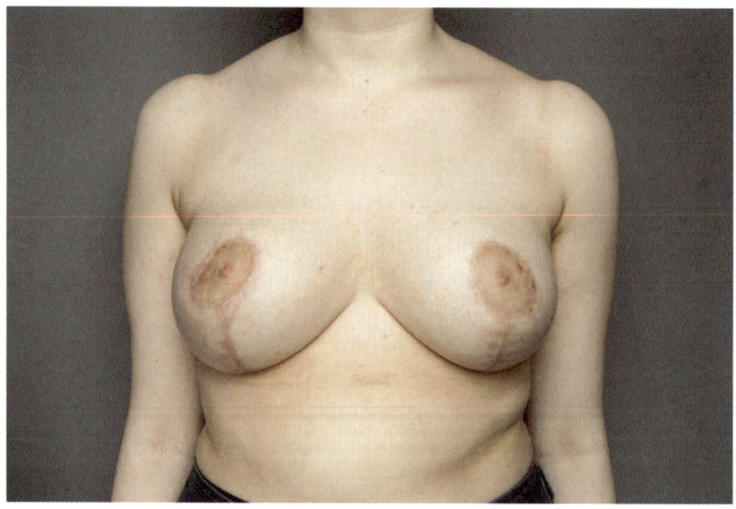

There's a definite difference between how I think about my breasts now and how I used to think about them. Before I had my reduction surgery I felt a mixture of distaste and shame towards my breasts. I used to get a lot of catty looks and jealous comments from girls and a lot of inappropriate comments from boys. Also, I had a lot of physical problems which were the main reasons for the reduction. They ended up taking off two kilograms of fat from my breasts.

I feel much better about them now. I don't think they are one of my best attributes, but I don't feel any shame or dislike towards them in the way I used to.

Because of the size of my breasts I used to sweat more, and I was embarrassed because I thought I smelled. I used to get very bad back problems. I still have deep grooves on my shoulders from my bras.

I've gone down about six cup sizes, I'm now a DD. That was the most I was able to have taken off without it looking disproportionate to my shape. I've always had a broader figure than other girls, sadly, much as I've always wanted to be petite. I've always thought petite girls are pretty. If I'd had more taken off, it would have made me look bottom-heavy. It was a balance between taking a good amount off and looking natural.

If I could choose any body shape, I would be 5ft 3in, very petite, and preferably a lot smaller on my chest. A lot of my friends when I was growing up were these smaller little girls and everyone thought they were pretty and cute. I'm not tall and beautiful, and I'm not small and cute.

I used to get very venomous looks from girls in the changing-rooms at school when we had PE. Some girls thought I was so large that I must have had surgery to enhance them. I was a 34GG, and I'm a size 10 to 12 everywhere else.

Occasionally I'd get rude and suggestive comments from boys, but I used to have more problems with them looking and staring. It made me feel extremely uncomfortable. I felt it was how people defined me. All through high school and college I was known as 'that one with the big breasts.' The breasts were all most people saw when they looked at me.

School was difficult. I was bullied from year four until year 11 when my mother became ill and subsequently passed away. Then people realised they couldn't legitimately tease me. They knew they'd get into trouble. Before that, I was teased because I'd always been more creatively inclined, and had less feminine interests than other girls, and because of my ethnicity as well. Especially after 9/11 I used to get racist comments, because my father is Muslim. One boy called me a mongrel because my mother was English and my father is Moroccan. I'd asked teachers for help before but I'd never really got any. I had that feeling of being abandoned by people, and people thought it was alright to take pot shots at me, my breasts being one of those things.

When I first told people I was having a reduction, the reactions from girls and boys were completely different. My very best friend was more excited than I was. She knew how much it affected me and how upset I was about it. She was really supportive.

Boys were the ones I had more problems with. They said things like,

'How could you do that? That's like slapping God in the face,' and 'How could you get rid of them? They're amazing!' and I thought, 'Yes, you probably do think they're amazing, because you don't have three and a half kilograms of them stuck onto your chest every day!' It was like boys were angry with me for getting rid of something they admired.

I'm asexual, I don't have a partner. I haven't had intercourse, although there have been times I've got close to foreplay. I've had sensations in my breasts when I've been with someone, but it hasn't been arousal. That's what asexuality is, it's the absence of arousal and an urge. I would say my breasts are sensitive and I get a level of feeling from them, but it hasn't encouraged me to go further. Because I had a bilateral reduction, where the nipple is moved to put it back in proportion, I've lost nearly all sensitivity. I've regained a little bit of feeling, but it'll never feel like it did before.

As long as surgery makes people happy and it's done for a good reason, that's OK. I don't think it should be done simply because someone thinks, 'Big breasts will make me look better,' or, 'I'll get more attention from men.' If someone was going up to a GG, like I was, I'd like to know if they are planning on spinal implants to support the weight! I don't understand why someone would want to be that big. I'd imagine they don't realise about the back problems that come with it.

The surgery lasted for about four hours. They remove a triangular sandwich of fat, bring the parts together, then move the nipple so it appears in proportion to the newly-reduced breast. I was kept in overnight. I was on strong painkillers for about three weeks. I gradually reduced my own dosage over that period. I wasn't able to wash properly for a while, I had to sponge myself down. I had to change the dressings and put iodine on the scarring for about three or four months. I couldn't raise my arms above my head. You can rip the scars, cause the wounds to open, and you could lose a lot of blood.

I was well prepared by the surgeons about what to expect. They told me all the risks: not being able to breastfeed, losing sensitivity in my nipples, the scarring lasting. I was told all of that before I signed the permission form.

It's quite a major procedure, but it was nowhere near as bad as I imagined. The scarring is a lot better than it was. It's fading very quickly. It's not red or irritated like it was. It will probably be almost fully healed in a couple of years.

I used to have to order bras from specialist websites to get the right size. I couldn't wear strapless bras or dresses. I look at going clothes shopping completely differently now. I can buy pretty underwear and feel nice about myself, it's wonderful. While companies make petite ranges, they never make anything that's specifically for busty women.

My best friend took me shopping for bras after my surgery. She turned around to me and said, 'I want you to see this, it will make you really happy.' She had found one of my old size bras and was wearing one of the cups on her head, and she said, 'Look how small you are now, compared to this!' Oh gosh, I felt so happy seeing that, knowing just how far I had come, from being a size you could wear on your head! It was hard work carrying all that around.

I struggle to understand why breasts are used everywhere. It's about 'sex sells'. They are used in advertisements even when it's not relevant. There's this 'perfect woman' image, in which she's supposed to have very large breasts, but small everything else, including her brain. I feel that having large breasts is glorified, mostly by people that don't have them. They are seen as this beautiful, amazing thing to have, when actually they are an extreme pain.

———————

Age 19 | No children

"I wish I had appreciated my body more before"

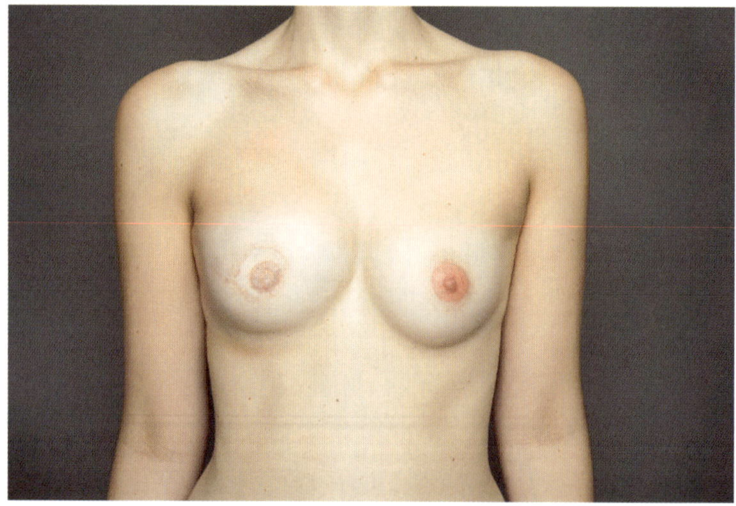

I was 27 when I was diagnosed with breast cancer. I wasn't fussed with checking my breasts, but I'd been for a massage and I felt uncomfortable on one side when I was lying on my front. I decided to get it checked out. The GP thought it would be fine, just cysts but she referred me to the breast clinic anyway.

The ultrasound showed a shadow, so I had a mammogram. They could also feel lumpy lymph nodes. There was a small one centimetre lump. They did a core biopsy with a needle. They give you a local anaesthetic, but it's quite painful. *(winces)* You know by the time they do that core biopsy that they are pretty sure. They said they thought cancer was likely, and I had to come back in two days for the results. I was in complete shock. I thought I would be told, 'They're just little cysts, you're fine,' and I'd be back to work. I'd told work I'd only be an hour.

However, the biggest shock was they couldn't just whip out a little lump. It was difficult to think about having a mastectomy.

I remember looking down at my breast in the bath before the surgery thinking, 'You're going to go, I will never get you back.' My husband is very pragmatic, he said, 'It's just a boob.' He was brilliant. But his dad had died of cancer. It connected him to those feelings again.

The lump was in a deep position, so they couldn't do a lumpectomy. I saw a plastic surgeon to talk about options. What we went for was own tissue reconstruction at the same time. The nipple came out, then the mastectomy, they took some tissue and blood vessels from my bottom and then took a bit of rib away to reconnect the blood vessels. I know, it's incredible, right? It doesn't always work, in which case they can take your tissue out and do an implant. When you are in recovery they listen every hour for blood supply. They know in the first 12 hours if it's worked.

It's a massively invasive procedure, but it is amazing, and it means I don't have to have surgery again. Implants need to be replaced every ten years. The scar on my bottom is really clean. You see that dip? *(points to bottom)* It's quite subtle, isn't it? It shows in a tight skirt. They just took tissue from one side, I'd thought they would take a little bit from each side, which would have been brilliant! *(laughs)* The first time I got up to go to the toilet I felt like the skin on my bottom would split open.

I had about eight months of chemo. It was like an endurance race. You get into the mode of the cycle, but you know you will feel cumulatively worse. I tolerated it quite well. If you can be well on chemo then I think I was. The worst part was my hair. I had the 'cool cap', which is like a bike helmet full of ice, and you wear it for an hour or two before chemo. It's brilliant, because it helps you keep your hair, but it's uncomfortable, like the headache when you eat ice cream and it hurts, except you have that for hours. Eventually I had to wear a wig, but I was never bald, which I would have found psychologically hard.

I was most worried about the surgery. I work in a hospital, my job involves looking at things that go wrong, so knowing I'd be under anaesthetic in surgery for eight hours …It's a long time. Would I get through it OK? The main thing was I just wanted to wake up. I miss morphine! *(laughs)*

I was never given my five and 10 year statistics. I don't think the odds are important. After all, the odds of getting breast cancer in my 20s with no family history were very small, so unlikely. So even if someone said it was very unlikely to happen again, it wouldn't necessarily reassure me.

About nine months later I had another little operation where they stitched and twisted the skin to make a bump for a nipple. Its gone flat now. They tried to tattoo a nipple on, but it wouldn't take. When a reconstructive nipple and tattoo go well and there's a good colour match nobody would notice. Mine isn't that good. They ran out of ideas, and at some point you have to think, 'OK, that's it.' They had a go.

I've always covered up, I was like that anyway. I've never let anyone see me in the changing rooms. Now, I don't want people to look and ask me questions if I don't know them. I don't want to have to tell them my life story. Like today! *(laughs)*

My husband or a family member came to each chemo session with me. My family felt like they were doing something, someone would stay for the week and do the meals, and it also meant my husband didn't have the added pressure of doing each hospital trip. We felt so supported by family, friends, prayer and support from the local church. It was one of the nice parts of going through something like that, you realise how many people love you. It was overwhelming in a good way.

My boss was brilliant. To start with I worked between chemo cycles. I work for the NHS and was on full salary for the whole year. I felt hugely supported.

The difficult thing for us as a couple was the effect on fertility. We saw a fertility specialist in the first week of being diagnosed and she thought she would take some eggs and get some embryos in the freezer. Later the same day we saw the oncologist and she wanted me to start chemo straight away so we had to choose at that point. That was a hard decision, one of the hardest things to deal with. We chose to start chemo. We'd been married for several years and we might have started trying for a baby soon.

They said there would be a 75 per cent chance my reproductive system would kick back in, but there was also a chance my body would go into early menopause. I haven't! I am confident I still have eggs. After the five year course of Tamoxifen we'll find out. I'll be 32, so still young.

I think hope is really important. I don't want to worry till I am 40. I find it helpful to just plan for the next set of decisions. The next decision will be how long do I try naturally after coming off the tablets before going back to the fertility clinic. Until you are at a decision point, you just don't know what you would choose.

It's easy to make everything about the cancer, but there are a lot of people who can't have children. We didn't know we would be able to have children, we just assumed we would. At least we know there might be difficulties. I'd love to go through having a baby, but I just want to be a parent. I would be keen to adopt, but I know my husband wouldn't.

During the treatment we were quite intentional about having sex even if we didn't feel like it. It was mind over matter. We were determined to keep as much intimacy as possible. I didn't enjoy it as much as when I was well, but psychologically and emotionally it was important.

He doesn't touch the reconstructed breast, I've told him not to bother wasting his time, because it's so numb. He only needs one hand now! *(laughs)* It's hard to think back to before, but my breasts never used to be a mega important part of sex.

Breast cancer hasn't changed how I feel about myself as a woman. I would have found it harder without reconstruction though. I call it my fake boob sometimes, or my 'bottom boob'. I don't feel less womanly. It's like I have a new body.

Overall, breast cancer has made me more grateful. I don't take much for granted. You are naive in your 20s about what life is going to be like.

If I hadn't had breast cancer I never would have done this project, but I think it's important to make my story available to a project like this. I've had quite a lot of surgery and I still like my body, that's a positive message for people. I would advise young women to get any concerns checked out. Also, I wish I had appreciated my body more before. I didn't like my bottom before, but I would be more grateful if I could go back in time.

———————

Age 31 | No children

"My nickname was 'Fried Eggs'"

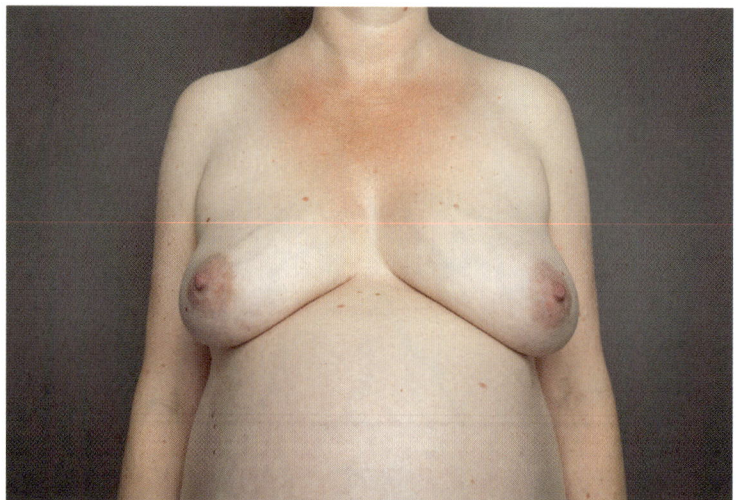

I don't think of my breasts as sexual objects. I don't get this business of, 'I'm a breast man', 'I'm a bottom man'. I find it slightly offensive: they aren't theirs, they aren't part of their body. It objectifies women, and it's offensive. I wouldn't go around saying, 'I'm a gonad woman'.

It was a shock seeing ow much my breasts grew the first time I was pregnant. The stretch marks afterwards distressed me slightly. My breasts are quite disfigured. I went from 34B to 34D. The more productive breast stayed a little larger. I always felt one worked better than the other.

All of that coming up again... I don't think I'll breastfeed quite as long for selfish reasons this time. I breastfed for a year first time. It becomes habit, and it's more comfortable the longer you do it. I will definitely breastfeed for three or four months, but I might stop around the time of weaning.

My partner has tried my breastmilk – expressed, not from the breast. Trying from the breast would feel slightly wrong. *(laughs)* He tried some of a friend's once too. She put some expressed milk in a cup for him. He said it was really sweet. It's natural curiosity, I don't mind at all. I tried my own too. In *The Grapes of Wrath* a woman breastfeeds a man. She loses her baby and she saves someone's life.

I saw my mum's boobs in the bath with her occasionally, maybe up to the age of about seven. She always put a flannel over her vagina for modesty, which is ridiculous. My mum was very old-fashioned. We never talked about breasts or growing up. I think I learned what I needed to at school.

My granny lived with us, and I remember looking at her when she was in her 80s, and her breasts were really long and saggy. She looked around and asked if I was looking at her 'funny old bags'.

My friends and I went out with these chaps, and they called one girl 'Pizza Face' because she had spots, another friend was 'Lamb Chops' because she had big calves, and my nickname was 'Fried Eggs'. I didn't particularly care, I thought 'Pizza Face' would have been more cruel. We didn't have names for the boys.

If I was starting a relationship now I would be more self-conscious about my breasts. I might not parade around the room naked in quite the same way to start off with. I'm not dating or in that situation, but if I were it would be slightly odd. I've been with my partner for a long time so he has seen them go through all the changes. Sagging and stretch marks are part of the ageing process, it's just how it goes. I expect my stomach will look wonderful after this baby! *(laughs)*

My daughter sees me naked all the time and is interested in my changing body. She's noticed my nipples getting bigger and prodded them. Mostly she teases me and tells me I look like an elephant. *(laughs)* That's fine.

———————————

Age 43 | One child, pregnant

"Breasts are supposed to have their own intelligence"

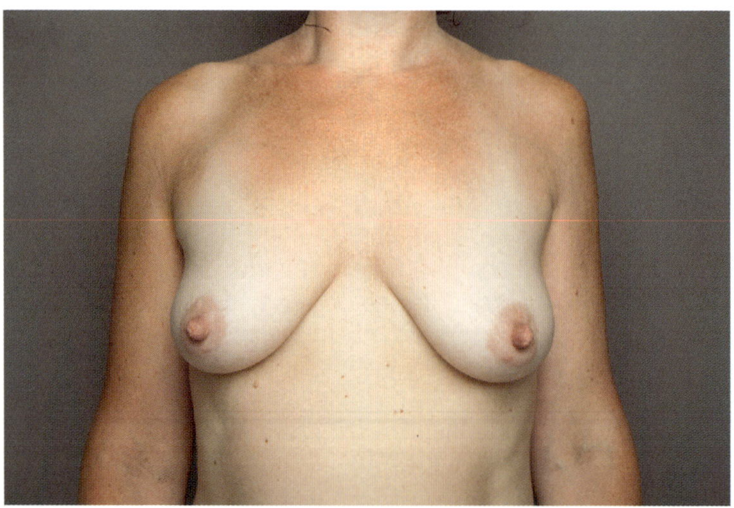

I read that breasts are supposed to have their own intelligence. When a baby is feeding, the breasts change temperature according to the temperature of the baby.

When my children were small we lived in a caravan. If I went to the neighbouring caravan in the evening, I would get a sense I had to return, and as I returned the children would be stirring. Only once did I return as a baby was crying. I would always get back as they were just waking up.

I quite like my breasts, but I feel they are a bit droopy and small for my size. I quite like the shape of them. I'd rather have proportionally bigger breasts, but it's not a massive issue. I envy other women's breasts if they are a C cup.

I do normally wear a bra, because I think if I don't I will lose the muscle tone and end up with really floppy tits. Even though I know that not wearing a bra is better for your tits – things to do with circulation flow and underwired bras.

I think I was quite excited when my breasts started growing when I was 12. My first bra was really sweet, I loved it. It was cotton with tiny lacy holes in it. Like the one I'm wearing today. How funny! *(shows me her bra)*

I used to work in a pub when I was 18. They called me 'Melons'. I think it was because we wore these tops which were balloony in the front. It annoyed me, but I also quite liked it. I liked that men were attracted to my breasts. I didn't agree that I had particularly big breasts, I thought the men were wrong.

I used to do crazy things. I'd get drunk and flash lorry drivers from the passenger seat of the car. Just for a reaction and to be naughty. I had the expected reactions; honking, and 'Phwoar!'

I'm happy to sunbathe topless, and I'd walk down the street in a topless protest. There's a naked cycle ride next week. I'd like to take part. I fancy doing a nude protest. I do cycle too.

When I told my 10-year-old daughter I was doing this today, she said 'Eurgh, that's disgusting!' I asked her, 'Why? Don't you like your boobs?' She said no.

When we're naked, we're all to be celebrated. Someone can look lovely in their clothes, their face is perfect, and then you take the clothes off and they have a scarred belly or breasts you wouldn't envy, something like that, and it puts everything into perspective. It's bare, naked reality. I think we need more nudity.

———————

Age 46 | Three children

"The breasts are located either side of the heart chakra"

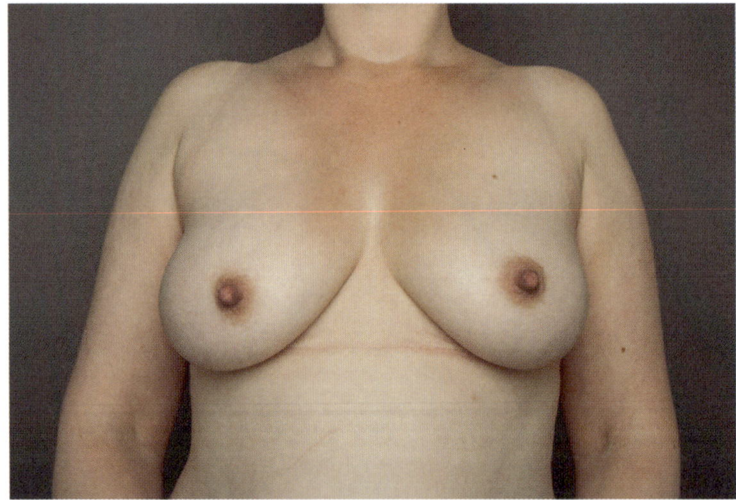

I've always felt my breasts are among my better physical attributes. I was relieved they didn't sag after breastfeeding; they kept their shape. I've been told that's not always the case.

This is the first time my breasts have been photographed and I'm aware now of a lopsidedness. I was surprised the nipples are in different places. It hasn't left me feeling negative, but it's interesting to know what they look like in reality.

When the time comes to get naked with people, my breasts have always been complimented, which is great. I've felt proud and enjoyed them and felt comfortable about people seeing them. I've been more self-conscious about my bottom half, thinking my legs are too short and fat and my bottom's too fat.

My deeper appreciation of spirituality has given me a feeling of pride as a woman: my breasts, my womb, the ability to have a child. I have a closer relationship with the Goddess through watching my body go through all those changes. I celebrate the female form. I'm proud to be a woman and have breasts. The spiritual side of my life has helped me to embrace and celebrate my natural body. If women happen to look conventionally beautiful then great – but if they don't then there is a beauty in all sorts of things. The definition of beauty needs to be re-examined in society.

The breasts are located either side of the heart chakra. If we think of the body as a map, the love area would be around the heart and breasts. This is where babies come, to the breast, and they can hear the heartbeat of their mum when they breastfeed.

I don't want to compare them to some ideal as defined by the porn industry, I'm proud of my breasts for what they are. I would never ever have cosmetic surgery. I don't believe in buying into bodily perfection, it doesn't exist. Paying for surgery is a form of brutalising the female form. Surgery is mutilation and it's to keep us investing and spending.

I think we're living in an age where many people under the age of about 40 have experienced the fallout of internet porn. The focus is on penetration, aggression, hardcore pumping – angry, nasty sex. It takes away from the slow, massaging, kissing, touching sex. There's very little appreciation of the breasts. The breasts are an erogenous zone and need to be explored as well as anywhere else. I've noticed men in the last 15 years go straight down to the lower part of the body, and ignore the breasts. If you like your breasts being touched then loving sex should include that. If a partner isn't touching my breasts I try to find ways to make that happen more. I'm less happy with my breasts being sucked since breastfeeding.

My mum had her breasts removed when she had breast cancer. It powerfully upset her; she said it destroyed her sexuality. After the mastectomy she never had sex again. I think I would be shattered if I had a mastectomy and I've worried it would make me feel the same, so my breasts must also be an important part of my sexual identity.

Age 36 | One child

"Most of the time we don't realise how beautiful women are"

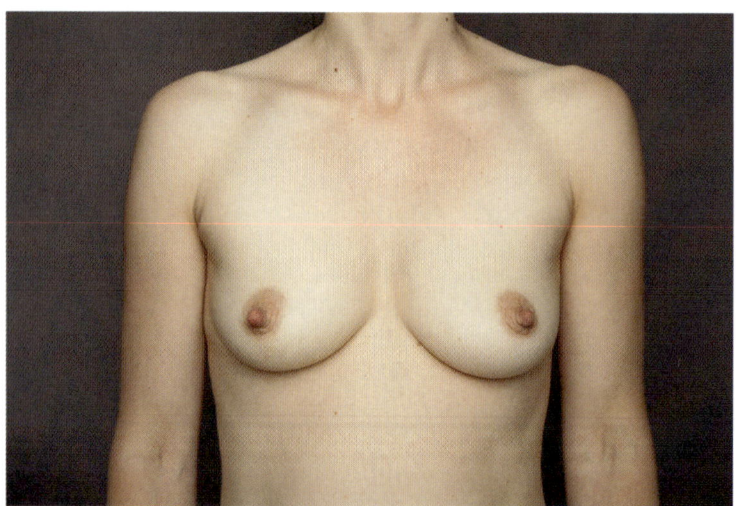

I think women's bodies are beautiful, the female form is beautiful. Most of the time we don't realise how beautiful women are. There aren't many women who have that self-confidence.

I've never been 'Wow, hey, look atme!' although I don't lack confidence and I don't particularly worry about my weight. I've always had small breasts, I'm 36A, maybe I could have done with a little bit more.

My parents are both blind. My mum has a beautiful body but she would never have shown it off. She has beautiful breasts, so does my sister. Mine have gone a bit saggier since I breastfed, but I am not worried about the form.

Being blind, my mum wasn't a confident person physically, although my parents didn't hide away. As a teenager I didn't want anyone to touch me, so I didn't hug my dad much as I grew up. If you are blind it's easy for someone to give you a hug and catch a boob. I found it awkward.

As a teenager I found people shouting at me in the street inhibiting. No one shouted out about my breasts, because they were small and neat and I am really quite glad about that. But I remember hating blokes who shouted at me and not wanting to wear short skirts because of that.

Having a child changed my attitude towards my body dramatically. You think, 'My god, I did that!' You breastfeed, these things are to give your child food, rather than just sexualised.

I fed my daughter for three years, and I would have continued except my partner wasn't so happy about it. He put pressure on me from when she was about two. I'm glad now that I gave up when I did though. I had a couple of miscarriages when I was still breastfeeding and I wonder if my body had too much to cope with. My husband blamed the miscarriages on the breastfeeding, he said, 'You gave it all to one for so long'.

You have this bond between you and the child when you breastfeed. I embraced it, as an older mother, and as someone who lost physical contact quite early with her mother. I am really into attachment parenting.

I didn't feel my partner was as involved as he could have been. He didn't say breastfeeding put him off sexually, although it is quite all encompassing. He couldn't see how to create a bond in a different way. He would argue that his reason for wanting me to stop breastfeeding was that I was too tired. He would say things like, 'She's draining the life out of you.' But it didn't feel like that for me, I had no problem with her feeding in the night, I would sleep through it, plus I would sleep in the day. I felt energetic, not tired. I think he felt pushed out. There are couples who both manage to enjoy it, but you have to be equally committed to it.

I would feed anywhere, but my partner started feeling embarrassed when she got to a certain age. His mother breastfed him for six months. She would say, 'Isn't it time she got her own bed? Isn't it time she finished breastfeeding now?'

My partner likes my breasts, but I think he thinks they are saggier since breastfeeding. He makes comments which really annoy me. He's called them 'saggy spaniel ears'. I was pretty angry with him. He does a lot of that sort of stuff. He is used to a lot of wind-up from his father, so he thinks making silly comments is funny, when it's not. He probably apologised after.

My breasts have been quite funny since I stopped breastfeeding. When I stopped I really noticed how sensitive they were, and I didn't want him to touch them sexually. I don't like being touched on my breasts too much, but when we're actually making love I quite enjoy it. Since having my daughter I am more sensitive, there is more of a connection between the two bits you know?

A friend of ours, her partner just walked up – not long after having a child – and put his hand down her top. I would have punched him in the face! That would be my reaction because I don't want my boyfriend to just come up and touch my boobs. But when you are aroused, yes, it's pleasant and nice.

There was an abusive situation when I was about 13 with a family friend. He had a bit of a fiddle with them, which was hideous. He was a much older man. It was horrendous. It's really scarred me.

He was a friend of the family and came to stay with us, with his wife and family. The wife was blind, but he was sighted. I was just 13, just started developing, not in a bra yet, I would have had tiny little boobs. I was at that age when girls start to bloom and look really pretty. He went to give me a hug. You just don't know at that age what's going on, he touched me there. *(indicates chest)* Later on the same day he came upstairs to me and was rubbing between my legs. I went and told my mum and dad. Luckily my parents completely believed me. What was really sad was the man's wife wouldn't believe it and dad was sure he was probably abusing his own daughter. She had the most severe eczema all over her legs, maybe stress.

I never ever discussed it with anyone, till quite late in life ... It makes me feel emotional now ... *(cries)* I wouldn't talk about it with my parents. I think dad realised I needed to talk about it, but I was embarrassed and that was part of the reason I didn't want him to touch me. I was like, 'Right, fuck off, all of you!' It marked me, even though a lot of girls must go through even more hideous things. It must be awful for people if they can't tell their parents.

The incident definitely affected my relationship with men. It took me a long time to want to have any kind of sexual anything. I didn't want attention from men for a long time. *(cries)* It affects confidence in your whole body. It was awful.

———————————

Age 41 | One child

"It's hard to tell the people you are closest to that you have breast cancer"

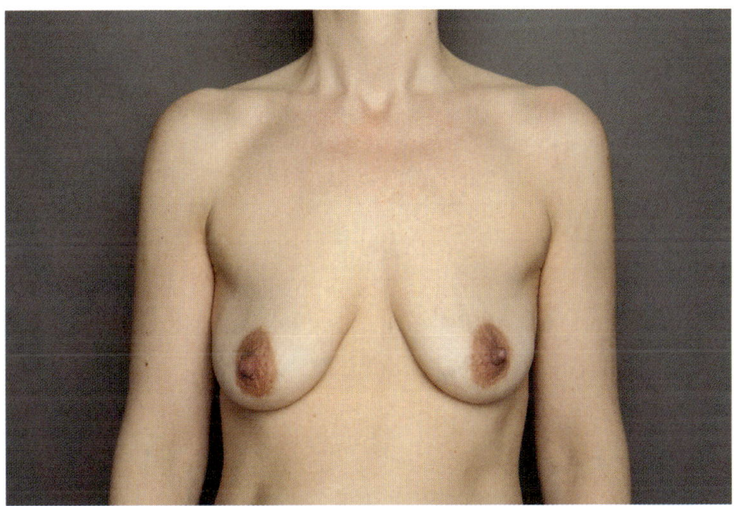

Last summer I felt a pea-sized lump in my breast and I was a bit concerned about it. I went to the doctor and was told it was fine, just to monitor it. Seven months later, at the beginning of this year, the lump had grown and was more solid and had started to be painful. So I went back to the doctor and she couldn't feel it. That made me wonder whether I was imagining it. But I was referred for rapid diagnostics.

A couple of weeks ago I went to the hospital and had an ultrasound. They couldn't see a lump. She said she thought it was all fine, but they sent me for a mammogram and a deeper ultrasound. So, it's quite a deep lump.

Using the pictures they took a biopsy from the lump. It was all the same day. A lovely doctor told me it didn't look good, it looked like it might be cancer. It's small, which is good news.

I went back two days later to get the results. It's cancerous. I was told it needed to come out. That's where we're at now. I'm booked in for surgery tomorrow.

There's nothing that suggests that I'm not still going to be here in 20 or 40 years time. The Royal Marsden just inspire confidence. All the contact I have had with different people has been excellent.

I'm having a radioactive injection today – the science of this is amazing, I have been flabbergasted – so they can see which lymph nodes the lump drains to. If the lymph nodes are affected by the cancer they decide how much of the lymph system to take out.

I won't lose a massive amount of breast tissue. There's no need to replace it with anything else. The scar will be under my arm.

I wasn't totally surprised. I knew I had a lump and my doctor didn't believe me. I knew I had it, but I was disappointed it wasn't a cyst.

At no point have I felt sad or sorry for myself. No. My husband was with me when we found out. Before, when I told him on the phone they had found a shadow, I was probably more emotional than I normally am, because I was worried about how he was going to take it.

It's hard to tell the people you are closest to that you have breast cancer. Part of me didn't want to be overwhelmed by care and concern. I appreciate it, but I don't want to feel there is more to worry about than there is.

I think my husband has done very well, but he has been upset and shaken by it. But it's all to the good in a funny sort of way. After you have been married for a long time you can become complacent about the other person. Sometimes, when life throws challenges at you, I think it forces you to appreciate what you have in your relationships, and refocus on the priorities. Although it's a rotten thing to have happened, it's a positive thing for our relationship.

It's easier to cope with something that's happening to you rather than watch things happen to someone else. I would be in a much worse place if something was happening to my children. I've got three children. The oldest is about to hit puberty and she is the most aware of what's going on and the most concerned. She understands the word cancer, but maybe doesn't understand how brilliant the prognosis is for restoration to full health. My job as her mother is to keep reassuring her that although it will be a difficult few months there is no reason to worry. The youngest is pretty oblivious to what it all means. The middle one knows of people who have died of cancer so she may have reason to be anxious about the word cancer. I hope that my confidence and being totally relaxed about it has helped her realise she doesn't need to panic. She's not suffering sleepless nights and she seems OK for now.

I haven't wanted to have long conversations with my mum and dad yet, and they have respected my need to deal with it in my own way. They are very supportive. I know they want to be helpful and do what they can practically, but for so much of my life I have been so independent of them, that it seems strange to emotionally involve them more now. In the past I haven't poured out my heart to them. It could be a trigger point for some people to say, 'OK, now's the time for me to start sharing my life with my parents'. They know that if I wanted to talk to them, I would. At the moment I don't think there's anything I need their reassurance about. I'm quite an analytical, rational, logical person.

I think that up until now, I hadn't fully appreciated the care that my friends and family have for me. You can take relationships for granted. When I've shared the news with my friends, the overwhelming reaction has been massive care and concern, offers of support, generosity of spirit and kindness. I feel blessed and privileged to have all those people there, sending texts, emails, coming up to me in person. It's overwhelming, but it's an honour to have a circle of such deep friends who want to look after me.

It's made me realise what a proud person I am. I need to be ready to ask for people to help me. Instead of being the one who does stuff for other people, I need to be on the receiving end of generosity. I have to learn to be relaxed and thankful for it. It's pride. I like to think I can do everything myself. Pride is when you are not ready to let other people see any weakness.

I am confident, because of my faith, that nothing happens outside of God's plans for us. Even though other people might see breast cancer as a mistake, or wrong, or out of his control, I would dispute that. I would say that God uses all things in life for his good and for his glory. If you know your Bible quite well, that is exhibited in the story of Joseph and his technicolour dreamcoat. God equips people to deepen their relationship to him, or enable them to be a witness to him to other people. It sounds odd that a bad thing enables you to know God's love better. I am convinced of that already through all the people who love us and are praying for us. Going forward, as a family we will learn great lessons about growing our love for each other, and also enabling us to empathise with and support other people better. We can use this experience for other people's good. Although it looks rotten, I am confident it is intended for good. It has a meaning, it has a good purpose.

I am very content in my own skin, it doesn't bother me what my breasts look like. But I am blessed with a body I am happy with. I'd rather change things about my face! *(laughs)* If I was having a full mastectomy I would be more upset.

The side with the lump has been tender so there have been limits as part of making love. I've guarded myself. He didn't know at the time. This experience will improve our relationship because our communication is going to improve. I'm not particularly fussed about my breasts sexually now; after breastfeeding their function became different. It seemed inappropriate ... there's a crossover. I don't know quite why, but the function of them changed. My erogenous zones are balanced throughout, I'm not particularly excitable just in that area.

I would encourage women to be aware of their breasts. I might have neglected my lump if it weren't painful, but cancerous lumps are normally not painful. My advice would be: even if it's not painful, don't ignore it. Maybe I should have gone back to the doctor earlier before it got painful. In any event, it's been found early so I don't have to kick myself.

Cynical, jumping-on-the-bandwagon breast cancer awareness by the media disgusts me. I mean *The Sun*'s 'Check 'em Tuesday' campaign. It's pretty cynical. I found the 'no make-up selfies' interesting too, it's come at a funny time for me. A number of my friends who know about my diagnosis have done it. They've bared themselves for public consumption and donated money, and it's touching. That turns it into being all about me, and I don't want to do that. I think they are doing it for a number of reasons, but one of them might be to support me, and that's a lovely thing to do. I don't feel in a position to do it myself at the moment.

———————————

Age 42 | Three children

"I'd like to look like a Victoria's Secret model"

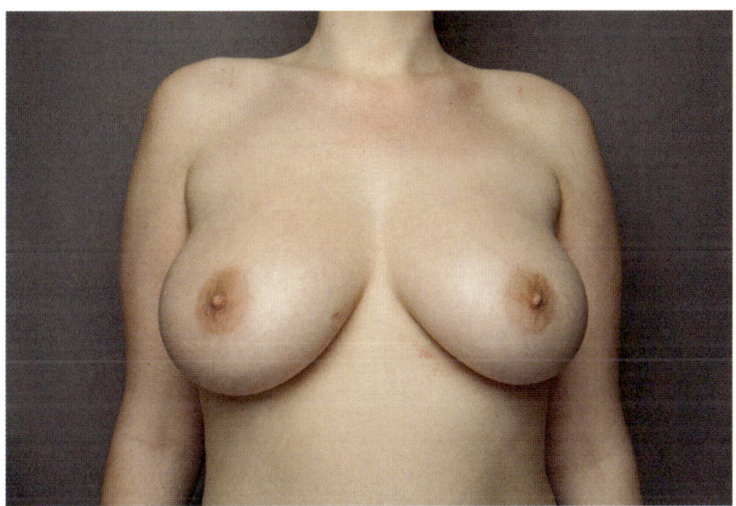

They're big, I like them. I used to be slimmer and didn't like them as much because they made me look bigger. I wanted to look like models, and they are all skinny with small boobs. I wasn't bothered about male attention when I was 15 or 16, I didn't think of my boobs as sexual then. But when I put on weight, I thought, 'Thank God for big boobs. There's something good about my body'.

I work in a pub, and if you wear anything even remotely with cleavage you get so much attention and looks. I don't hate it, but it's annoying after a while. I don't blame the guys, but some of them are perverts. I can't help it if my boobs are big. I'm not really a feminist, it doesn't bother me.

I haven't had a boyfriend but I have seen people. Boys like my breasts. I've been told they are amazing. I think some guys have been drawn to me because of them, because they've complimented them rather than other parts of my body. My breasts aren't erogenous. I don't find someone touching my boob amazing.

We're always on a Tumblr page about boobs. People send in pictures of their boobs and the moderator tells everyone they are lovely.

Have you heard of Snapchat? It's an app that's designed purely for sending pictures. You decide how many seconds you want the other person to see the photograph for, then it's gone. They can print screen, but if they do you get a message telling you they've done that. I use it for sending silly pictures to friends. Some people send pictures of boobs. It's fun. I've got a friend who asks me to send him pictures of my boobs, but I haven't done it, just in case he captures the screen.

Guys like big boobs. Rugby lads go on about them. The guys at school were real lads, and I hated it. They were so horrible about women. Just one physical imperfection would be talked about. I think it's why I haven't had a boyfriend. It's put me off. I care too much about someone saying mean things about me behind my back.

Most young guys have really warped ideas about women from porn. All the lads at school used internet porn. It definitely affects their expectations. They expect someone to be slim with big boobs. They like the fake look. I think they would rather say no to a girl who's not that good-looking and have no one. They'd rather not go out with anyone.

We all remove our pubic hair. It comes from porn, because guys don't like it. I think it looks neater. Some boys remove their pubic hair too. I thought it was weird when I saw that. A lot trim it. If you had a bush, they'd probably shag you anyway because, as they say, 'Any hole's a goal', but they'd probably talk about you afterwards.

I want to be a lot thinner. I'd like to look like a Victoria's Secret model. I know it's not natural to be like that, but I can't help it. In a way I want girls to look at me and think 'Wow, she's got a good figure', rather than guys. Girls are quite competitive about their bodies. I've never been happy with how I am. None of my friends are happy with their body. I've never met a girl who's happy with her body.

———————

Age 19 | No children

"My breasts have always been a turn-on"

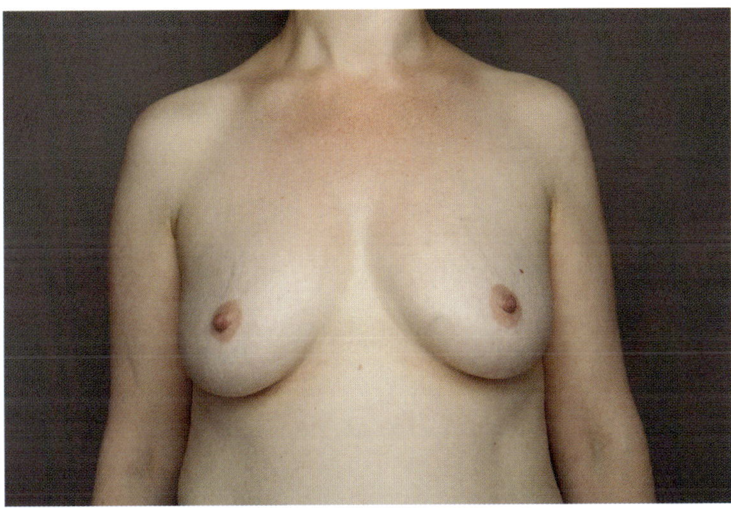

I really like my boobs. I feel quite sexy about them when I'm in a relationship.

If I'm on a date and wearing a nice top then I feel sexy. I like them being touched sexually. I haven't been in relationship for a while though. Before having a child, they were an important part of my sexuality.

My breasts have always been a turn-on for men I have gone out with. I think that's partly because I've always been confident with them. I couldn't imagine them not being part of sexual life. I had a boyfriend once who wasn't that into boobs. He was from a culture where boobs are out all the time and they are seen as for the kids. I had to encourage him to touch them to give me sexual pleasure. It wasn't like he didn't touch them, but there was a significant difference compared to other relationships I've been in. I liked his attitude.

I had bad boob trauma after I gave birth. No one told me about that side of having a baby; it was more distressing than labour in a way. I couldn't breastfeed properly. It was excruciatingly painful, but I was insistent I wanted to make it work. At La Leche League a woman came and helped me and got the baby to crawl up to my boob. She said my baby needed to learn to gravitate to me and I had to just let her learn to do it. She put the baby on my stomach and she nuzzled her way up because she could smell the milk. It was really cool actually! I had to help her latch on a little bit.

I wasn't breastfed for the first six to eight weeks because I was very premature. After that my mum only breastfed a little bit, not every day. I think that affects the bonding, as well as the immunity and nutrients. I know other people who have relationship problems with their mums who weren't breastfed. I am really close to my mum, but she's not a nurturing maternal mum. If anything is wrong with me in an emotional way she can't handle it. If I'm honest I haven't thought about these connections before.

I don't like padded bras. What's the point of making your boobs look bigger than they are? I've got friends with big boobs, and men look at them all the time. I'm glad I don't have them for that reason. And I wouldn't want to get sweaty underneath. I'm lucky with mine actually.

Padded bras for girls who are still growing are fucking outrageous, disgusting. At 12 they are still children, they don't need padded bras. Frilly little bikinis don't really sit that well with me either. My daughter wears an all-in-one jumpsuit with sleeves. She's got short hair and people think she's a boy.

When I was younger I looked at my mum's boobs, and said, 'Why are they so saggy?' And she said, 'Well it's your fault, you and your brother'. So I did have some awareness about what breastfeeding would do. She also didn't wear a bra for a while though. She's the same size as me. So I always wear a bra.

Age 36 | One child

"80 per cent of the time they are a feature of sex"

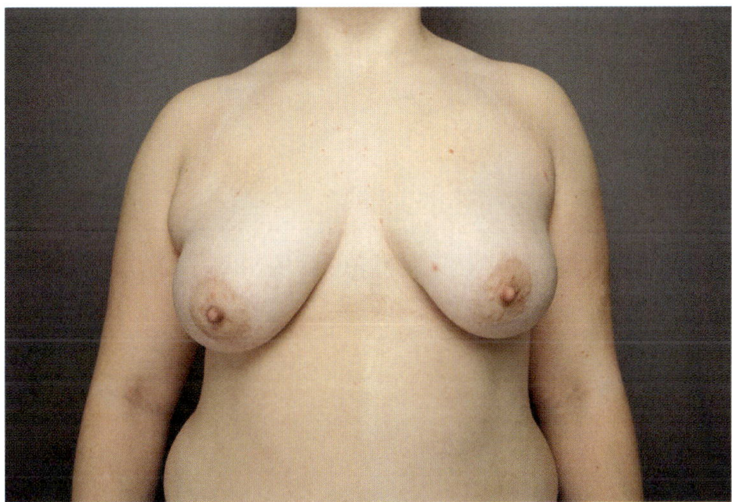

My breasts are quite big, but then I'm quite a big person. They're in proportion to my body.

I was 11 when they started growing. It really hurt. They were like little marbles. I couldn't lie on my front. I was at boarding school while I was developing. I asked my matron at school. She was really scary, really old, but I asked her about it and she said it was normal. I was about 13 when my periods started at school. I was on the trampoline *(laughs)* and I had to run off.

I'm a bit of a girl's girl, I have lots of female friends and we talk about everything. At school we spoke about everything all the time. We're still really close, all of us. When you're 11 it's weird, you don't want to talk to your mum about things like that.

I'd like to try and breastfeed if I have a baby. I think it's good for the mum and brilliant for the baby. I'm a nanny. The child I look after wasn't breastfed. Mum didn't even try, she was straight on the bottle. She wanted the dad to help out with the night feeding, and didn't want to express, so they went straight on to the bottle. They had a maternity nurse before me.

I know my boss felt pressure to go back to work. If she took too long then a man would wiggle his way in and take her job. She only took six weeks of maternity leave. I think it was a factor in her decision not to breastfeed.

My partner likes my breasts. She's jealous because mine are bigger! They are quite a big part of our sexual life, because we don't have willies! *(laughs)* My breasts give me a lot of sexual pleasure. I like nice touching and stroking. I would say 80 per cent of the time they are a feature of sex.

Men are obsessed with them because they don't have them. They poke, they want to touch them rather than please me. Whereas women really want to please you. And because they have them, they know what to do. Men think they know what to do, but they don't. They touch them, flick them a bit, lick them, they are all about the nipple. That's all they do, it's like a tick box. If you watch porn, that's all they do with breasts. I had sex with four men when I was younger, checking what I was missing. Women are a lot more gentle, and they know what they like and what it feels like for them, so they treat your breasts better. Women are better, I've always said!

I don't really get them out. I'm not dressing to impress men. Loads of my straight friends have them up to their chin. They look awful! I think, 'God, love! Have some self-respect!' Then they complain that they're getting harassed, and it's like, 'Well put them away!' There's one girl in particular, she'll go out in a corset and men will literally talk to her breasts.

Men love breasts, they're fascinated with them. Guy friends have said they'd love a pair for the day, just to see what they were like. It's funny how men feel about breasts. It's a typical teenage boy thing, it's all about boobs.

———————

Age 26 | No children

"I don't touch my breasts if I'm masturbating. It's all about speed these days!"

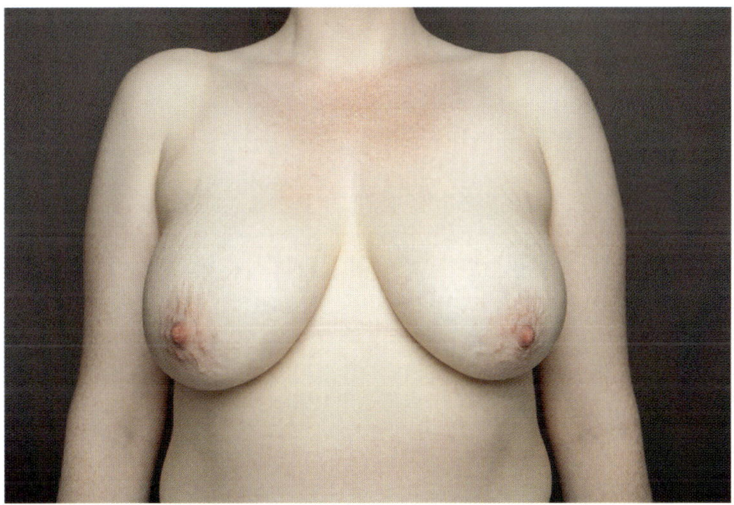

My breasts grew suddenly as a teenager, which was embarrassing as I felt very different to everyone else. I was an ugly duckling when I suddenly blossomed, slimmed out, grew breasts and long hair. I was surprised by the attention. I went from being completely ignored by the boys at school, to being this buxom young lady, 'Oh hello, who's this!' The boobs got the boys interested.

I ws a prefect and had to wear a tie which hung between my breasts, which was not flattering and attracted attention. I got a lot of physical touching, boys sitting next to me touching my knee.

My boobs were felt by a boy before they were seen by a boy. I was about 15 the first time they got felt. It was during the throes of heavy petting, and it was fairly erotic. I was self-conscious about it, it was part of me that hadn't ever been touched before, not since I was a child, but by the time you have boobs your parents aren't touching you there anymore.

I remember once boys found nipples they never went anywhere else, 'Ooh, this is the tweaky bit.' Very fumbly. As an adult now, I think, 'Oh god'.

My breasts are a prerequisite to foreplay. I would feel a bit put out if someone went for 'down there' straight away. They are the appetiser, get things warmed up, then once I am in the throes of things I don't need it. I know women who say their boobs aren't erogenous at all, but for me they do help the sensation.

Breastfeeding was horrendous at first, so painful. But I was bloody-minded and determined to do it. After that it was nice, very relaxing. My daughter was a hardcore breastfeeder, she breastfed till she was three years and four months old. That's quite a long time in the grand scheme of things.

Then I went on to become a breastfeeding peer supporter, and now I help other women breastfeed. It's changed my opinion of breasts. I know so much about breastfeeding that I think of breasts' first job as being milk production and their secondary job is a sexual one. I know they are an erogenous zone for a lot of people and that's their primary thing.

I used to find my breasts unattractive and now I actually find them more attractive, because they did a great job. They may not be the best-looking boobs in the world, but who has the best-looking boobs in the world? It doesn't matter what boobs look like when you breastfeed. I see a lot now, and the more you see the more you become desensitised. That's why I was happy to take part in this project. Breastfeeding has changed my relationship with my breasts.

I've given antenatal talks to pregnant women and we talk about how to prepare. You can't prepare though really! Mastitis is just a word till you've had it, but you can prepare by knowing you might have problems. A woman recently knew she was becoming engorged so she kept putting baby to breast and prevented it, because she was prepared.

Breastfeeding should not hurt very much. When I did my peer supporter training they said it might be uncomfortable, but if it hurts it means the baby hasn't been latching on right for a while, it hasn't got a good mouthful. But nobody expects the discomfort. There is not enough support for breastfeeding mothers.

I have to go to training every six months to check my advice is up to date and I am not going against the WHO guidelines and whatnot. We were sent up to date information by email about the recent stuff about sharing beds with babies.

I wasn't prepared for the intensity of feeding. I thought before having a baby that they would feed every three or four hours but that's not true, they feed when they want to feed, and that might be every 20 minutes in the beginning.

Since being a breastfeeding peer supporter I am even more angered by stupid men thinking that its OK to see women's breasts as objects. You get your boobs out to breastfeed and you get tutted at or asked to go elsewhere, or be more discreet. I hear about this a lot from women I support. And it's not OK to see boobs as only for titillation. I think women need to take back ownership of boobs. They should be sexual objects for us, not for men. Breasts should be on women's terms, not men's terms.

I hear women say they won't breastfeed because their partner won't like it, because he sees their breasts as his. It angers me so much. I want to say, 'Go home, give him a slap and tell him they are your breasts!' but of course as a peer supporter I can't say that, I have to be empathetic and maintain my professionalism.

Previous partners have described my breasts as theirs. It's weird and disturbing that men think they own part of a woman. Maybe it's because they don't have them, I don't know.

My breasts were completely off limits in our sex life when I was breastfeeding. I was really scared of squirting milk everywhere, that would have been the ultimate turn-off for me. Once I was sitting in a restaurant and it squirted out and hit the table! I could reach you with my milk from here. *(over a metre away)*

My daughter's partner and I separated when she was about two and we hadn't had sex for a year before that. I started a new relationship while I was still breastfeeding my two-year-old. I did wonder how to broach that I was worried about milk leaking during sex. How would I explain that to him? I wondered if it would put him off sex, especially as I was breastfeeding someone who wasn't his child. In the end, we only went on a few dates, it fizzled out. I suppose he might have liked it, but then that would have sent me for the hills!

I don't touch my breasts if I'm masturbating. It's all about speed these days! It's about time when you have kids. Maybe I would touch them if I had a spare half an hour. *(laughs)*

Age 34 | One child

"Breasts are a homing device for men"

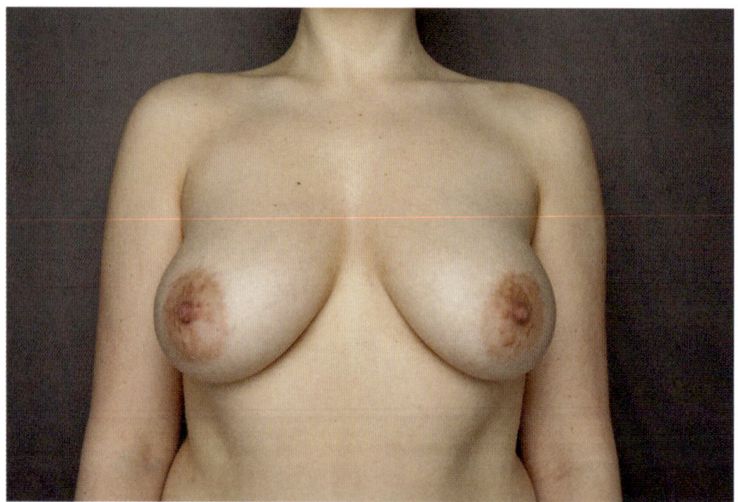

I've grown into my boobs. I like them more now than I ever have done, and I think that has a lot to do with turning 30. My husband loves them and that's made me love them.

What is it about men and breasts? They're like a homing device for men, they find them incredibly arousing. We don't look at men's bits and say, 'Wow, yeah, I've got to stare at that and touch it with my face.' There's definitely something maternal, but I don't know how many men would admit it. My husband was breastfed. I think his mother had the same size breasts as me, maybe a bit bigger.

Is it nature or nurture? Are they told they have to adore them by society? Or are they programmed by their biochemistry? The female physique is beautiful, and that's regardless of sexy images everywhere. I think we are genetically programmed to be attracted to women's bodies. I like looking at other women's boobs, breasts make women look beautiful.

I was embarrassed by them at school. They grew before I was mature enough to deal with them. I was 15 or 16, but men treated me like I was a woman because of my boobs and I didn't know how to cope with it. It's almost like they're flashing beacons and they attract men even if you don't want them to.

I've always thought that I've got slightly larger nipples than normal and that my breasts are the wrong shape. I thought they had to be perfectly rounded and upright, a false shape. I've tried to emulate this with bras, but I thought that they had to look like that when I took my bra off too. I felt there was something wrong with me for ages.

I've had lots of comments. I was once asked if my boobs were real, and in my head it was, 'Wow! That's a compliment. I have a bikini on, and they think my boobs are fake. I've succeeded, my boobs look perfectly round.' It was one of those sculpted bikinis, like a bra.

When I see photoshopped pictures I feel numb. From studying photography I know how images can be changed. The pictures shape my conscious aspirations for my body. I want to be skinnier, which is really sad. I want to strive to be better. There is this feeling that breasts are something we are supposed to worry about. We are constantly told that women worry about what they look like, that they have to buy products to make themselves look better.

With 36D boobs you can't get away with a little camisole slip, and certain clothes are not acceptable. None of my friends would go out with a big cleavage. I would like to say people can wear what they want, but if I saw a group of women like that, I probably would make an assumption about their antics for the evening: using their boobs to make themselves more attractive to whoever they want to pick up for the evening.

If you went outside without a bra on people would probably think you weren't normal. Unless you have dressed your breasts in a nice cocktail dress that you can't wear a bra with, you have to wear a bra. If I went out with a T-shirt on, but no bra, and I didn't have my hair down and make up on, people would think I was slightly mad. Maybe it's because of false representations of breasts in the media, but we hide them. It's like Victorians covering up piano legs, we fetishise breasts.

My husband thinks my boobs are sexual. They are only mildly sexual, from my point of view. My nipples are really sensitive, to the point of being painful. I'm terrified that if we have a baby I'm not going to be able to breastfeed.

I'm scared because my mum had massive boobs after having children. Before she had children she was a similar size to me, but since having children they're huge. I think I would have a reduction if mine got that big. Everyone is so scared of being the person who doesn't look nice.

When I was 21, I was woken up on an aeroplane by a man groping my boob. His words were, 'Mmm, very nice.' I rang the bell, the lady came, and she tried very hard to find me somewhere else to sit, but the plane was full, so she swapped me round so I was on the aisle seat and he was on the window seat. He wasn't reprimanded. It was a bad experience.

One night I was walking home and I was wearing a short skirt and tight top – 'inappropriate clothing'. A man walked up to me, grabbed my arm really hard and put money down my top and told me I was coming home with him. My instant reaction was to take the money out of my top and throw it. I managed to get away and ran. In retrospect I should have kicked him in the balls, kept the money and ran, but I didn't want the money.

That incident made me feel like I was inappropriate. A male friend said, 'You have to look in the mirror, that's why that happened.' I think it was a freak incident, but it wouldn't have happened if I was wearing jeans. Women's clothes do give off signals. It's not your fault, and it's not an excuse, but it is a communication.

My dad said if I was ever in the wrong place at the wrong time I wouldn't want to be wearing inappropriate clothes.

We live in a male-dominated society and it's totally unfair women can't be topless. There have been other cultures where societies were female-dominated but it's been suppressed and taken away from us. I wouldn't want to sit in a park with my boobs out, because of unwanted attention, I'd feel self-conscious. People would think you were mad. I've never sunbathed topless, even though I live really close to a nudist beach.

I am tempted to do the nude cycle ride. It's a yearly tradition, and I've always wanted to do that. It looks fun, there's a sense of camaraderie between the people taking part.

I feel like I am having a bit of a revolution in my life. I went to hot yoga for the first time and I had a naked shower with other women. I'd sweated with these women and turned purple, and the shower just felt nice. It was amazing because it was totally normal, there was no staring, and it felt really 'womanly'. There was no judgement.

So, then I heard about this project, and I thought I had to do it. First a naked shower with other women, now this, next the nude cycle ride!

———————————

Age 30 | No children

"He was kissing away when breastmilk came out"

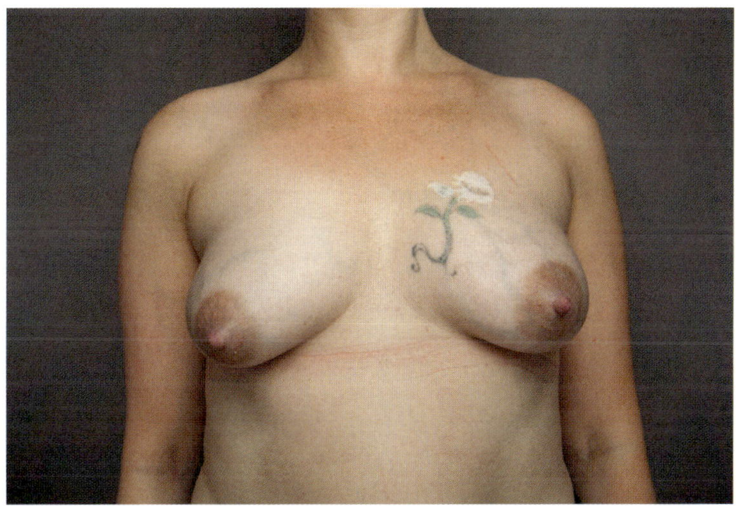

At the moment I feel really good about my breasts because they are a bit fuller and I've always felt quite negative about small boobs. We're kind of conditioned to want big boobs.

They are small and pointy, not round, and that round shape is quite important.

I've always been shy and insecure. You want to be pretty for boys and I didn't think my boobs were big enough or nice enough. I used to read a teenage girl's magazine called *Starlet*. You look at the pretty girls, and think that's how you should look. Media is a reflection of society, society is a reflection of media. I still went topless on the beaches though. I'm Swedish and we're comfortable with being naked.

I used to dream of winning the lottery so I could have a boob job. I don't feel like that now. I have totally changed my mind about getting a boob job. Image is not as important as it was when I was younger.

I didn't breastfeed my first two kids, it wasn't even on the radar. I'm quite ashamed of that now. I'm on my third marriage; it's just the way life worked out for me. My third husband is quite a lot younger than me so obviously I wanted another baby and I knew I would breastfeed.

Since my first two babies I've been to university and trained as a psychiatric nurse. I've read a lot about psychology, early years, attachment theories, breastfeeding, the bonding experience. Also I thought this might be my last child so I was determined to experience breastfeeding for myself as well as for the benefits for the baby.

I know it sounds strange but before I didn't think my boobs were for breastfeeding. Bottles were everywhere in our family. What your mum does is a big influence as well as what's around you. There weren't as many posters in the health centres then.

Breastfeeding has affected the bonding. I'm not saying that I didn't bond with my other two children – we are very close – but I feel extremely bonded with my baby. You can't measure bonding really, but I'm enjoying my baby so much more this time round.

A friend of mine who breastfed both her children was saying, almost apologetically, that it's not a bad feeling, it's actually quite nice. Not to the point of having an orgasm, but nice. For the first three months I had no idea what she was talking about, but now I see what she meant, it is nice. For me, it's like when you have an itch and you need to scratch – breastfeeding relieves an itch.

Breastfeeding has made my breasts feel more sensitive in a good way. It feels a bit weird talking about sex and breastfeeding in the same sentence, but I suppose breastfeeding has made them become more a part of sex. I also feel better about my boobs psychologically because of breastfeeding, and I think that has helped make them more of an erogenous zone.

My breastmilk dripped when we were playing around! I could feel it coming and I thought, 'Will he be disgusted by it?' He was kissing away when breastmilk came out. I've never been a squirter, it just dripped. He stiffened up a bit then he carried on. I thought he would be grossed out, but he wasn't at all. We didn't talk about it afterwards. I would have liked to know what he thought about it, but I don't think he would have wanted to analyse it. He'd always said he wanted to try breastmilk, and now he has!

For my children breastfeeding is natural, it's part of our family. My son will say, 'Are you going to feed the baby before we go out? Will it be one boob or two boobs?' Like, how long is it going to take? It's the most natural thing in the world. I hope he will grow up to encourage his partner to do it.

I asked my daughter what kind of mum she thought she would be. She said she would definitely be 'a natural mum, a bit like you, carry the baby in a sling, breastfeed, have a home birth'. My heart just burst, because if I have done anything right in my life, it's her saying that. Maybe I didn't breastfeed her, maybe I didn't bond with her the first two days, but now she thinks that.

I was 22 when I got the tattoo on my breast. I started treatment to remove it a few years ago. I like tattoos, but didn't want one on my boob anymore. I was embarrassed about it and felt it looked a bit tacky.

I was sold a treatment which is apparently better than laser. You put something on your skin and the ink goes to the surface of the skin and forms a scab, and then the scab falls off. That happened, but I lost pigment in my skin as well. So I thought I would try laser. I had one laser treatment, which mainly removed the stem of the rose. With laser it goes almost completely; it will take another four treatments probably. But I got pregnant and had to stop. I'm quite upset about it especially as I am starting to like my boobs. I would like to wear a top with a cleavage but I can't because my left boob is ruined.

I won't get the pigment back, so I might tattoo over it. I'm getting back into tattoos.

There's an image I really like: an outline of a woman breastfeeding. I know it sounds airy-fairy, but I want it because I love breastfeeding so much and am so passionate about it. Breastfeeding has changed the way I look at motherhood.

―――――――――

Age 40 | Three children

"They were so sensitive it was like having two clitorises on my chest"

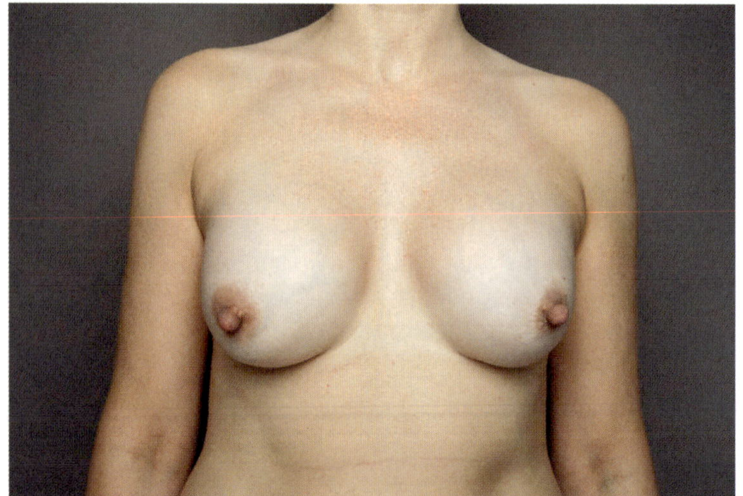

I had my breast surgery when I was 34.

I've always been a very body confident person. I exercise and take care of myself, but the one part I couldn't do anything about was my breasts. When they were small and I was younger they were quite pert, but they didn't fit my frame. Fit my frame? How ridiculous is that. They didn't fit my frame compared to images I had grown up with.

I breastfed for ages, so although I had these perfect little boobs to start with, they lost a lot of that tissue and became these little spaniel's ears. I just didn't want them seen. In the end I was in gel bras all the time. If I wore a T shirt with no bra I looked like I had nipples but no breasts. I didn't like to have sex without a bra on because I thought they were that bad.

I grew up with a lot of images. My dad wasn't a massive porn user but there were pictures of women with exposed breasts in the mainstream media when I was growing up in my home. My mum had massively negative feelings about her whole body, but particularly her breasts, which were small. After my dad left, the first thing she did was get a boob job. Most women get a haircut, but she had a boob job. So that's my legacy: breasts are supposed to look a certain way, and if they don't then you can fix them.

Body confidence is a double edged sword. If you go the gym you are quite focussed on your appearance. How do I put this without sounding big-headed? I was lucky enough to be relatively attractive. I wasn't Cindy Crawford, but I would turn heads. I had positive feedback from men and women about my appearance and that becomes part of your identity. So when part of your appearance doesn't fit in, it eats away at you.

I can't remember noticing my breasts being particularly erogenous before I had breast enhancement, although my sex life was a bit rubbish on and off throughout my married life. I'm now divorced and in another relationship and now I have a fantastic sex life.

They warn you that your nipples may lose sensitivity, but I had the opposite effect. For a while it was ridiculous – they were so sensitive it was like having two clitorises on my chest. It was not convenient. After a while they settled down, but they are still very sensitive. It used to be around the time I ovulated, but now I have a coil in. But yeah, very sensitive. Breasts are nearly always involved in the build-up to sex, they are a big part of what turns me on. You could touch my breasts alone and that's enough to get me started. If he gets hold of my nipple, and he can be quite rough with them, that's an instant turn-on for me.

Your breasts are so firm after the surgery, it was like the woman in *Austin Powers* shooting bullets from her breasts. They were in your face. But they've settled down into something quite natural. To start with they felt alien, not part of me, but now it's like they've always been there.

I fed my son till he was two and a quarter and my daughter till she was three and a half. My husband was very supportive of the extended breastfeeding. He asked a funny question about whether it was going to turn our son into one of those men who walks around with his hood up and looks like he's stumbling over his feet, like one of the weird kids at school. I said, 'No, they're the ones who were never breastfed.' My children are very rounded people. Breastfeeding was one of the best experiences of my life. I didn't attempt to elongate it in any way, I just went with them.

Although I had negative experiences of what breasts should be growing up, I also remember my mum feeding my brother and one of my aunties feeding her baby. I felt besotted, and thought, 'I so want to do that.'

Breastfeeding is sensual. It's awkward to talk about isn't it? It's so intimate. I know people are uncomfortable with this. Babies stroke you while you are feeding them. My son used to play with my hair while he was breastfeeding, my daughter used to tickle my back. It was a lovely intimate experience breastfeeding my children. I think we are so messed-up in society now. Women are presented as being sexual for men, and we are frightened of talking about sensuality and intimacy. Actually there is an intimacy with your children, and it is not wrong. The two things are separate but they overlap in some ways. Breastfeeding affects your hormones and your sex drive – you can lose interest in sex – but maybe it's also because the intimacy has been taken over by the intimate relationship with your baby.

I was lucky that I had a positive experience with breastfeeding. I've read about the politics of breastfeeding, I have taught about breastfeeding, talked to people about cultural influences, how we sexualise breasts in this country and how unhelpful that is for breastfeeding initiation.

I don't regret the breast enhancement. I wouldn't want to go back to how I felt before I had it. I wouldn't change it and I do really, really like my boobs. I can put anything on and they look great. The only thing I have an issue with is that my nipples, which were already fabulous, are sitting on the end of these fabulous boobs. So they are a bit more prominent. I have to be careful about tops because my nipples are really in your face. I think when you can see nipples, it looks great. I feel very, very sexy when I put a vest on without a bra. God, I love going without a bra, who the hell likes wearing a bra all the time? I haven't got one on today. I don't need one. It's great to be able to do that. You get stories in the paper about celebrities, 'Ooh, look, you can see her nipples.' Get over it, we all have nipples!

I was 14 when my mum had a boob job. It lodged in my head, 'I could do that one day.' I am racked with guilt that I could do that to my daughter. At 11 she already has the same size boobs I had in my 20s, so I think she's going to be bigger than me. She's a huge feminist, she's fantastic. She's asked me if she is going to get shouted at in the streets by men. I stopped and thought, 'How do I answer this?' I said, 'Yes. But you can decide how you want to respond to that.' We tried some different responses out. She wanted to say something like, 'It's so uncool to shout at people in the street.' I said she could say something like, 'It's 2013 not 1970', but she said that would suggest it was acceptable in 1970, and it wasn't. I just got hold of her hand. She's wonderful.

I know my son has watched porn. We've talked about it openly. I can't stop my 15-year-old son from watching porn. I just try and equip him with what he needs to know to dismantle it. He's got into arguments with friends about the way they talk about women, so I don't worry about him too much. He doesn't want to be identified as a feminist in a school in a very working-class area, but he is a feminist.

My daughter has seen porn too, and so have most of her friends, on their iPods. I was shocked when I found out my daughter had seen it. I felt like I had failed. She had typed in the word 'vagina' because she wanted to see what a vagina looks like. If you type 'vagina' into Google... a whole world of evil opens up! It broke my heart. I'd already suggested looking in a mirror and having a feel to see what it's like.

Breasts are fascinating. We have a mixed-up culture: you can see pictures of breasts all over the place, but it's not OK for women to breastfeed in public in some circles. We have such a weird relationship with our breasts. The more women who tell their story about how they feel about them and what they are really like – the wonderful things, and the difficult things – and the more girls growing up who read those things, the more open dialogue we have, the better. This project is great.

Age 39 | Two children

"My grandma always said a good handful is enough"

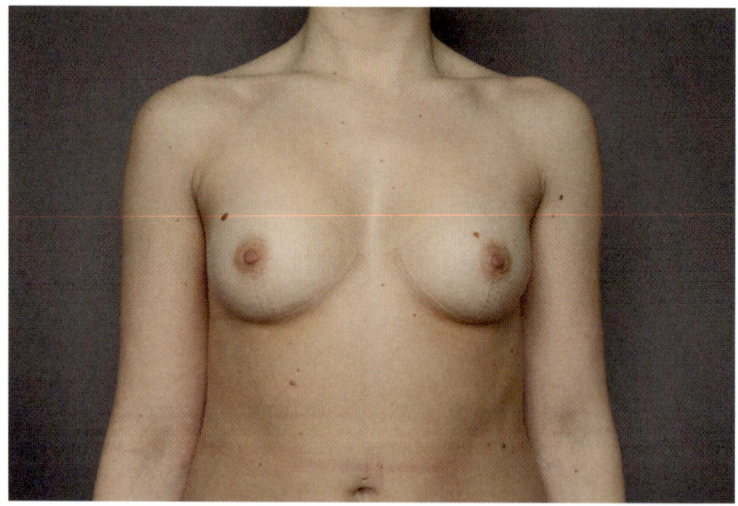

I quite like my breasts. I like that they are petite. My grandma always said a good handful is enough, and I have a good handful, so that seems just about right.

I've always had thing for nice underwear. I can remember when my breasts first started growing, when I was about 12, because I remember the first bra I ever had. It was a baby blue Gossard bra. When I was younger I wanted to make them look bigger so I used to buy the padded bras. I don't like padding anymore.

Clothes fit me well the size I am. My boobs seem to be in proportion.

I'm a size eight, but I'm curvy. I would say my best asset is my bottom, not my top. My partners have been bum men, more than boob men. Normally I will wear a tightly fitted pencil skirt or dress, and I'll get comments for my bum.

Without breasts I would feel less feminine, but I don't like them being touched. Sexually they don't do anything for me. I like my stomach being touched a lot more than my boobs. The sensation of my breasts being touched isn't as pleasurable as the rest of my body being touched. If my partner goes for them, I might cover them with my elbows or ask him to stop. He understands.

Breasts are sexy because curves are sexy, they're part of the female form. I think men are interested in them because they don't have them.

My auntie had breast cancer. If I had to lose a breast to stay alive, of course I would do it. No hesitation. Especially with what my auntie went through.

I go to the gym and exercise regularly. I go spinning or running two or three times a week, and do weights to tone. And I eat healthily, very, very healthily, and I try and keep track of what I eat. We can live longer lives if we eat healthier, are active, and keep our brains active. There are so many nasties out there like cancer. If I know I am trying my best to look after myself I know I am doing what I can to prevent those things happening to me. I've always felt like that.

I feel a lot more confident when I've taken care of myself. I'm happy to show people my body because I know I've looked after it. Whereas, over Christmas when I've had lots of cheese and chocolate I'd be a bit more shy about showing my body because I'd be concerned about about dimples here, and cellulite there.

Even a year ago I'd have been thinking of my body very selfishly. If I didn't look thin, or I didn't look healthy, I'd lack confidence and self-esteem. But recently my partner and I have been talking about starting a family, and as we've talked about my body as a vehicle for something amazing to happen, my insecurities have flown. Before I would have said I don't want to have children because I don't want to lose my body. But I kind of have to if I want to have children!

Age 24 | No children

"My breasts have pleasurable feelings that I wasn't aware of before"

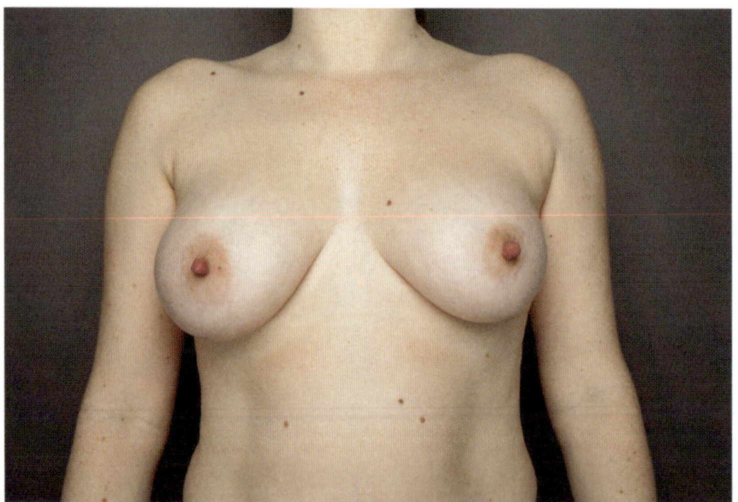

My breasts are quite large at the moment, slightly bigger than I feel comfortable with. It's interesting that the first thing I've said is on the negative side. They can look a bit buxom. But why the hell shouldn't they?

I was a late developer. There was one boy in my class who was a bit of a bully, and he called me 'Holland'. *(laughs)* It didn't exactly roll off the tongue! It was so rude and out of order, I felt awful and embarrassed. Maybe he thought he was being funny. I think he fancied me later on.

I definitely thought I was straight at school, there wasn't any question about my sexuality till my early 30s, when I had a relationship with a woman. My breasts were nowhere near as significant in my relationships with men as they are now as a pleasure zone. My current partner is very aware of her breasts as an erogenous zone, and I have learned I feel the same. A lot of time can be spent on them. I think it depends where I am in my cycle. Sometimes they are unbearably sensitive. But as a general rule I like them orally stimulated. There is variation, she might like a bit more of a tug or pull, but I don't. The relationship I am in now is the most long-term, loving and committed I have had, and I do think that has a bearing too, it intensifies everything.

When I was with men, I could take or leave stimulation of my breasts. In fact a few times I was irritated by it, they would be too rough, or my nipples felt too sensitive, and I didn't like it. But I've also had great, loving relationships with men in the past, and very satisfying sexual experiences too.

Breasts are presented as being for men's gratification. It's so rife, so commonplace, to see images of oiled up cleavages, sexual poses, selling any number of things, not just bras. I'm so used to it, I don't even stop and think about it anymore. If I stop and analyse it, it's scary. I could write a whole essay on the subject.

Through my job, I know girls are 'sexting', then it's sent around school, and put on Youtube, and they're bullied and harassed. There's a lot of distorted thinking. It would have been unthinkable when I was at school.

I'm more conscious of a man's gaze than a woman's gaze. You can be having a conversation with men about work, but they are half listening and looking me up and down. I don't like that. 'Come on, concentrate. What the hell!' I think men are more likely to look at breasts than women.

I feel self-conscious about my nipples being erect and noticeable. Going to work, or to a meeting, I've put two or three layers of tissue paper in my bra to take the edge off. If my nipples were showing I would worry that men and women might look and it would make me uncomfortable and anxious. Although, maybe I am sexually objectifying myself? I know I'm not sexually aroused in those situations, more often than not I'm chilly.

I sleep on my side, and I get creases on my chest, I think the skin is ageing, getting a little thinner. I get these deep crevices, and it's not consistent with my skin everywhere else. What I have found helps, is this *(shows me a rolled up T-shirt)*. Every night, I wear a tight tank top and I wedge this in my cleavage and I sleep like that. It stops the line forming. It's pretty vain, but it's not uncomfortable.

I have a friend who's a fashion designer, and she once went quite far down the line inventing a bodice thing that you would wear at night to hold breasts apart. She said, 'People will pay for this. There are lots of older women who don't care how uncomfortable it is, they don't want creases.' It was like a reverse bra, a separator, a contraption to wear at night. I don't want to develop the idea, I don't want to be that person who brings the corset back! That's my confession. It's not very feminist.

———————

Age 37 | No children

"My milk went when Hitler marched in"

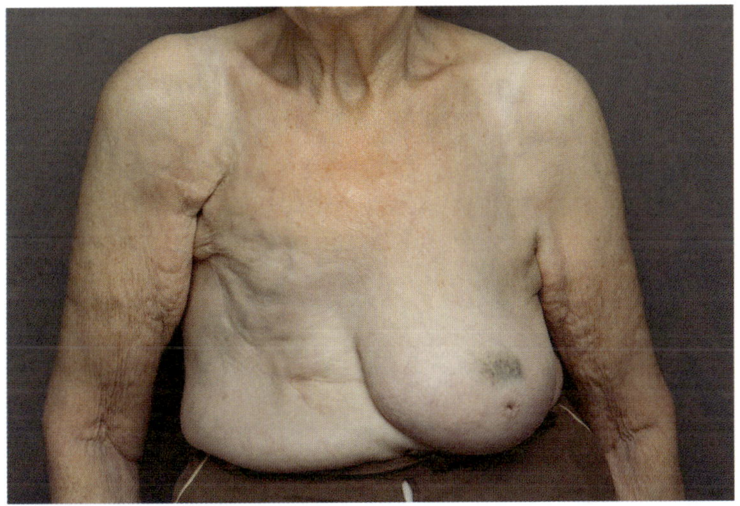

I'm afraid my daughter was born a week before Hitler marched in, and my milk went. It was the shock. We were Jewish. I intended to breastfeed her, but in the end she grew very well without.

My husband was taken on Kristallnacht, the day everybody was taken. He had gone out, against my advice. The authorities wanted me out of my flat. I went to the SS headquarters and told them in no uncertain terms what I thought of them, 'I'm not going to leave my flat and you can kiss my arse!' *(laughs)* Maybe it was foolish, but attack is the best defence. My husband was in Dachau and somehow I had to get him out.

My husband's boss was an ex-Nazi, but he was a very nice man, and he was fond of us. I asked him what to do, and he said, 'Go to the Gestapo'. I thought that was a good idea. My parents said I couldn't, but I said, 'I'm not afraid of the Devil! And if it helps, I will do it'. I rang up and made an appointment.

I saw a middle-aged man and we got talking, about this and that, like us now. After half an hour he said he had to go, but he said, 'I tell you something, I promise I will get your husband out, in three weeks, but I want something from you'. I knew what he wanted, but I said, 'Oh, what can I do for you?' 'I want you to visit me twice a week, I love talking to you.' 'What days do you want?' 'Tuesday and Friday.' I was quite prepared for anything. What's my little thing, if it means getting him out? It's unimportant. Getting him out, that's the important thing. But the man really only wanted to talk. I entertained him, I had prepared some topics – like Sheherazade! *(laughs)* And after three weeks, to the day, my husband came home.

We came here as refugees with no money at all, so we had to start right from the bottom, with a one-year-old child. The English were very lucky not to get me as a domestic, because I had never done anything, I had a maid at home. I started as a secretary and worked in the rag trade in a showroom in the West End.

My boss wanted me to get into the stores, but that was not an easy task, especially when you look like me. The representatives from other firms were elegant, tall, chic, and there was me, a little nothing. I knew I didn't have a chance, and my boss was very dissatisfied; he said it was my dress. I said, 'For what you pay me I cannot dress any better'. That was it, I left.

When I was 52 I went to the doctor, and said, 'There's a lump in my breast'. I'd had a hysterectomy four years earlier, but there was nothing there, it was benign. This time I thought it would be cancer. In those days they did not take a biopsy, if there was a lump it was taken out, that was standard, and the whole breast was removed. It was benign and I didn't need the radiotherapy treatment I'd been about to start.

In a way I felt relief that it wasn't cancer. I could have sought legal proceedings, because I was disfigured, but in those days you didn't think about those things. My husband didn't mind. I said to him, 'How do you mind having a wife with only one breast?' He said, 'Would you mind if I lost a leg?' I said, 'Of course not!' 'So there you go'. We had a very happy marriage, and there was no ill effect at all. That was our marriage, everything was talked about and that is why we had 52 happy years.

My breasts were important, they were erogenous. My husband and I had a very good sexual relationship, as well as the friendship. Nothing changed after the mastectomy, our sex life didn't change until my husband had an operation for his prostate. I consider I was blessed. 52 years, how many people are blessed with that? Not many.

After my husband died, I got my independence which was very important to me, and I could do what I liked. There is always something positive. It's the way you look at life.

I fell over last week, that's why I have a bruise on my breast. *(laughs)* It hurts. But again, it'll go. I always manage my falls by relaxing myself. I never hurt myself, except bruising. I don't fall over much, the last time was over a year ago. I don't use a stick yet.

When my nipple inverted suddenly about 10 years ago, I immediately went to the clinic to have it examined. I know it is a sign of cancer, but it can also be a sign of old age. It doesn't bother me.

I was conscious of the mastectomy and wouldn't have exposed my chest. I would never have gone topless anyway, never, even in my younger days. Don't forget, I was born in 1912, things weren't quite as ... We had nudist clubs, but that wasn't for me.

My breasts were never of any importance to me. I was always small, I didn't have a good figure, I didn't consider myself very good-looking, I was average. But I was vivacious and always had lots of friends and boyfriends. My body didn't bother me because it wasn't important. My figure has hardly changed. My mother-in-law said, 'She's a very nice girl, but where does she keep her organs?'

I'm very careful with my appearance. I wear a prosthesis. I forgot it once on holiday. I had to use loads and loads of plastic bags! *(laughs)* If I go swimming I have a costume with an insert. I used to swim every day until three years ago. When I was 97 I would swim 20 lengths in one go, but my physiotherapist said it was too much.

I am still interested, and still learning. I've had quite an interesting life. I still go to the opera, bridge. When I heard about this project I thought it was a good thing.

Age 101 | One child

'No Less a Woman'

There are so many different emotions attached to the tragic realities of having had a double mastectomy. Many cultures are unaccepting and terrible things happen to women both physically and emotionally. After reading Laura Dodsworth's *Bare Reality: 100 Women, Their Breasts, Their Stories*; in which 100 women bravely share un-airbrushed photographs of their breasts alongside honest, courageous, powerful and humorous stories about their bodies and their experiences, I knew I wanted to work with her somehow.

We both share in the idea of making something that allows women undergoing breast cancer to have something to be proud of, something with no shame attached. We wanted women to know that you can still be feminine, have your sensuality, have all of the things that are attached to being a woman and that part of your body can still feel beautiful on the outside, as well as the inside. Together with Laura Dosworth and the Hello Beautiful Foundation we have created the #NoLessaWoman campaign to continue supporting women around the world.

Stella McCartney

"I didn't get the chance to grieve for the baby"

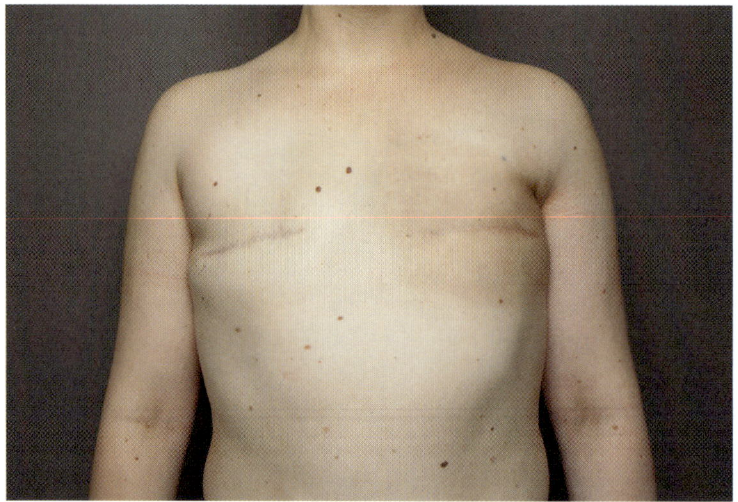

I feel more normal-looking when I wear prostheses, but the bras for them are not very comfy or pretty. They don't seem to be for younger people. I love the mastectomy bra Stella McCartney designed for breast cancer survivors. It's so comfy and pretty. We need more of these.

To be honest I wasn't too bothered about losing my breasts, because I just wanted the cancer gone. I was a size AA before the mastectomy; I was too small to have a lumpectomy, so you wouldn't think there would be much difference, but my chest actually goes in now. In some tops you can see the concave shape. Not all clothes look right with no breasts. Some days I feel upset if I try on old clothes. Of course, I'd rather that, than have cancer.

I've got no breasts, I'm in the menopause and, when I was bald as well, there was just nothing that made me feel like a girl. For about a month I couldn't get undressed in front of my partner.

I haven't thought much about whether to have reconstruction, because for a while they thought the cancer had spread to my bones. Touch wood, I am clear, but I had four months of thinking I might have bone cancer. I don't know how I coped. I cried a lot, and took anti-depressants.

My mum was in pieces. She always says, 'It should be me.' My sister wishes it was her because she already has a daughter. I was pregnant last year and we lost the baby. The doctors think the pregnancy hormones spurred on the cancer, because I had the oestrogen-sensitive cancer. My nipple had changed, which they thought might be from the pregnancy, but they gave me an ultrasound to be sure, and that's when we found out. It's been a horrible eighteen months. I didn't get the chance to grieve for the baby, because there were only four weeks between the miscarriage and the diagnosis. They can't guarantee that the cancer won't come back if I try and get pregnant again. I'm too scared to risk it.

My partner and I are much closer now. He's my best friend and I am more in love with him than I ever have been. He kisses my scars.

I'm a nurse. You get used to giving bad news when you're a nurse, but I have great empathy for the other side of it now. I really want to work in chemotherapy – who better to give chemo than someone who's had it?

I've been stripped of everything, literally. Hair, eyebrows, eyelashes gone, ovaries shut down. I've been to the lowest point. Anything after that is better. This is going to sound strange, but I am more confident now.

The day I found out I didn't have bone cancer I was so excited. I say 'yes' to everything now. Like this! I love life. I absolutely love it. I feel like I have a second chance.

―――――――――

Age 33 | Double mastectomy

"I can't run away from my body"

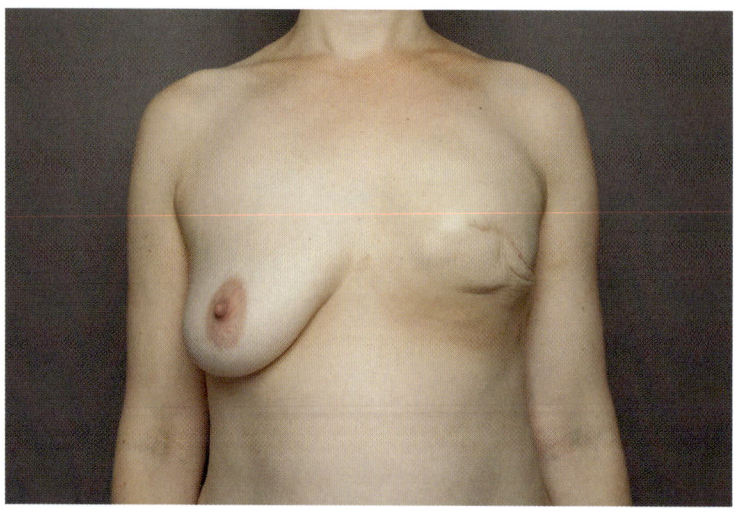

I like the photograph in the first edition of *Bare Reality* of the woman who has a tattoo where her breast used to be. I'm a bit jealous of that! So, when I saw you were looking for more women for this project, I thought it would be really cathartic for me.

After I had my surgery it took me time to show people my scars. One of my daughters said, 'Mummy, I never want to see you walk around the house without clothes on again!' But they have got used to it. I've shown my friends now as well. Some people say it's not that bad, because they are trying to reassure me. But I showed a friend after we had a couple of glasses of wine and she burst into tears. I thought, 'Oh God, it must look really bad!' *(laughs)*

There were only two weeks between the diagnosis and the surgery; I didn't have time to think about what was happening. The cancer was quite far advanced. I remember the nurses showing me pictures of other women who had had the same sort of surgery and I was absolutely horrified that none of them had a nipple. I remember thinking, 'Holy shit! Where the bloody hell is the nipple?' I found that hard to deal with. I don't know why.

I was given a stick-on nipple to wear. They show you a selection box of 12 nipples. I did think about getting a comedy one and surprising my husband with a massive one or a teeny tiny one. You have to find some humour in this somewhere! At first the nipple helped, it made me match. But then I couldn't see the point, it kept falling off and I lost it on the consultant's couch! I was too embarrassed to phone up: 'Have you found a nipple?' *(laughs)*

I've always liked my breasts. I breastfed two children, and I was happy to be able to do that. I felt like my breasts had been treacherous getting cancer.

I'd love to be that woman who doesn't care about her scars, be cool with it, but I don't feel that way, and it's been 15 months. To start with I was glad I had the surgery, I wanted the cancer gone. Now, I'm completely at odds with my body and what's happened to it. I would like to have the sort of body someone would glance at and think it's a normal female body, one that has the composite parts. At the moment it doesn't feel like part of me. It's a mutilation. *(cries)* I want to be more normal. I look at old photographs and I'd give anything to go back to that feeling of invincibility.

I'm not going to be that perfect cancer patient who eats her healthy food. If I am going to pop off any time soon, I want to feel alive, and sometimes kick and scream about it if I want.

I think I'm at a particularly difficult stage, it's harder than having the chemo. I'm tired and emotionally rumpled. What I want is not to be in this body any more. I want to run away, but I can't run away from my body.

———————

Age 38 | Single mastectomy

"You are still a woman, beautiful inside and out"

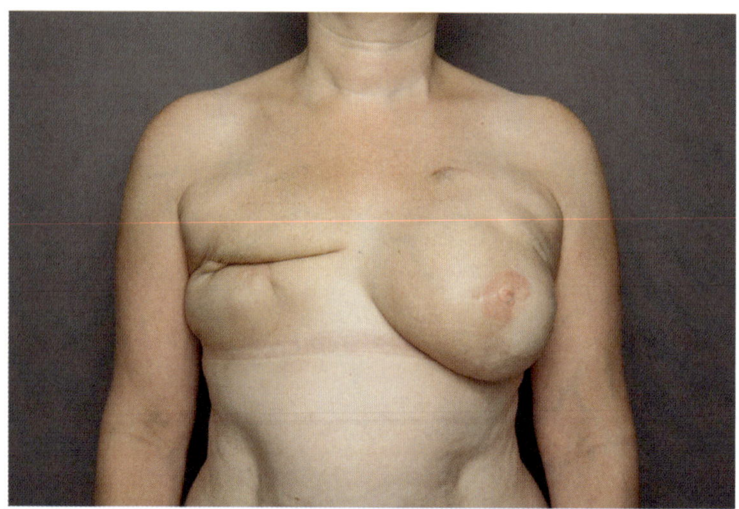

I want women to know if you lose a breast, you are still a woman, beautiful inside and out. That is how I feel, and it's how my husband has made me feel. I cried the first time I saw it, but now I don't mind. I want women to know it's not as bad as it seems. You're still the same person.

My husband has been there for me 100%. He's made sure I always feel like a woman. When I lost my hair I wore a little sleep hat or wig, and he used to flick the wig off, make me laugh, and say, 'It doesn't matter, you're still you.' There's a lot of humour, and he's very emotionally supportive. He would hold me all through the night during the worst times. I couldn't fault him.

Last year we thought it might have gone to the brain and that was the hardest time. I remember sitting, rocking on the floor, terrified. All I thought about was not being there for my daughter and husband. I had an MRI on Christmas Eve and found out I was clear. We just burst into tears.

In the end it was the best Christmas I have ever had. Every day I feel like I am living the last day of my life. I appreciate everything: the trees, breathing the air, the people I love. Thinking you might die changes how you feel about life. I appreciate people more, particularly my daughter. She is 20, but she's still my little baby.

She was amazing when I lost my hair. When my hair came out in clumps she held me while I sobbed. The lovely thing is we've spent a lot of time together. She came to my treatments with me. It was like having a best friend with me. I'm very proud of her.

I have the gene, so my daughter will have to be tested. She's not going to rush it though. She's very vigilant. If she has the gene she will have risk-reducing surgery when she's older.

I've had three mastectomies. After the reconstruction surgery the wound started opening up. I had to go back in a few times. The implant was bursting out. I couldn't look at it; my husband had to change my dressings for me. They couldn't start my chemo on time, because I just had this hole in my body. And once it did start they couldn't give me the sixth chemo because of the infection, they said it could kill me.

They will have to do more surgery on my breasts, so I'm toying with having another reconstruction. I'm used to how I look in the mirror, and my husband doesn't mind, but buying clothing is frustrating. I'd like to be able to wear a nice summer dress.

Despite what I have been though, I am lucky. I am here, with my family and friends, and that's all that matters.

Age 43 | Three mastectomies

"I love my wig now, it's part of me"

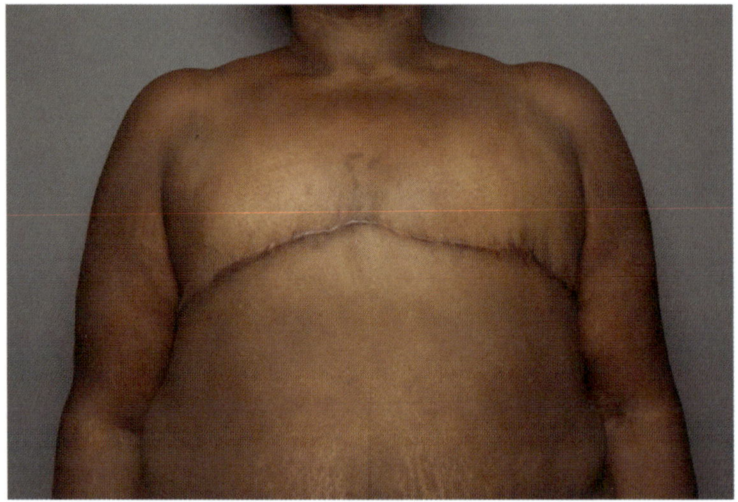

My hairdresser made me a wig in case I needed chemo. In the end I didn't need chemo, but the hormone treatment thinned my hair out anyway. I love my wig now, it's part of me. It makes me feel like who I was before the surgery.

I had very, very big breasts before the surgery – size 38KK. From KK to nothing... All my adult life, my breasts have been a big part of me. People used to see them before they saw me. I had to learn how to dress for them, what styles suited me. They made me a woman I guess. Having a bilateral mastectomy took that all away from me.

After the surgery, and after my hair thinned out, I couldn't even look at myself in the mirror. I felt like I had lost my femininity, the things that made me a woman. The wig has replaced both my hair and breasts.

Cancer has taught me that life is short. I'm in my mid-40s and if I want to be glamorous every day, I will. I make an effort every day. My hair is part of the way I feel glamorous.

I had bleeding from my nipples and they found pre-cancerous cells. There's a family history, so as a precaution they removed all of my milk ducts. My husband didn't think twice, he said, 'They've got to go.' I was worried it would impact on our relationship, but it didn't. He's an amazing man. He loves me for who I am.

We've got a little boy who's eight now. The mastectomies affected him more than anyone else in the family. He loves his 'mummy cuddles'. After my breasts were gone, cuddles weren't the same for him. He asked me not to come to school without my prostheses because he didn't want his friends to know my breasts were gone. I hated having to wear the prostheses, they are very uncomfortable, but I wore them every day for him. (cries) I didn't want him to be bullied, I didn't want him to be sad. But they were heavy and my scars became sore and inflamed. I learnt that if I wore patterned tops he didn't notice. So I started wearing busy floral prints. One day he noticed and said, 'Mummy, you're not wearing them. You look OK actually! You don't have to wear them anymore, Mummy, because I don't think anyone will notice. I didn't.'

I've found that in the black community, women don't talk about breast cancer that much. I've known women who have died from breast cancer in the Caribbean rather than go to the doctor. I think it's cultural. I wonder if people think that there is a stigma, that cancer is a bad thing. My mum has just been diagnosed after finding lumps in her breasts. She lives in the Caribbean. She said to me, 'If I go to the doctor, everyone on the island will know.' So I had to arrange for her to fly to a different island and have the biopsy. I want this to raise awareness.

———————

Age 45 | Double mastectomy

"I'm proud cancer didn't beat me psychologically"

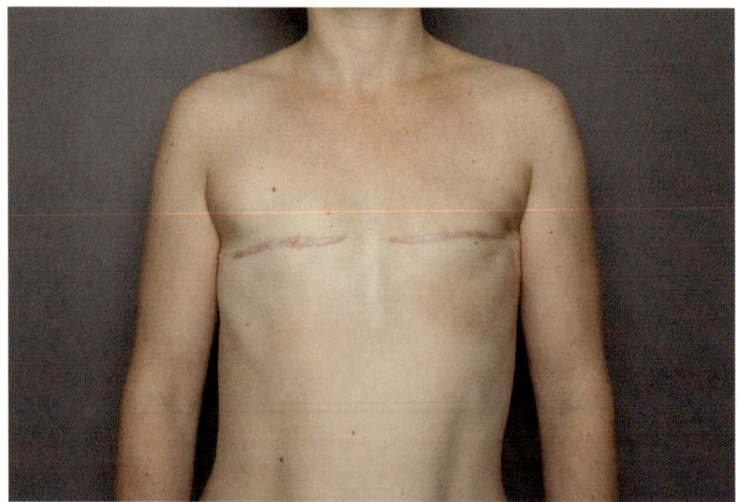

My mother died of breast cancer six months before I was diagnosed. I was pregnant with my daughter when cancer was found in her brain, lungs and liver. She became slowly sicker and sicker before my daughter was born. She asked the doctor if she would see the baby. We didn't think she would make it, but she held on. Luckily she got to meet her, but by that point she was already quite ill. She held her once, she understood.

I breastfed my baby. Around the time when my mother died, one side stopped producing much milk. I could express 10 ounces out of one side, but only two out of the other. The health visitor thought it was probably just the shock and grief. Of course, in hindsight, it was the tumour. I kick myself now, but at the time there was no reason to think it was cancer. Despite my grandmother, mother and I all having breast cancer, we don't have a genetic factor. When I was finally diagnosed it was very big and had spread to my lymph nodes.

It was a car crash time. I was so cross when I was diagnosed. I remember thinking, 'I don't have time for this.' I had to juggle my mum being ill, having a baby, mum dying, going back to work. It seemed so unfair. I was determined not to let it affect me. I carried on working and even cycled to chemo. There was another woman at the hospital who cycled to chemo, and I thought, 'Right, I can do it too.' I've been strong enough to get through it. I'm proud I had the resolve not to let cancer beat me psychologically.

I had size AA breasts before. I wasn't aesthetically attached to them. I'd rather stay alive and eliminate the risk. I didn't go through reconstruction because I didn't want to spend any more time in hospital and have more operations. Maybe if my mum hadn't just died I wouldn't have been so worried about dying. But I felt they were causing too much trouble in the world. They were responsible for taking mum, responsible for what was happening to me, and I didn't want them anymore. From the point of diagnosis they were gone in my mind.

My surgeon and oncologist are still worried I made a rash decision, and ask if I am sure I don't want reconstruction. The longer you wait, the harder it is to have reconstruction. Having a reconstruction is the default decision. I don't know why they worry so much.

I desperately want to get back to how it was. But everything feels different. I remember the night I was going into labour, and I went to bed. I remember how our bedroom felt that night. I want to get back to that feeling. Now when I go to bed I don't have that feeling, instead there is a risky, scary feeling hanging over me. I hope I will get past it in time, feel less scared. Maybe.

———

Age 34 | Double mastectomy

"My scars are like smiley faces"

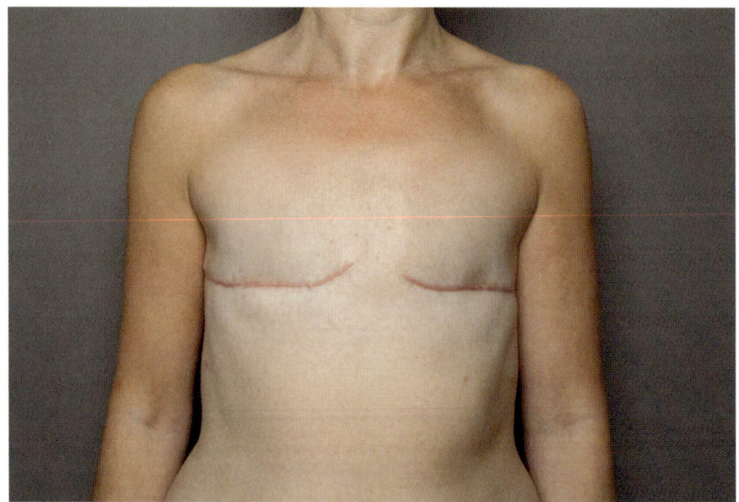

At the time of being diagnosed I'd never seen a mastectomy scar. That really frightened me. I didn't know what the future held. I didn't know what I would look like after my surgery. We don't see the scars, and we need to see the scars. For me, the fear at the beginning was the worst part. And it took me two weeks to look at the scars after the operation. I even hid them under a shirt in the bath. I know it was ridiculous. But I know women who have waited months or even years before looking at their scars. The one in eight women who are going to get breast cancer need to know what to expect, to take the fear away.

People are embarrassed by breast cancer. I don't know why. Because they're breasts? The breasts are gone! When people lose limbs that isn't hidden away in the same way as mastectomy scars.

After the initial panic, I felt strong, ready to fight this. I also want to be a positive role model. There is a lot of breast cancer in my family. In the event that my daughter or niece has to face it, I want them to see that life gets better again. I've been volunteering to do lots of crazy things – this project is just one of them!

I used to get stressed and now I go with the flow. I worry less about trivial things. I've fought a massive fight and I am proud of my body. I used to pick it apart, like most women do: didn't like this part, didn't like that part. Now I would encourage women to appreciate their bodies the way they are. I've gone through so much, and I'm still standing. I wouldn't have chosen to have this, but I am proud of my scars. They are like smiley faces.

I breastfed my children when they were babies, so my breasts had done their job. Before the mastectomies, my kids ran around singing, 'Bye bye boobies, thank you for the dinners!' as a joke.

I had a friend who said she thought breastfeeding was perverted. That made me really sad. If there are people in society who feel that way, then something is really, really wrong with society. That's what breasts are there for! I do understand some people choose not to breastfeed, and that's fine, but it's certainly not perverted. It shocks me that people feel that way.

We need to change attitudes. Get it out there. Talk about it. I've never been extroverted, never been one to stand in front of a camera. But I want people to know that having breast cancer isn't as bad as you would imagine. It's frightening, painful and gruelling at times, but it's manageable. Thousands of women are managing it every day.

Cancer is a lonely place. You can be surrounded by love, family and friends, but still feel alone on your path. That loneliness stems from fear, so we need to talk about it and normalise it. I got to 44 and I'd never seen mastectomy scars, even though I knew people who had them. Sadly women are diagnosed every day. We need to help take away the fear.

Age 44 | Double mastectomy

"Cancer has been a beautiful gift, but in ugly wrapping paper"

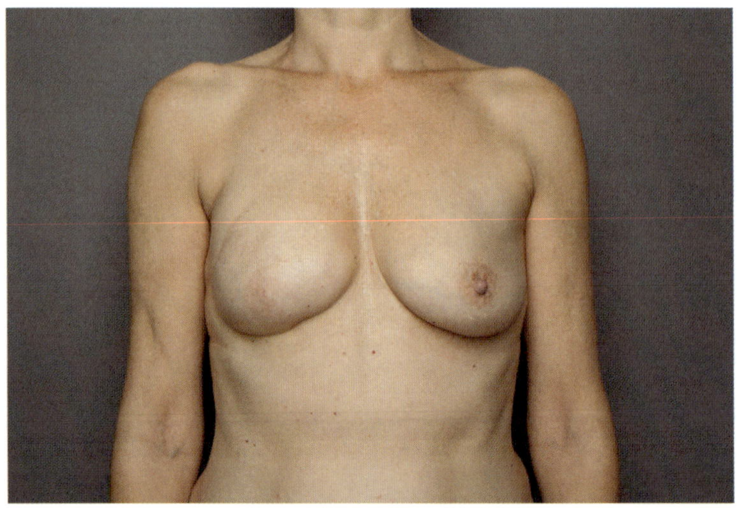

I'd just turned 40 when I found a lump during a shower. The news that I had to have a breast removed took my breath away. The sentence 'We have to remove your breast' was horrible, but of course you would do anything to survive.

It was a long saga. I spent most of that year on treatment: surgery, chemotherapy and radiotherapy. The following year I had three attempts at reconstruction. For some reason my body wouldn't accept the implants. I woke up and they were upside-down on my body, they wouldn't settle. I have never heard of this happening to anyone else

– it was bizarre! After the second time, the surgeons used the flap technique, using my own body to reconstruct a breast. They didn't choose this technique in the first place, because I don't really have enough body fat. There was a risk of failure, and then there would have been no options. I really crossed my fingers this would work! Finally, I had five years of hormone treatment.

I am now totally happy with the results. It is numb, but it feels warm, just like a natural breast, whereas the other one was hard and cold. Also, if I gain or lose weight, it does the same.

I used to have a high-flying job as an engineer, a cartographer. I loved my work. Then I was diagnosed with cancer and everything went on hold. I struggled after treatment to go back to my work. I identified myself very strongly with work and my role, so I felt like I lost my identity during that time. I was in limbo, I couldn't move on, as though everything had been taken away from me, not just my breast. Then I got in touch with a life coach and it was a life-changing experience. I realised it was what I wanted to do with my life, it became my calling. A completely different career!

I used to map the world, and as a coach I help people to map their lives. So there is still a relationship with what I used to do, I am still a cartographer in a way.

Then I had this lightbulb moment. Why not use my coaching skills and my personal experience with breast cancer? I found a partner, a GP who is a breast cancer survivor, and we set up LYLAC: Live Your Life After Cancer. We support people when they come out of treatment and they need support, to help to map their lives, build confidence and plan for the future.

Because of cancer I have changed, my job has changed and there have been positives. Sometimes we need these wake-up calls in life. I can say now that cancer has been a gift to me – a beautiful gift, but in ugly wrapping paper.

Age 52 | Single mastectomy

"This whole journey was meant to happen"

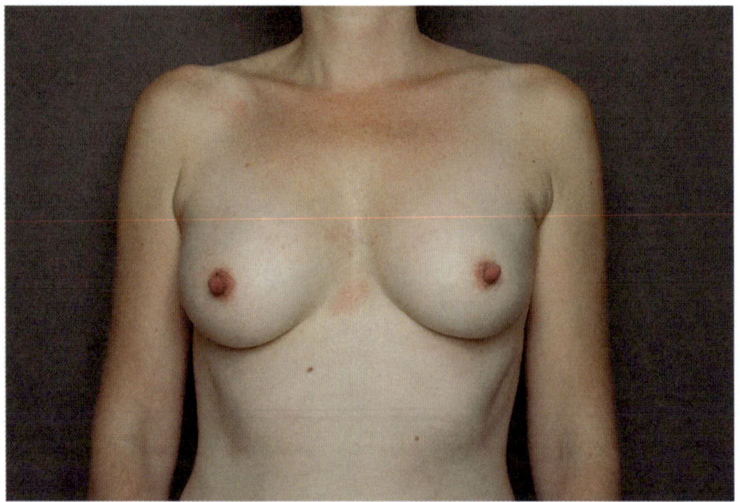

One morning, just by accident, I brushed my breast in the shower and felt a lump. I already had an appointment to see the doctor that very day. I feel like I was meant to find it.

When I went for the results of the mammogram and the biopsy, there were two doctors in the room, so I instantly knew it was bad news. I could see a load of notes on the desk and I made out the words 'breast cancer'. I found myself making polite conversation, 'This room is so pink isn't it?' and chatting to the doctors to make them feel better!

I'm a spiritual person, I've always had faith, and I feel as though this whole journey was meant to happen. I see it as a blessing rather than something bad. Given the choice to have my life back as it was before, or go through it all again, I would choose the cancer. I've learnt and developed so much and I can use that to help other people. It feels like this is what I'm meant to do in life, my direction, my path.

The day after I was diagnosed, the nurse sat me down and said the worst things. She said it was going to be awful, I'd be depressed, sit at home, watch daytime TV eating crisps, give up work and give up on life. That is what she told me. Really. She was trying to be helpful but she told me I would be so depressed I would find it hard to fit into society. I thought, 'Wow, this is crazy.'

The day I finished my treatment another nurse said, 'You must be so depressed and tired, get back into work when you can.' I'd never given up work or given up on life. So, right from the beginning, I knew I needed to help change things, and I set up Hello Beautiful.

Hello Beautiful is all about educating people about a healthy, happy and non-toxic lifestyle. Having cancer and setting up Hello Beautiful have been a positive transformation for me, and I want to give that to other people. I think being around positive people is very helpful.

I used to be a stressed person. Now I'm more relaxed and I enjoy the small things in life. I've changed how I eat, what I put in my body, and I feel so much better. You need a healthy body and healthy mind for your whole body to work. I'm not perfect but I am a lot better than I used to be.

Cancer has given me a new creative outlook. I have created lots of new artwork and I make casts of women with breast cancer. Hello Beautiful holds 'art therapy'-style workshops in schools and hospitals. Cancer can be a very inward experience, so art can help people open up, talk and get through it. Breast cancer is close to your heart, literally, and connected to a lot of emotions for women. I love being able to help women.

———

Age 39 | Lumpectomy

"Agonising about what we look like is a waste of our time and talent"

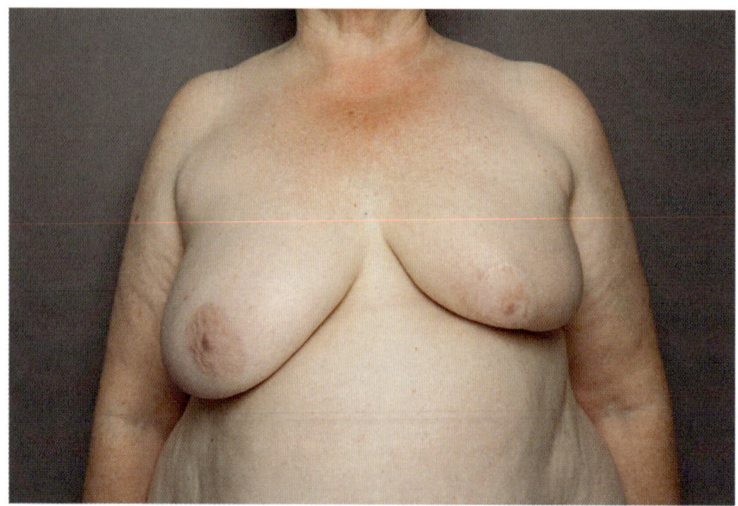

I was so mad busy at Christmas that I forgot all about my mammogram and didn't go. Luckily, I was sent a letter about a new appointment. It was devastating to find out I had breast cancer. I had a lumpectomy. After that, they found out there was a bit more, so I had to have another surgery, similar to breast reduction.

Even though you know some people are cured from breast cancer, others die. It took a while for the seriousness to sink in. I had chemotherapy and radiotherapy and am on hormones now. I'm really grateful to the health service, all the doctors and nurses. I could have had the other breast reduced to match, but I didn't want another operation. No one is going to stare at my breasts and think they are odd. If they do, then that's their problem!

You can't open a magazine or newspaper without seeing someone's idea of 'perfect'. It makes me angry. People are so much more than what they look like. I know it affects men too, but there is so much for women to agonise about. Agonising about what we look like is a waste of our time and talent.

I've modelled for a life drawing class. It was a wonderful experience. The artists were enjoying looking at my body in a non-sexual way. It was eye-opening. Everyone's pictures were all so different.

I also did a nude photo shoot for an art exhibition called Happy in My Skin. I was a little bit nervous, but there is safety in numbers. We stripped off, put our dressing gowns on and went down to the sea. It was a lovely hot day and of course there were loads of people there! We threw off our robes and ran into the water. We were jumping up and down and hugging each other and it was indescribably joyous. We are all unique and we all realised there is nothing wrong with us. I don't know who decides who is 'perfect'.

So, I felt fine about this photograph. I am more nervous about talking. I think I am very ordinary. I don't have a special story. I like gardening, I like to spend my money on plants. When they grow, thrive and spread that gives me real joy. I like the cinema, theatre, meeting friends, and I have two wonderful daughters. I'm interested in doing things and not thinking about what I look like. So my relationship with my body hasn't really changed.

The idea of having photographs of real women, not celebrities, on Stella McCartney's website is mind-blowing. It's such a positive step in the right direction. I think it would be good to see real women in adverts as well. I wish there was less talk in the media about what women look like. For example, politicians – who cares about her shoes, trousers, top, where she bought them and what they cost and what they look like? It makes me cross.

Age 63 | Lumpectomy and mammoplasty

"I tell myself I am going to live till I'm 90"

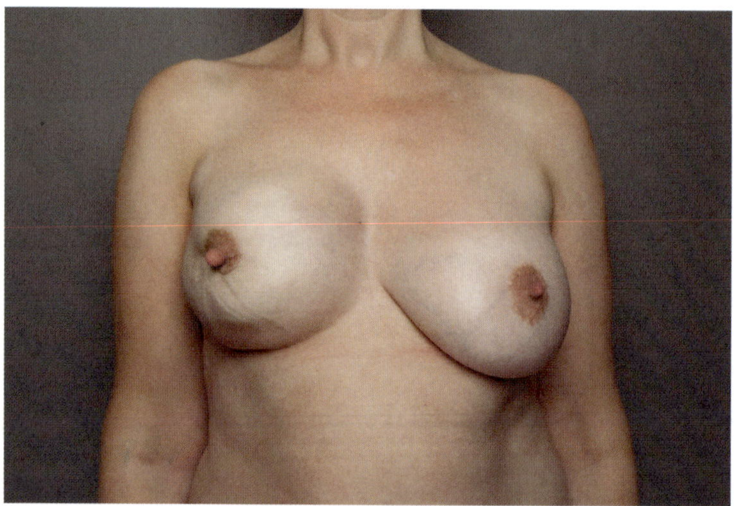

I couldn't feel a lump, I had a pain under my arm. My boss's mother had just died of breast cancer so she insisted I go to the doctor. It turned out I had a 5cm tumour with legs, like a little spider. It was painful because the little spider legs had started to go under my arm.

The lump was very close to my bone so I am regularly checked for bone cancer. They think I am going to be OK. I'm now going to go down to six-monthly MRIs and bone scans. Worrying about the cancer spreading has been the worst thing.

I had a really rough time mentally. I struggled with the fear of dying, mainly because of my boys who are four and nine. I used to think about dying every day. I was so scared I couldn't sleep. (cries) My partner had to hold my hand all through the night. You can believe every day you are going to die, or you can believe every day you are going to live till you are 90. You know what? No one knows. Every time I get a negative thought I tell myself I am going to live until I'm 90.

You've probably heard the chemo stories. Your hair falls out, your eyebrows fall out, your nails fall off, your bones ache. It's fucking horrendous what happens to you. Oh, and the sickness. I was in hospital for a week each time in recovery.

But I want to talk about the success. I've radically changed my life. I think you have to. I changed my stressful job. I green juice every day. I exercise as much as I can – yoga, little runs, walks in the park, meditation. I've massively reduced my alcohol intake, but every now and then I have a blow out, because, fuck it. I forgive myself that. Do I really believe all this makes a difference? I'm on the fence, but I don't want to look back and think I didn't do everything I could to help myself.

Life has gone by in a blink. It makes me sad. So now, I really live in the now. I'm a better mum, a better wife, my friendships are closer, I have more empathy. Everything is more meaningful. If I had never had this experience, who would I be? You have to say, 'I am bold, and strong and I am going to live through it.'

My partner has been brilliant. We've been together 11 years and we just got married. We're in love again! We're so solid.

You always think you have another day to do something. You know when your kid says, 'Can we play? Can we read a book?' The dads do a lot of the fun stuff, while we mums make dinner or whatever. This has made me spend more time with them. I'm more conscious of their feelings and listen to them. I will sit down and read a book now. My oldest son knew what cancer was and was very scared. He became angry with me for being ill. I have had to woo him back, make him feel comfortable, make him feel it's safe to love me.

If in doubt, don't leave things because you're busy. If I hadn't gone to the doctor about my sore arm I might not be here today. It's that simple. I wanted to do this to increase awareness. It can happen to anyone.

It's unfortunate you have to go through something as big as this to know you have to live in the now. All those things you realise on your deathbed, I know them now, and I take them with me. My life will have more purpose now, and that's a good thing.

Age 42 | Mastectomy

"We won't know if my fertility is affected until we start trying"

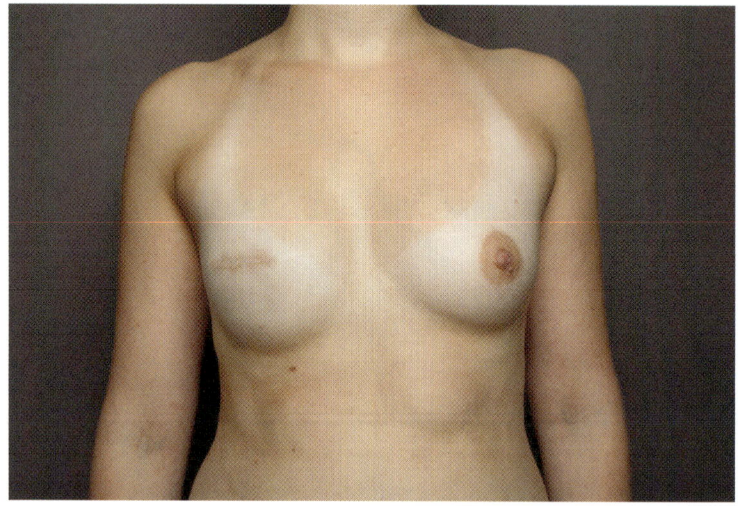

I was diagnosed when I was 27 and had just got married. I want to have children someday, so I went through the first stages of IVF before chemo.

We won't know if my fertility is affected until we start trying. I'm on hormones at the moment, in a temporary state of menopause, and I need to stay on these drugs for five years at least. So I don't even want to think about it at the moment.

We have eight frozen embryos. We have turned it into a cute little joke, where if we end up having to use those, we can say to them, 'Well you were conceived when we were in our mid-twenties, so if you're naughty it's because we were too immature then!' But hopefully they are an insurance plan and we won't have to use them. It would be a long drawn-out process, and I don't want any more procedures. If things could be a little more natural from now on, I would appreciate it!

In the fertility clinic I was surrounded by all these lovely couples who were trying to get pregnant. Someone asked me how long I had been trying. Not a day in my life! That was a challenging start to the whole cancer process.

I didn't have a great relationship with my breasts before all this. My remaining nipple is half inverted, and the other was completely inverted. I was bashful about them because I thought I didn't look normal. The more 'perfect' media breasts I saw everywhere, the more bashful I became. In fact, I thank my breasts for stopping me from being too sexually promiscuous when I was young, because I was too ashamed of them to do anything sexually! I didn't loathe my breasts, I just didn't want to flash them about. When I met my husband I didn't care though, because he was amazing and loved me no matter what. I used to worry about whether I would be able to breastfeed one day... If I am able to get pregnant I'll have to see if I can breastfeed with one breast with a half inverted nipple!

Sexually, I don't know if I will ever get used to the reconstruction. If my husband touches it, it shocks my brain, and it interrupts that lovely little place you enter... My husband and I couldn't have been closer during everything, but sexually things just stopped for a while. You kind of become sad puppies together. It's all love, but sexually we went into hibernation.

People are afraid of cancer, but it's so common now. I know this sounds strange, but there's nothing really to be afraid of. Going through treatment is not as bad as you think it's going to be. People find their own ways of dealing with it, their own way of owning the experience, whether it's wearing a wig or not wearing a wig. Choosing something like that can give you a feeling of control.

____

Age 28 | Single mastectomy

"Cancer was like an unwanted house guest"

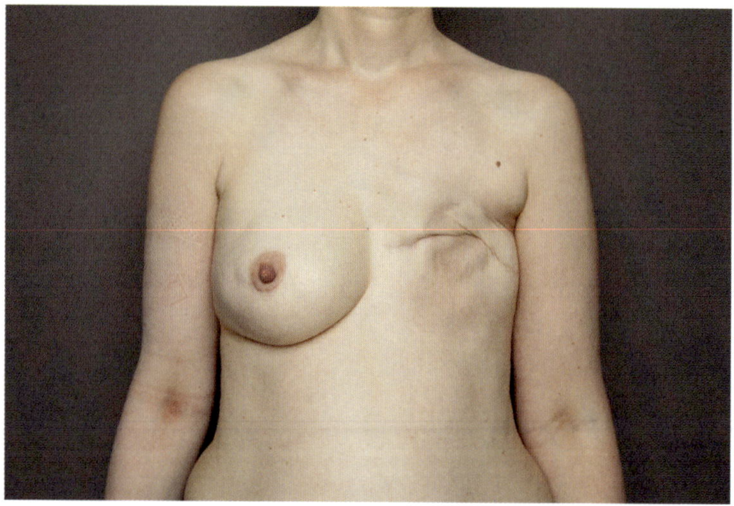

I have a long and complicated breast cancer history. Lumpectomy, bilateral mastectomies, reconstruction, recurrence of cancer, third mastectomy and two rounds of chemo.

When I had the bilateral mastectomy I thought about what my breasts meant to me as a mother, a woman, a lover. Up until that point I had taken them for granted. I am a feminist and don't see myself as defined by my breasts, but losing them was terrible. If I wanted to live, for my daughter, that was the sacrifice I had to make.

I didn't want to remove them, I wanted to keep them if I could, and that's why I had reconstruction. After cancer was found again and I lost one of the reconstructed breasts, I was devastated. I felt like I had worked so hard to overcome my genetic destiny, only to fail. I'd tried to be one up on cancer, had the risk-reducing surgery, but I couldn't outwit cancer. When the reconstruction failed, I felt like I had failed.

My scars represent all the pain I have experienced. My body is a map. Every scar tells a story of vulnerability. On the one hand I have learnt a lot and take some positives from the experience, but cancer is also a deadly disease, which causes pain and loss. I feel like I live this dichotomy.

Cancer was like an unwanted house guest: it made a mess, had parties, then went. I shut the door behind it and thought, 'Phew, thank goodness you're gone, don't come back.' But when I found out I had the BRCA mutation I felt like the cancer was part of me. I didn't simply acquire it, it came from within. I think we are taught to believe in our culture that we have more control over our bodies than we do. When you are breastfeeding, your milk comes in and your body knows what to do, it has a will of its own. When cancer arrives in your breast, it can feel like your body has a will of its own in a different way.

When you go through treatment for cancer your body becomes a source of pain, rather than pleasure. Surgery involves cutting, chemotherapy involves what feels like poison going through you, radiotherapy involves burning to your skin. Your physical sensations take on a different meaning. And while that is going on everyone wants to hug you, to kiss you, but actually you don't want to be touched. So it's not just about breasts, it's about what touch means to your whole body. At a very fundamental level cancer affects your relationship with your whole body. You have to relearn that touch can equal pleasure, not just pain.

Only my daughter sees me naked. I don't hide from my husband, I could go to greater lengths, but he hasn't seen me naked. My chest has to be covered. It took me a long time to look at the scars myself. I couldn't let just anyone photograph me. The *Bare Reality* book was wonderful and inspired me to take the leap. I bought it to help my daughter make sense of her body as she goes through puberty, to understand what real women's breasts look like and mean to them, rather than the sexualised images young people come into contact with.

Today has taken courage. I feel my body has a story and I want to give my body and story a voice. My pain has been a secret. I hope this will help other women know you can survive pain.

Age 46 | Three mastectomies

Why Create *Bare Reality?*

When I was a little girl, my dad had a pink, satin Sam Fox cushion. It lived in the back seat of his car for a while. The cushion fascinated and intimidated me and remains a vivid childhood memory.

Why create *Bare Reality?* Why spend a year meeting strangers, photographing their breasts and interviewing them? Inspiration for creative projects can be traced to recent events in our lives, attributed to the influence of our families, friends, experiences and environment, and perhaps to our DNA. Now it's now my turn to bare all. Although I feel vulnerable relinquishing my anonymity, I think it is the only way I can participate fully in my own project with integrity and honesty.

Growing up, I never thought my breasts were very attractive. They didn't seem to measure up to the breasts I saw all around me. I grew up believing my breasts were objects that should be 'perfect' and desirable for men, and that they fell a long way short. I absorbed the notion that women should be passive and sexually pleasing to men. I think I shared these preconceptions with many women, but I recognise parental influence.

My father was a sex addict. Before continuing, I have to say that he was a wonderful man and he loved me very much. He had more positive than negative influences on me, but life is complicated. You don't make lemonade without lemons. He had a topless calendar on the wall in his study. Pictures of topless women in his wallet. Alongside *The Times* and *The Observer* he also bought *The Sun, The News of the World* and *The Sport.* He had a large collection of porn videos and magazines; I didn't watch and read these, but I was aware of them and saw the covers. He also had lots of girlfriends and partners, before and while being married. I could say more, but it is his story, not mine.

He never told me I should look like the models, although of course I understood I should make the best of myself, and he encouraged me to be academically successful and pursue a professional career. The inference from my father's collections and attitudes, as well as wider culture and the media, was more subtle. I internalised the notion that breasts were my sexual calling cards, and that they were for men.

So, I have always been fascinated by the dichotomy between women's personal lives and how they are depicted by the media; between how we feel about breasts privately and how they are presented for public consumption.

In recent years, I've noticed how breasts appear more and more in the media, alongside an increased sexualisation of the human body. To me

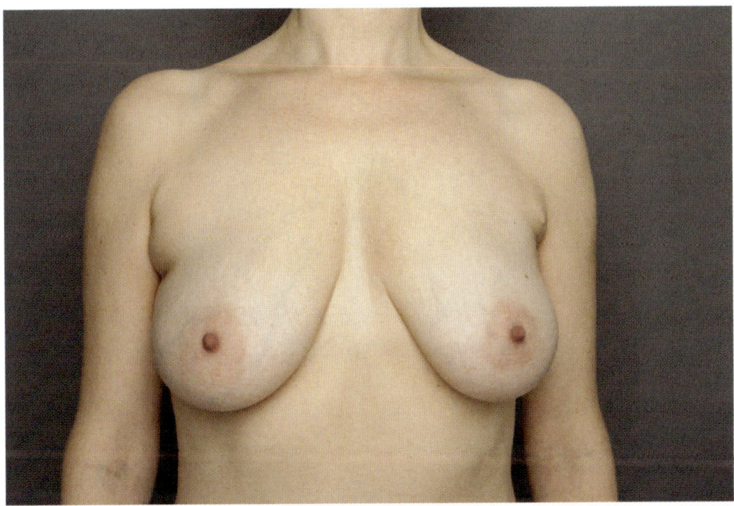

this is a one-dimensional view of womanhood and a pale shadow of what female sexuality is and can be.

Art has often flattered women and adhered to the culturally-desirable aesthetics of the time, from prehistoric fertility goddess statues to Botticelli, but never before has the human image been so altered and controlled. The breasts we see in films, on TV, on the Internet, in newspapers and magazines are often surgically enhanced, professionally lit, and photoshopped. Airbrushed breasts, belonging to models and actresses, not only create an unflattering comparison but present an unobtainable ideal. If a model can't live up to the ideal of perfect breasts, how can anyone else?

We see images of breasts everywhere in the media and yet images of 'real' breasts, and actual breasts themselves, are almost never seen. Breasts aretaboo, hidden away beneath clothes and bras.

I've grown up, matured and altered. And in the course of creating *Bare Reality* I have seen 100 women's breasts. I know they come in all shapes and sizes, none us are 'perfect'. I am fortunate to feel relatively at peace with my body and breasts, especially since creating *Bare Reality*. I am lucky my breasts are healthy. But still, like many in *Bare Reality*, I feel self-conscious about my breasts and their 'imperfections'.

Recently, I came across on article online called 'The Third Boob'. Finally, I understood one aspect of my breasts which had always created insecurity: it wasn't fatty tissue between my left breast and armpit, it was what is known as an 'accessory breast', or polymastia. When I breastfed I never leaked a drop of milk from my breasts, but I did leak from the supernumerary nipple on the accessory breast. I'd never heard of this happening to anyone else before I read 'The Third Boob'. My GP and a consultant breast surgeon confirmed that this level of additional breast tissue plus a third nipple is abnormal and agreed to remove it for me.

Genetic throwback to our ancient mammalian past, mark of the witch, or indication of extra femininity? It's certainly ironic that I had a little third breast all this time without realising. Was it partly responsible for generating my interest in breasts and how we feel about them? It made me feel abnormal - did it prompt a need to take a closer look at myself and other women? I suppose if the third nipple had been darker or raised it would have been more obvious, but I find it strange looking back that I didn't know it was there. The act of creating *Bare Reality* is responsible for this late realisation. The physical discovery is matched by (and perhaps could be said to represent?) an emotional and artistic evolution.

I've surprised myself – I didn't think I would have a cosmetic procedure, but I'm glad the third boob is gone.

Prior to that, having babies led to a major evolution in my attitude towards my breasts. Breastfeeding was empowering. There were difficult times but, following gynaecological troubles, it gave me a sense of peace and achievement as a woman. I finally liked my breasts for fulfilling their biological purpose, if nothing else. Breastfeeding could also create a pleasant sensation. That oxytocin rush and the sweet bonding with a baby were so relaxing.

I've noticed some women are embarrassed to acknowledge that breastfeeding is sensual (I do not mean sexual) as there is an uncomfortable crossover between breasts being used for feeding, and being seen as sexually attractive, and feeling erogenous.

In common with other women who took part in *Bare Reality* I experienced mixed reactions while breastfeeding my babies in public. I perceived disapproval and heard tuts from strangers. I was asked when I would start giving my first baby 'proper food' when he was only six months old.

I've received comments from strangers about my breasts. At times I felt this was what I wanted. After all I had 'dressed' my breasts and my body to inspire male admiration. At other times it felt seedy and unwanted. When I was younger I didn't believe I deserved the compliments, I thought there was something wrong and embarrassing about my breasts, and that they didn't meet Western culture's diet of 'porn breasts'. I've experienced a number of instances of sexual harassment in relation to my breasts. A male boss used to stare at my breasts while talking to me, always. I wanted to poke his eyes out. A gynaecologist once offered me a breast check right after a vaginal examination – unnecessary, inappropriately-timed and shocking.

Over the years a tension built within my psyche. So many motivations came together and crystallised. In creating *Bare Reality* I wanted to re-humanise women through honest photography and interviews, present our breasts as they really are and burst the 'fantasy bubble' of the youthful, idealised and sexualised breasts presented by the media. More than that, I was compelled to explore what it means to be a woman, and make women subject, not object. When we talk about breasts we talk about intimate aspects of womanhood.

In *Bare Reality*, 100 women speak for themselves, telling their own stories. Their photographs are honest, but not unkind. They represent reality.

Bare Reality has changed me, and changed how I think and feel about women. It has transformed my relationship with my breasts. Quite simply, I like myself more as a woman, and I like my breasts more. In retrospect it is clear to me that *Bare Reality* has been a very personal exploration of what it means to be a woman. Talking to 100 women has helped me deconstruct cultural myths and define being a woman on my own, fresh terms.

Surprisingly, my breasts and nipples are now significantly more erogenous and a more important focus in lovemaking. They never used to be very important to me sexually. I believe this is connected to a greater acceptance of my breasts, my body and of myself as a woman. It's an unexpected outcome, but it correlates with observations from the project. If women like their breasts then they are more likely to find them erogenous. Or conversely, perhaps it is that if their breasts are sexually important they are more inclined to like them. Not a single woman who strongly disliked her breasts also thought they were important as an erogenous zone. It would appear that this is about more than basic nerve endings: our relationship with our breasts is connected to sensual feeling in our breasts.

I am deeply grateful to the women who have taken part. Their stories have moved me, opened my eyes, inspired me, and healed me. They bared their breasts and their souls. I am honoured that they shared so much with me. I feel tender about my own experience as a woman and full of admiration and warmth for female experience.

I hope that you have been moved by the wonderful women who took part. I hope *Bare Reality* has transformed you in some way.

This is how we look. This is how we feel.

Age 41 | Two children

Methodology

I sought to include a variety of women who would broadly represent the female population of the UK, in terms of ethnicity and sexual orientation. I also wanted to represent women of all ages (18 was the minimum age for participation), career, life experience, shape and size. It's important to remember that *Bare Reality* is an art, not an academic, project. As well as meet the stated criteria, I was looking for willing participants in a sensitive project, who would have interesting tales to tell.

The participants were given information about the project and its aims, and signed a release form. Interviews were recorded, then transcribed verbatim. In the editing stage, word choices were not changed, although the text was shortened and rearranged to improve the flow.

The photographs were not altered in photoshop, and were shot so they could be viewed consistently, comparatively and non-sexually.

A discussion guide was used to help structure interviews where useful, but not strictly followed.

Breasts Discussion Guide

1. Your breasts

What do you think of your breasts?

Do you like them?

What is your bra size?

When did your breasts first start growing?

How did you feel at that time?

How did your growing breasts change how people perceived you or treated you?

Do you always wear a bra?

How would you feel if you were braless on an ordinary day?

How have your breasts changed with age and how do you feel about it?

2. Children and breastfeeding

Do you have children?

Did you breastfeed your children?

What was it like?

Did you experience any pleasant physical sensations during breastfeeding?

Are you glad you did / didn't breastfeed?

How important do you think breastfeeding is for babies?

What proportion of your friends and acquaintances have breastfed their babies?

How did pregnancy and breastfeeding affect how your breasts look and feel?

Were you breastfed?

Did you ever see your mother's breasts and do you remember what you thought of them and what she felt about them?

3. Partner

Do you have a partner?

What does your partner think about your breasts?

What are other people's reactions to your breasts?

Are your breasts an important part of having sex for your partner and for you?

Do your breasts give you sexual pleasure either during sex or masturbation?

4. Breast enhancement

Would you ever consider breast enhancement surgery? Why?

Has anyone ever asked you to have breast enhancement surgery?

Have you ever considered doing anything else that might enhance your breasts, like exercise or using creams? Do you wear push-up bras?

What do you think of the growth in breast enhancement surgery?

What do you think of padded and push-up bras?

What do you think of padded and push-up bras for girls with growing breasts?

What would you say to your daughter if she wanted breast enhancement surgery?

5. Media and Society

Have you seen many women's breasts in real life situations?

How do you feel about seeing bare breasts in casual situations, such as changing rooms etc.?

What do the women you know think about their breasts?

How do the breasts you have seen in real life compare to the breasts you have seen in films, on TV and in magazines?

How do you feel about how women's breasts are portrayed in the media?

What do you think society considers the ideal pair of breasts to be like?

What do you think the ideal pair of breasts is like?

What do you think about the fact that women cannot go about bare-chested like men can?

Why do you think there is a taboo about bare breasts?

6. Compliments / harrassment

Do you receive many compliments or comments from strangers about your breasts?

Have you ever been sexually harassed about your breasts?

Have you ever been teased about your breasts?

Do you feel the way men treat you has been affected by your breasts?

Do you use your breasts to gain men's attention or to control them?

7. Health

Are your breasts healthy?

Do they change during your monthly cycle and, if so, how?

Do you examine your breasts?

Have you had breast cancer?

Do you know anyone who has had breast cancer? Any experiences you can tell us about?

What would it mean to you if you had to lose a breast?

8. Further thoughts

Do you think your breasts have had an impact on your life, for instance, the sorts of partners you have attracted, the type of job you have, your success in your career, the kinds of clothes you can wear?

Is there anything else you would like to add?